Safety for the Forensic Identification Specialist

2nd Edition

Nancy E. Masters

MASTER CONSULTANTS

13386 International Parkway
Jacksonville, FL 32218 • USA

This book contains descriptions of processes utilizing chemicals or combination of chemicals which may be hazardous to the user's health. It is strongly recommended that proper precautions be taken when using hazardous chemicals or combinations thereof. The author and the publisher assume no responsibility for the use or misuse of any of the chemicals, procedures, methods or ideas described herein resulting in injury and/or damage to persons or property.

Lightning Powder
13386 International Parkway
Jacksonville, Florida 32218 • USA
Tel: (800) 347-1200
Fax: (800) 366-1669

www.lightningpowder.com

Publisher's Cataloging in Publication Data

Masters, Nancy
Safety for the Forensic Identification Specialist
1. Laboratory Safety. 2. Criminalistics. 3. Material Safety Data Sheet. 4. Crime Lab.
I. Title 363.258 Library of Congress Catalog Card Number: 95-75630

Current Printing (last digit)
10 9 8 7 6 5 4 3 2

PRINTED IN THE UNITED STATES OF AMERICA

Some of the material appearing in this publication has been previously published in the *Journal of Forensic Identification*.

Acknowledgments

The opportunity to write this publication has proven to serve as a humbling experience like no other. Both frightening and exciting, it has led me through the computer crazies as well as the ecstasies. I have awakened with inspiration in the middle of the night only to have forgotten everything by morning. I have fought frustration and anxiety to accomplish completion. I feel this material is desperately needed by most forensic identification specialists. Without that belief to prop me up and propel me on, I may have dug in and never finished the project. Regardless of my feelings, none of this could have materialized without the support and encouragement of a number of people whom I am also privileged to count as my friends. I can only acknowledge a few here, but my appreciation is with everyone who encouraged me over the last few of years.

Helen Axford, Companion and Confidant, who saw me through the most difficult of times, always cheering and cheerful. Without such constant support and understanding, I would have lost the vision.

Ruth Borger, Librarian, California Department of Justice. She rescued me numerous times with her tips for survival and kind words of encouragement. A special "thank you" to her for sharing her talents in the editorial review she made of this work and her "sourdough starter".

Mike Carrick, Former Director, Lightning Powder Company, Inc. My deepest appreciation for giving me this opportunity. His confidence in my ability to complete such an effort helped to nurture my commitment. He has been admirably patient.

John D. DeHaan, Criminalist, California Criminalistics Institute. He always supports me in all endeavors, urging me onward and upward. And he taught me that achievement comes with effort, commitment and perseverance. There is no accomplishment or honor or reward in mediocrity. He is a special colleague and even more special friend.

Joseph T. Latta, Executive Director, International Association for Property and Evidence. He provided me with the opportunity to give instruction to evidence and property room personnel throughout the United States. This is an area in law enforcement where safety related issues have long been ignored. I offer my deepest appreciation to Joe for recognizing the need for, and actively supporting, such training.

Rod Oswalt, Industrial Hygienist, California Department of Justice. A technical review would not have been complete without his assistance. He kindly and generously gave of himself, his time, and his knowledge. His perspectives and insights were invaluable. He gave me the gift of "peace of mind".

Thomas Valentine, Criminalist, California Department of Justice. He has bolstered my confidence from the days of my first foray into the world of safety. He has always been generous with his time and resources. His years of hard work provided me with a foundation for developing some of my material. A special "thank you" to him for his technical review of this material.

Kathleen D. Saviers. An incredible amount of work is required to prepare a manuscript for printing. Kathy single-handedly took this manuscript, transferred it into another computer language, formatted it for inclusion of photographs and graphics, and polished it for printing. Without her perseverance and dedication, *Safety for the Forensic Identification Specialist* would never have rolled off the presses. I am forever indebted to her for her professionalism and advocacy of this project.

About the Author

Nancy E. Masters has worked in the field of fingerprint identification in excess of thirty-five years. She has participated in the development of curriculum for courses in Latent Print Techniques, Specialized Latent Print Techniques, and Latent Print Comparisons. She was an instructor in these courses, which are presented by the Department of Justice's California Criminalistics Institute. She has served as the Safety Officer for the Bureau of Forensic Services Special Forensic Sections. During this assignment, she wrote safety documents and procedures and conducted training of personnel on safety issues. She assisted in the writing of California's first *Clandestine Laboratory Manual of Instruction and Procedures*. In 1987 she received the California Governor's Employee Safety Award. Ms. Master's has been published internationally as well as presented papers at forensic conferences and international symposiums in the United States and Israel. She has instructed evidence and property room personnel throughout the United States in safety related issues. She continues to give consultations in latent print technologies, methodologies and safety and conducts latent print examinations of casework in private practice.

Nancy Masters is a Distinguished Member in the International Association for Identification where she served as Chair and Committee Consultant on the Safety Committee. She is also a long-standing member of the Editorial Review Board for the *Journal of Forensic Identification*. As a past member of the California Division of that organization, she was appointed to serve on the Ethics Committee and Science and Practices Committee. Currently, Nancy is a member of the Pacific Northwest Division of the International Association for Identification. Additionally, Ms. Masters is a Fellow of the Fingerprint Society of Great Britain.

Forward

This publication is intended for those individuals working in the fields of forensic latent prints, questioned documents, and photography, specifically to the area of latent prints. The information provided does not include all the provisions for a complete criminalistics laboratory. The field of safety is immense and numerous texts have been compiled. It is beyond the scope of this work to cover safety at all types of laboratories and crime scenes, however some basic protocols should be followed in all laboratories and at all crime scenes. There are also provisions which should be made for laboratories which are task specific (such as DNA laboratories where radioactive materials are routinely handled).

I intend to provide much needed information to individuals working in facilities which have not traditionally been equipped as a complete chemical laboratory. Additionally, laboratories or "processing areas" that were built ten or twenty years ago may now be inadequate, and some newer facilities lack personnel trained in the safety aspects of facility usage or in the necessary protocols for performing their duties.

Many states do not have their own Occupational Safety and Health Administration (OSHA) and are entirely under the auspices of federal OSHA regulations. I have avoided making the material in this publication specific to California. All cited codes and mandates are based upon federal regulations that states must meet.

Safety has evolved from being totally ignored to a top priority status. As knowledge develops, more questions and issues arise. We have only recently become aware of the hazards associated with fungal spores that can grow in our work environment. Consequently, I have included an additional section to address the topic of *Aspergillus*. While the original work was intended to address laboratory safety, current need and awareness dictated that I also write new sections on Crime Scene Safety and Evidence and Property Room Safety. These three new sections have been included in this edition.

The purpose of this publication is to provide forensic specialists the requisite knowledge which will enable them to both accomplish their tasks in the safest possible manner and in a safe work environment.

Table of Contents

Introduction

The concept of occupational safety is not a new one. For years, working people, from bus drivers to airline pilots to welders to physicists, have been concerned with choosing the best available safety techniques. Immediacy of the hazards they face have made police officers increasingly aware of the dangers of their occupation. Unfortunately, the inherent dangers facing the forensic identification professional have not received a commensurate amount of recognition and attention. Quite often, practitioners as well as their management have been lax.

There is a common myth that certain individuals are "accident prone." No scientific evidence exists to support this idea. Fifty years of research fails to confirm anyone's propensity to mishaps. [1] Individuals control circumstances. Man is really the most powerful means of preventing an accident. [2] Therefore, it is imperative that safety protocols be established, supported, and enforced.

In the 1960's, the federal government enacted legislation for all American workers. The 1970 Occupational Safety and Health Administration (OSHA) Act was written to prevent work-related injuries, illness, or death. Contained within this act is an "employee bill of rights" titled as Public Law 91-596 which lays out general employee safety. (For a complete listing of those employee rights see Appendix A.) The most current federal legislation which regulates laboratory safety is governed by OSHA Regulation 29 CFR 1910.1450. This standard is a basis for all chemical hygiene plans.

In 1989, California state government recognized the need for an Injury and Illness Prevention Program and signed into law Senate Bill (SB) 198. Stats. 1989 c.1369 mandates that CAL/OSHA compliance officers emphasize safety programs in addition to enforcing strictly CAL/OSHA safety standards. The law requires each agency or department to have written operating guidelines which identify workplace hazards as well as investigation of accidents, illness and exposures. The law also requires documentation of employee safety training and a communication system allowing employees to discuss safety and health problems freely.

In 1990, the California legislature passed Assembly Bill (AB) 2249, also known as the California Corporate Criminal Liability Act, which added Section 387 to the California Penal Code. Some managers unaffectionately refer to it as the "Be a Manager Go to Jail" Act! Stats. 1990 c. 1616 makes it a *criminal* offense, punishable by state or county jail and/or fine (not to exceed $25,000 per individual or $1,000,000 per corporation) for any manager who knowingly conceals a danger which poses a serious health risk to workers in industries regulated by the Division of Occupational Safety and Health, Department of Industrial Relations or an appropriate agency. The concealed danger must be one that is not a readily apparent hazard but one that is hidden and has a substantial probability of causing injury, death or a serious exposure. Another element of the crime is the failure on the part of the manager to take positive action to ensure correction of the unsafe practice or condition or to notify the employees and regulating agencies. Present interpretation would indicate that this law does not apply to governmental agencies. However, it is expected that governmental agencies will follow the spirit and intent of the law. [3] Many states in the US. have laws commensurate with the California statute.

There exists a tremendous body of available safety knowledge which is not always used. Consequently, the same types of accidents occur over the years. [4] The results of such accidents can be measured not only in property and equipment losses, but more importantly in human suffering: injuries, disabilities, and deaths. Over 11,000 people die from on-the-job accidents every year, and a worker is injured every 18 seconds. [5]

Essentially, accident prevention depends upon behavior. [6] Humans are not born with knowledge. The supervisor as well as the bench person must learn different facts and functions. [7] One of the stumbling blocks to the implementation of various aspects of the OSHA Act by law enforcement agencies has been a failure of these agencies to understand the requirements laid upon them.

Individuals must be "safety-minded" in order to have a proactive health and safety program in the work place. This attitude goes hand-in-hand with a personal commitment to and responsibility for safety concerns, compliance with laboratory protocols, and hazard awareness.

Written protocols must be developed which include:

- standard laboratory practices
- respirator protection
- hazard communication programs
- Right-to-Know information

Complete and current Material Safety Data Sheet (MSDS) collections must be available in the laboratory at all times. Once the written programs are in place, all employees must receive training on the written procedures.[8] None of these conditions can be met without total management commitment, including the funds required to support the programs.

Interestingly enough, in 1973 a safety professional made a proposal to assess criminal penalties on the employer for injuries incurred by an employee. [9] In 1985 that proposal was taken to heart when the courts held an employer responsible for the death of his employee. The employee worked in a Chicago area film recovery plant where X-ray film was processed for the recovery of silver. The employee died from cyanide poisoning. The employer was held both civilly and criminally liable and sentenced to a term in prison! [10]

Now in the twenty-first century states such as California have legislation defining the punishment for a manager's breach in responsibility. Centuries have passed in which workers were totally expendable. The time is finally here when employees are protected under the law. But how can an employee or employer do the "right thing" without knowledge of the elements of the law and a safe work place? Perhaps the following pages will assist in teaching these elements.

1
Roles and Responsibilities in Safety

Prior to any actions being taken to develop a safety program, decisions must be made as to "who is responsible for what." Intentions and genuine concerns accomplish nothing unless management assigns specific people to specific roles in the safety program. With responsibility must also come authority to complete and oversee the necessary tasks. A program which fails to establish the lines of action and control is a program in name only. This section enumerates the various duties of the laboratory manager, safety officer and the employee.

The Laboratory Manager is responsible for the health and safety program. If the forensic identification section is not contained within a regulation laboratory, then the supervisor of forensic services would fill this role. This individual sees that all work practices conform to the chemical hygiene plan and health and safety policies. S/he prepares procedures for response to accidents which may involve employees exposed to toxic substances. S/he must determine and write into policy control practices for the handling of hazardous substances and make and maintain inventories of hazardous substances. S/he must specify areas for handling of toxic substances and possible or known carcinogens. The manager also prepares a safety plan which defines the use of hazardous substances. This individual administers the safety program.

The Health and Safety Officer is responsible for monitoring all aspects of the safety program and providing health and safety information to all employees. As detailed in Stricoff and Walters' *Laboratory Health and Safety Handbook*, the requirements of the safety officer include:

1. Assisting the laboratory manager in defining hazardous operations, designating safe practices, and selecting protective equipment;

2. Making copies of the approved safety plan available to technical and support staff;

3. Obtaining, reviewing, and approving standard operating procedures, detailing all aspects of proposed laboratory activities that involve hazardous agents;

4. Ensuring that all personnel obtain medical examinations and the protective equipment necessary for the safe performance of their jobs;

5. Ensuring that technical and support staff receive instruction and training in safe work practices and in procedures for dealing with accidents involving test substances;

6. Monitoring the safety performance of the staff to ensure that the required safety practices and techniques are being employed;

7. Conducting formal laboratory inspections quarterly to ensure compliance with existing laboratory policies and government regulations;

8. Arranging for workplace air samples, wipe samples, or other tests to determine the amount and nature of airborne and/or surface contamination, and use data to aid in the evaluation and maintenance of appropriate laboratory conditions;

9. Documenting and maintaining compliance with all local, state, and federal regulatory requirements;

10. Developing rules and procedures for safe practices, assisting in the development and review of health and safety plans; consulting, advising, and making recommendations on all health and safety matters;

11. Developing health and safety training plans and programs, conducting training courses, and establishing safety references;

12. reporting to the laboratory manager incidents (a) that cause personnel to be seriously exposed to hazardous chemicals or materials, such as through the inoculation of a chemical through cutaneous penetration, ingestion of a chemical, or probable inhalation of a chemical, or (b) that constitute a danger of environmental contamination;

13. investigating accidents and reporting them to the laboratory manager;

14. investigating and reporting in writing to the laboratory manager any significant problems pertaining to the operation and implementation of control practices, equipment, or the facility;

15. disposing of unwanted and/or hazardous chemicals and materials, and;

16. ensuring that action is taken to correct work practices and conditions that may result in the release of toxic chemicals.

It is evident from the above requirements that the position of safety officer is a full-time commitment. Management approached me to fill the position of safety officer for "approximately six months of part-time responsibility to get the safety program off the ground." The six months of part-time related activities, in actuality, resulted in two and one-half years of full time commitment.

The reader can appreciate the need for one individual, experienced in forensic identification work, to dedicate himself or herself to the position of safety officer. If your department does not currently have such an individual, a tremendous amount of ground work must be done to get "on board" with a safety program.

Ultimately, safety in the workplace is the responsibility of the employee. Every individual is responsible for his or her own safety as well as the safety of his or her coworkers. Many identification specialists have been lax in educating themselves about proper procedures, following laboratory protocols, and demanding the safe work environment to which they are entitled by law. How does the employee assume responsibility for workplace safety? By developing an understanding of, and acting in accordance with, the safety requirements established by his or her laboratory or department. S/he must also use the safety equipment and wear the personal protective equipment necessary to perform any assigned tasks. Additionally, the employee must have a commitment to reporting to his or her manager or safety officer all facts pertaining to every accident that results in exposure to toxic chemicals, and any action or condition that may exist which could result in an accident.

This last requirement is probably the most difficult as it may require reporting how coworkers or supervisors breach policy. As unpleasant a task as this may be, keep in mind that safety begins with you.

Some employees are concerned that if s/he complains, a supervisor will either "stonewall" or retaliate. Such concerns are legitimate because they have happened. However, the time for safety has arrived. It is one of the greatest concerns in labor today. If a complaint must be made, make it verbally to the responsible authority, and document your conversation on paper. Note the date, persons involved in the conversation, and content of the discussion. If no action is taken in a reasonable amount of time (3-6 weeks), then put the complaint in writing. Once a memo is generated, bureaucratic protocol requires a response. Keep a copy of your memo as part of your documentation package. If still no action is taken or response given in a reasonable amount of time, generate another memo up the chain of command and attach a copy of the first memo. This should result in action. If not, you are justified in making a complaint to OSHA. A few last words to the wise: have complete documentation of any events, conversations, and written complaints; be sure of your facts, and give your management a fair and reasonable opportunity to respond and effect necessary change.

2
Written Policies

A positive, workable and enforceable health and safety program requires written protocols. These policies are the backbone and the basis for all procedures needed to fulfill requirements set forth by federal standards. The standard known as 29 CFR 1910 (Code of Federal Regulations) is the basis of legislation requiring employers to have and maintain a chemical hygiene plan. This legislation applies to all employers whose employees engage in the use of hazardous chemicals as defined by the code. By definition, this embraces the "individual employed in a laboratory workplace who may be exposed to hazardous chemicals in the course of his or her assignments." [1] As a result of such legislative requirements, a number of written policies are necessary to complete the chemical hygiene plan. Illness and prevention programs as well as hazard communication programs must be provided. The following paragraphs will make mention of some of the policies which must be written and maintained.

The OSHA Standard on hazard communication was the requirement put forth in 1985. In California, it became known as the Right-to-Know Law. Essentially, the purpose of the standard was "to ensure that the hazards of all substances produced or imported by manufacturers or importers are evaluated, and that information concerning their hazards is transmitted to all affected employers and employees." [2] The transmittal of information was to include container labeling and other forms of warning, Material Safety Data Sheets and employee training. The law required all employers to provide information to their employees about the hazardous substances to which they may be exposed.

The hazard communication standard must be a written plan which is understandable, accurate and concise. It must include definitive information on how the employer will meet the various requirements (labeling, Material Safety Data Sheet compilation, and employee information and training). An employer must make an inventory of all chemicals or hazardous substances in the workplace. This inventory process provides an excellent opportunity to determine the need for Material Safety Data Sheets not on file and for any necessary labeling to be accomplished. The inventory can apply to an entire worksite or to segregated work areas. The employer must write a plan of how to notify the employees of hazards they might encounter while performing non-routine tasks. The plan must also explain how the employer will inform contractors of any possible exposure hazards. This statement should include any suggestions relating to appropriate protective measures to be taken by the contractor's employees. (This circumstance occurs when a janitorial staff is contracted to do floor waxing, etc. or carpenters, plumbers, and electricians are contracted to perform remodeling work.) The employees must receive information and *training* on all hazardous substances known to be present in the workplace to which they may be exposed under normal conditions of use or in a reasonably foreseeable emergency. This provision applies to janitors and secretaries as well as persons working in a laboratory environment. All of the requirements enumerated in this standard are also embodied in the current law.

A chemical hygiene plan must contain the above elements. It should provide all necessary information on hazards in the workplace. This will include the compilation of a Material Safety Data Sheet (MSDS) collection for **all** chemicals in the workplace. The Material Safety Data Sheet is one of the most important methods for providing information to employees about the nature of the substances in the work environment. Another equally important means of transmitting information is through the labeling of substances. Material Safety Data Sheets and labeling will be discussed in a later section. There must be a written policy which states when and how these elements will be accomplished.

Other means of disseminating hazard information to employees is by providing training about the physical and health hazards in the workplace, of the methods and observations to detect the presence or release of a hazardous substance, and of the methods and procedures to protect the employee from exposure at the worksite.

Information and training on any hazardous substances must be provided at the time that the employees are initially assigned to their jobs and also immediately after any new hazard is introduced into the workplace. Training must include information on the hazard communication standard, including employee rights. Employees must be taught how to read and understand MSDS's and warning labels. The employer must identify any tasks, procedures, or operations involving hazardous substances.

The operative word is *training*. Simply supplying a manual of written procedures to the employee and having them "sign-off" that they have read the material does not qualify as training. Employees must have training sessions in which the information is provided and discussed. They must have an opportunity to express their questions and concerns. These training sessions may include the use of video tapes, questionnaires, safety exercises, and question and answer segments. The employer should keep detailed records of the training provided all employees.

Every laboratory should have a written safety manual or manual of laboratory protocols. This must include the general safety policy, standard laboratory procedures, use of personal protective equipment, and should include the procedures and chemical formulas used in the preparation of any reagents. For the forensic specialist, this means that the manual should explain, step by step, how chemical preparations are mixed and applied to evidence. An individual with no training should be able to read the manual and understand how to proceed when entering the laboratory. More specifically, written policies should be developed to detail the department's standards for the following:

1. **Fingerprint powders and chemical reagents –** Why, when and how they should be used and what the exposure hazards are. How a person avoids exposures. What an employee does in the event of an exposure. Where an employee goes for medical assistance.

2. **Flammable chemicals** – What they are and how to avoid accidents and exposures. What the handling and storage requirements are. How to avoid accidents in using flammables.

3. **Explosive and reactive chemicals** – What they are and how to avoid accidents and exposures. What the handling and storage requirements are. How to prevent accidents in using these chemicals.

4. **Corrosive chemicals** – What they are and how to avoid accidents and exposures. What the handling and storage requirements are. How to prevent accidents in handling corrosive chemicals.

5. **Toxic chemicals** – What they are and how to avoid accidents and exposures. What the handling and storage requirements are. How to avoid accidents in handling toxic chemicals.

6. **Chemical spills** – What procedures to follow in the event of a spill. How to clean up chemical spills and when to attempt clean up versus calling for assistance.

7. **Waste disposal of hazardous chemicals** – How to dispose of chemicals that result from chemical processing or spills without violating any regulations or creating a hazard for others who may handle the material. What waste is considered hazardous and who retains legal responsibility for that waste.

8. **Personal protective equipment** – What equipment to use to prevent exposure to hazardous substances. How to use the equipment and which type or style is appropriate for each procedure. How to maintain or dispose of the equipment safely.

9. **Fume hood and other ventilation methods** – When and how to use ventilation devices. How to maintain the hoods and when to test them for face velocity. How to clean hoods of contaminate buildup. Who completes such cleaning of ventilation equipment.

10. **Respiratory equipment** – What types of respiratory equipment to use for each procedure. How to fit, test, don, doff and maintain equipment. What the correct cartridges or canisters are. Who should and should not use respiratory equipment. Regulations about wearing mustaches, beards and contact lenses.

11. **Noise protection** – When to wear ear protection. What type to wear. Which ear protectors meet requirements for adequate protection from various noise levels.

12. **Firearms safety** – When and how to handle a firearm. Basic rules and regulations of handling weapons. How to render a firearm "safe." When not to accept a firearm into the facility.

13. **Emergency procedures** – Procedures established for dealing with medical, police or fire emergencies. How to safely leave a burning building. Systems for clearing the facility in an emergency. Where to report after evacuation. Where to find the fire prevention plan. How people receive training on the plan. Whom to call when a coworker experiences a heart attack or electrocution. Procedures for dealing with a bomb threat.

14. **Natural disaster procedures** – Procedures established to protect employees in an earthquake or tornado. What to do and where to go for safety. Systems for clearing the facility. Where to report after evacuation.

15. **First aid and CPR** – Who knows first aid or CPR. When to call someone for first aid or CPR and what to do if no trained personnel are available. What first aid equipment is available in the workplace, where it is located and how to use it.

16. **Crime scenes** – Processing crime scenes, including clandestine laboratories, is hazardous. What preventive procedures to take to avoid the inherent dangers. What strategies to employ to decrease these hazards. What protective equipment to use in which circumstances. What to do when someone is injured at a scene. How to get immediate police, fire, or medical assistance.

17. **Biological specimens** – What the hazards of these specimens are. What the routes of exposure are and how to prevent exposure. How to package and/or dispose of these specimens safely. How to store specimens. Who is eligible for medical monitoring or vaccinations.

18. **Employee vaccinations** – Who may be vaccinated and against which viral infections. Who pays for the vaccinations.

19. **Employee health screening** – Who is screened. Whether the employer provides the baseline or only subsequent screenings. Which tests are performed.

20. **Medical and employee records** – Which medical and exposure records are maintained. What the access and retention requirements are. Who prepares and stores the records. When and to whom to release the records.

21. **Laboratory cleanup schedule** – What the schedule is and who is responsible for cleaning up. What records to keep to document the process.

22. **Inspection** – What the schedule is for laboratory inspection. Who is responsible for the inspection. What the requirements are for passing. Procedures for surprise inspections. What measures enforce necessary corrections after inspection.

23. **Environmental monitoring** – Which procedures and equipment to use to monitor the laboratory environment. What the schedule is for monitoring the environment. How to clean the laboratory if an overload of contaminants is found.

24. **Defensive driver training** –Who has permission to drive departmental

vehicles. When to use the vehicles. What training is provided in defensive driving to avoid accidents.

The above list is by no means complete. Many other policies can be developed and written. In fact, Doug Walters and R. Scott Stricoff put it rather succinctly when they noted the content of the hygiene plan must include the following items:

- Standard operating procedures (SOP's) to be followed when laboratory work involves the use of hazardous chemicals.
- Criteria to determine the need for, and the nature of, exposure control strategies to reduce personnel exposures. These strategies include engineering and administrative controls and the use of personal protective equipment.
- A requirement that control measures, including lab hoods and other local exhaust ventilation, be properly selected, designed, installed, and maintained, along with procedures to ensure satisfaction of the requirement.
- Information and training procedures.
- A provision for medical consultation and evaluation.
- Circumstances under which a particular laboratory operation will require approval prior to implementation.
- Identification of personnel responsible for implementation and maintenance of the hygiene plan.
- For work performed with carcinogenic materials and other particularly hazardous chemicals, additional protective measures. [3]

All departments containing or using equipment or materials that may pose a health hazard to the employee must have a written chemical hygiene plan with the above elements. The employee must know the written plan and must be trained about hazards in the workplace. Additionally, each department must designate an individual to develop, implement, and monitor the program. In other words, **every department needs a safety officer.**

3
Material Safety Data Sheets

Material Safety Data Sheets (MSDS) are required by federal standards. Under the Federal Hazard Communication Standard, manufacturers must evaluate the hazards of each product. A written evaluation (MSDS) must be prepared if 1% or more of the product is a hazardous substance. The product container must also be labeled with its identity, manufacturer's name and address, and appropriate hazard warnings.

The manufacturer, importer, or distributor of any chemical substance **must** supply an MSDS for every chemical substance sold. Some products are exempt from labeling and/or MSDS requirements. Following are *some* of the exceptions:

1. Any pesticides as defined in the Federal Insecticide, Fungicide, and Rodenticide Act (7 U.S.C. 136 et seq.) when subject to labeling requirements and regulations under that act by the Environmental Protection Agency (EPA). [1]

2. Any food, food additive, color additive, drug or cosmetic, including the components of the ingredients of those products, as defined in the Federal Food, Drug, and Cosmetic Act (21 U.S.C. 301 et seq.) when subject to the labeling requirements and regulations under that act by the Food and Drug Administration (FDA). [2]

3. Any beverage containing alcohol, wine or malts not intended for industrial use, as defined in the Federal Alcohol Administration Act (27 U.S.C. 201 et seq.) when subject to the labeling requirements and regulations under that act by the Bureau of Alcohol, Tobacco, and Firearms (BATF). [3]
4. Any consumer product or hazardous substance as defined in the Consumer

Product Safety Act (15 U.S.C. 2051 et seq.) and Federal Hazardous Standards Act (15 U.S.C. 1261 et seq.), when subject to a consumer product safety standard or labeling requirement of those acts or regulations issued by the Consumer Product Safety Commission. [4]

5. Hazardous waste as defined by the Solid Waste Disposal Act, as amended by the Resources Conservation and Recovery Act of 1976, as amended (42 U.S.C. 6901 et seq.) when subject to regulations under the act by the E.P.A. [5]

6. Tobacco and tobacco products. [6]

7. Foods, drugs, or cosmetics intended for personal consumption by employees in the workplace. [7]

Some of the above regulations help the lay person to build a knowledge of labeling and MSDS requirements. When compiling MSDS collections, it is often difficult to determine whether a data sheet is necessary to meet compliance. This information will help the novice determine the need for a MSDS for photocopier toner but not for insect spray used to kill ants invading the lunch room.

It is also helpful to understand how the manufacturer makes a hazard assessment for the data sheet. Library research is sufficient as long as it contains a complete and accurate compilation of the required information on each product. The manufacturer is not required to do any actual flammability or toxicity testing. They are required to add any new significant information regarding chemical hazards or protective measures to the MSDS within three months. For this reason, laboratories should periodically update their MSDS collection. Newer MSDS's will reflect more recent toxicity studies and findings, increased risks to employee health, or new protective measures which can be implemented.

When a product is purchased, the MSDS should be received with the shipment. If the source of the product is the distributor, an MSDS should accompany the product if the distributor received one. If not, request a data sheet from the manufacturer. All manufacturers must comply by supplying either an MSDS or a written statement explaining why no data sheet is required. (This may occur in rather surprising ways. I requested a data sheet for a brand of typewriter cleaner which contained a known hazardous solvent. The supplier sent a letter stating that it is exempt from compliance because it is a state department.)

There are several elements of the Material Safety Data Sheet. It is divided into sections which contain specific information. The data may appear in different formats or be arranged on a page differently from one MSDS to another. All MSDS's must be written in English and contain the following information:

1. The name and address of the manufacturer and any emergency information and/or telephone numbers. This information is usually at the top of the MSDS and can be invaluable in the event of an accident or emergency. The date the sheet was prepared must be provided and may appear at the beginning or end of the document.

2. The identity of the substance as used on the label. (There may be exceptions to this requirement based upon trade secrets.) It must note whether the hazardous substance is a single substance or part of a mixture. The exact chemical name and common name must be included for all hazardous ingredients in the mixture. An example of a chemical name is "2-propanol"; however, it is commonly known as "isopropyl alcohol." This section also contains the Chemical Abstract Service (CAS) number. (The CAS number is one which the service assigns to every chemical for consistent and reliable identification.) The chemical formula is included in this section and looks like this for 2-propanol; C_3H_8O or $CH_3CHOHCH_3$.

3. The physical and chemical properties of the hazardous substances such as the vapor pressure, boiling point, flash point, solubility, and melting point. This section should also contain a statement about the appearance and odor of the substance. It may read "solid, odorless," "colorless to pale purple, pungent odor," etc.

4. The physical hazards of the hazardous substance including the potential for fire, explosion and reactivity data. This section will include fire and explosion data, flammability factors such as the explosive limits, flash point, fire extinguishing techniques and fire fighting procedures. It will often state unusual fire hazards such as the emission of toxic fumes or whether or not to use water to subdue, etc.

5. Reactivity and incompatibility data. Any incompatible chemicals will be listed, as well as any hazardous reactions which result from contact with other substances. This section also contains information on decomposition products and possible polymerization. (Polymerization means that two or more like molecules join to form a more complex molecule whose molecular weight is a multiple of the original but whose physical properties are different. [8])

6. Health hazards of the substance, which include routes of entry, signs and symptoms of exposure, and "any medical conditions generally recognized as being aggravated by exposure to the substance." [9] Any established permissible exposure limits or threshold limit values are noted here. Acute and chronic effects of exposure are detailed as well as first aid procedures.

7. Any known precautions to take in the safe handling and storage of the substance. This includes the use of personal protective equipment such as gloves, chemical goggles, rubber boots, respirators, etc. Any control measures or engineering controls, such as ventilation systems, should be mentioned. This section, or an additional section, will also discuss procedures to be taken in the event of a spill or chemical leak. Recommendations for personal protective equipment use and special precautions are detailed. Information on waste disposal may be included.

MSDS's must be available to employees. Employees should review these data sheets before a chemical is handled so the employee learns about the hazards in advance. It is a good idea to review the available information periodically, especially if a person does not work routinely in the laboratory. MSDS's should be maintained in a common work area and/or the laboratory. Maintain a master file of the original sheets to replace damaged or soiled copies, update information, and write safety protocols.

Once the MSDS has been read and understood, and all the necessary information assimilated, is the employee ready to proceed into the laboratory? Not necessarily. There are still a few considerations to keep in mind:

- MSDS's frequently note only the **minimum** standards or precautions for the safe handling of a chemical. An employee or employer may determine the need for more stringent policies.

- No blank spaces should occur on the MSDS. Sometimes information is not available to the preparer; however this must be indicated in the appropriate space. If a blank space occurs, contact the supplier and question it regarding the missing data.

- Never assume that a chemical is harmless because a particular health hazard is not mentioned on the MSDS. Sometimes the preparer of the data sheet did not have access to relevant test results. Additionally, new studies are performed and completed from year to year which may change current information. Do not be lulled into indifference about potential hazards of a chemical because a reading of the MSDS makes it appear innocuous.

- Never assume that a minor exposure or incident does not require attention. If a designated medical or health professional is not available for consultation, take immediate steps to follow the first aid procedures listed on the MSDS.

The Material Safety Data Sheet offers one of the first lines of defense in preventing an accident or exposure in the laboratory. It is also one of the first building blocks in developing a knowledge of the chemical substances which may endanger the individual in the workplace. Demand that MSDS's be made available. Always read them before proceeding in the handling of unfamiliar chemicals. Even when familiar with certain substances, periodically refer to and review the pertinent data sheets to refresh your memory. If any questions arise, consult a supervisor, designated safety officer, an appointed medical or health consultant, the supplier, or the manufacturer. Accident prevention will be enhanced by not leaving anything to chance.

4
Chemical Hazards

Chemical hazards are one of the two major laboratory hazards in the workplace. (Biological hazards, posing the other greatest threat, will be discussed in Section 5.) Keep in mind that the workplace extends to crime scenes or any other area where you are working in your official capacity. An officer shared one recent horror story. She was told to transport containers of ether which had crystallized. She wondered why her escort vehicle maintained a rather large distance between them. At the time of the incident, she had no idea of the explosive hazards of crystalline ether.

The National Institute for Occupational Safety and Health (NIOSH) has defined hazardous materials as "a substance or mixture of substances having properties capable of producing adverse effects on the health or safety of the worker" and, in addition, are "toxic, flammable or reactive." A NIOSH study of these hazardous workplace materials resulted in a finding of thousands of hazardous materials identified only by trade names (not chemical names), many unrecognized material hazards, many unrecognized exposures and a lack of uniformity and completeness in the labeling and identification of hazards. [1] There are numerous systems for classifying hazards, some quite complex. Classify chemicals by the predominant type of hazard they pose. The resultant classification will serve as a guideline for properly handling, using, storing and disposing of these substances.

Additionally, chemicals are often hazardous because of circumstances under which they are used (e.g., with boiling water), rather than because of their inherent properties (e.g., as with sulfuric acid). [2] This is an important concept for the employee to grasp. A person can read the MSDS and feel that s/he understands the hazards associated with a particular substance. However, s/he may not understand further hazards caused by handling, combination effects with other chemicals, or the environment into which the substance will be placed.

For the forensic identification specialist, most chemical hazards can be separated into four different categories. These classifications are

1. **Flammables**. Fire makes these materials hazardous. This type of chemical is commonly used in the laboratory, usually as a liquid. Some frequently used flammables are acetone, methanol, ethanol, petroleum ether, and hexane.

2. **Reactive**. Certain situations make these substances reactive and/or explosive. With explosives, a detonation or ignition source is necessary to begin the reaction. In the case of reactive chemicals, an uncontrolled reaction takes place as result of an interaction with water, air, a reducing or oxidizing agent, or some other type of chemical. The results are the same. A sudden and violent reaction releases substantial amounts of heat and gas. An example of this type of reaction is seen when water is poured into acid(s).

3. **Physical**. This hazard results in a physical destruction of body tissue from contact with chemicals which are corrosive. Such chemicals can be acids *or* bases. In either instance, these substances are caustic or can burn, eat away, or destroy tissue as result of chemical action. Such burns are usually more severe than those received from extremes of heat. Fumes of corrosive chemicals, in sufficient quantities in the air, can also cause serious damage to mucous membranes if inhaled.

4. **Toxicity**. These substances impair or destroy normal bodily functions through chemical interaction with tissues. This may occur at relatively low doses. The severity of the effect can vary from mild to lethal and is dependent upon the particular chemical, the sensitivity of the individual, and the amount and length of the exposure. The type of toxic effect the substance has on the body can include one or more of the following categories:

    a) poison – a substance which interferes with or destroys the body cells' ability to function properly. This inability causes sickness or death from either acute or chronic exposures.

    b) mutagen – a substance which causes changes in the genetic or chromosomal composition of the cells (i.e., DNA structure).

    c) teratogen – a substance which will affect the fetus in the womb of a woman. In other words, these chemicals cause abnormalities or birth defects. An example is thalidomide, given to pregnant women in the early 1960's as a sedative and sleeping pill. It was later discovered to cause severe malformation in limbs of developing fetuses exposed to the drug during very early intrauterine life. Thousands of infants were born without arms and/or legs.

d) carcinogen - a substance which causes cancer. [3] Most cancers develop over a period of time as a result of prolonged and repeated exposures to these substances. Examples of some known carcinogens are tobacco smoke, benzidine and asbestos fibers.

All chemicals should be handled as though they are hazardous. The degree of hazard may be unknown, so handle each substance cautiously until further information arrives. Herein lies the value of the Material Safety Data Sheet.

When first introducing chemicals into the laboratory or latent processing site, the forensic specialist and management should consider certain factors. When assessing the chemical or procedures using the chemical, consider the following: temperature sensitivity, impact sensitivity, flammability properties, pressure development, reactive energy, reaction rate, effects of volume or mass, concentration, contamination, catalysis (the speeding up of the rate of a chemical reaction by a catalyst), peroxide formation, effects of air and water, compatibility, and chemical structure. [4]

When assessing a potential hazard, the following energy sources must be considered for their impact on the chemicals or procedures: flames, sparks, hot surfaces, friction, compression, impact, vibration, light, spontaneous combustion, and rapid pressure changes. [5] Ignoring the aforementioned factors could result in a devastating accident.

Flammables

Flammable and combustible liquids are present everywhere in the laboratory. (See page 21 and Appendix C for the definition of flammables.) For this reason, the forensic specialist must be familiar with the subject of flammables and the characteristics of each solvent being used or stored in the work area. Many chemicals classified as flammables may also be corrosive and toxic. For instance, acetone is a well known flammable but also toxic to the skin and toxic through inhalation. Remember that any given chemical can have more than one action or hazard associated with it. When working with flammables, protective clothing and good ventilation are a must. Keep only minimal amounts in the working area and contain these in approved cans and cabinets. No flames or ignition sources of any kind are allowed where flammables are in use or stored. Flammable liquids should be well labeled with both FLAMMABLE and DANGER signs. Always store these chemicals in a well ventilated area. Make sure the refrigerator is explosion-proof if you store any flammables in it. If you must heat a flammable chemical, do so only with hot water, steam, or an electric heating mantle. Approved metal safety cans are best for transporting flammable solvents. If the solvent is in a glass container, then place it in a cushioned safety carrier. See Figure 16-3 on page 124.

If an accident occurs, take immediate action. Rinse well with water any spills on the skin. If a flammable is accidentally ingested, induce vomiting with syrup of ipecac. [6] If a person's clothing should catch fire, smother the fire with a fire blanket (or follow whatever policy has been established by your department to handle such an incident), and get medical help immediately. (Figure 4-1) Do not clean the skin with solvents. Any spill rags used for cleanup should be immediately placed into safety cans.

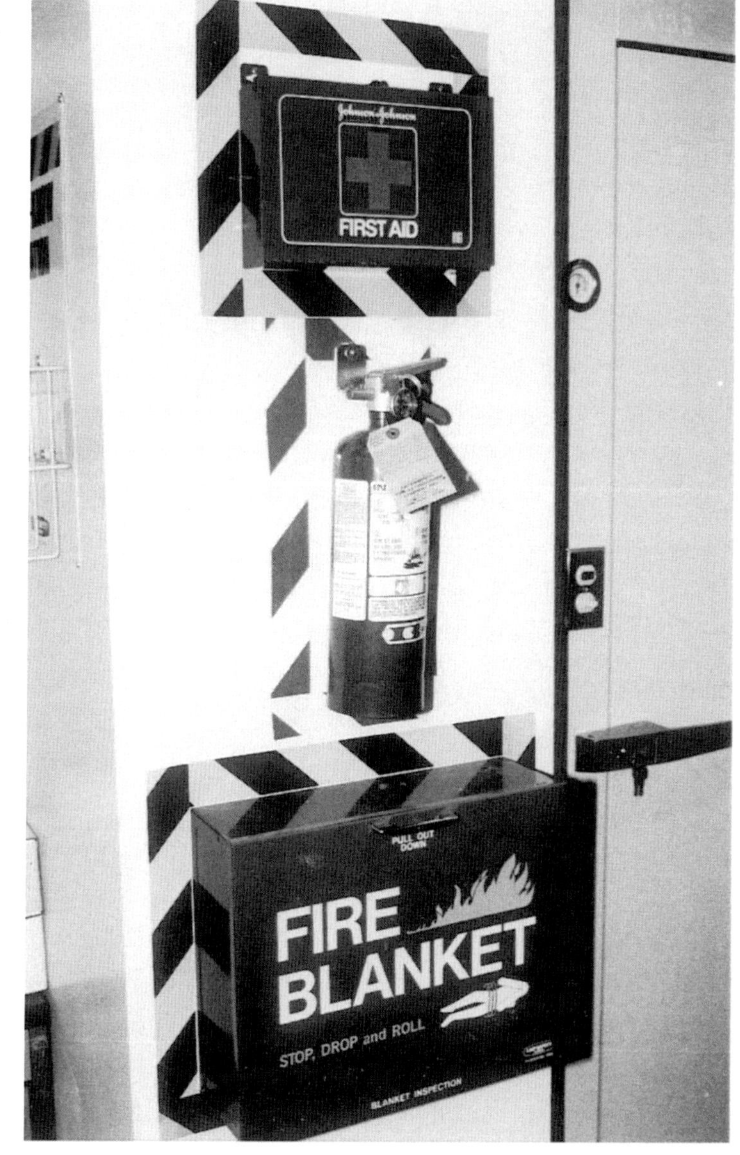

If a flammable solvent is contained in a metal container and is being poured or transferred into another metal container, clean the two contacting surfaces of dirt, paint, rust or other contaminating debris and then bond the two metal to metal surfaces before pouring. Otherwise, a static spark can create ignition. If one container is glass, bonding is not necessary.

Reactives

Explosives include materials which under certain conditions of temperature, shock, or chemical reaction can decompose so rapidly that either large volumes of gas or so much heat is released that the surrounding air is forced to expand very rapidly, resulting in an explosion. Generally speaking, keep all flammable chemicals such as organic compounds (those containing carbon - these include acetone, ethanol, methanol, petroleum ether) away from oxidizing agents (such as acids). Those materials with flash points at or below room temperature should be considered extremely dangerous. The term *explosive* defines primarily a set of conditions and not a type of chemical. Most explosives will be found under other hazardous categories as well. [7] The forensic identification specialist uses these chemicals which have explosive potential: acetone, ethanol, ethyl acetate, hexane, heptane, methanol, petroleum ether, and xylene.

Oxidizers are chemicals which contain oxygen available to react with reducing materials to yield an overall net energy release. They supply oxygen to support combustion of normally nonflammable materials, yielding heat, and are explosively sensitive to heat, shock, or friction. They also pose a toxicity hazard. Generally, the following chemical types are oxidizers: compounds ending in *-ite* or *-ate* or with the prefix *per-*, oxoacids, peroxides, halogens, halogen-nitrogen reacted compounds, and reacted mixed halogens. [8] An unplanned or greater than expected, even explosive, energy release of some oxidizers poses a very serious hazard. Containers of oxidizers should be labeled both DANGER and OXIDIZER. Perform work with oxidizers in the fume hood with the sash lowered as far as possible. Always wear protective clothing. Keep in mind that hydrocarbon greases or oils must *never* be used with oxygen or halogens.

While most forensic identification work does not require the use of many oxidizers, it is a good idea to become familiar with these chemicals and how to handle them. Do not permit smoking, open flames and other sources of heat near peroxides. Avoid friction, grinding, and all forms of impact, especially with solid peroxides. Use polyethylene bottles with screw-cap lids, not glass containers with screw-cap lids or glass stoppers.

Corrosives

Corrosive agents used in the forensic identification laboratory can be described as acids or bases that damage flesh with first-, second-, or third- degree burns up to twenty-four hours after contact. [8] Some corrosives destroy live tissue as they penetrate it and will produce pain, itching, skin discoloration, or fumes. Other such chemicals cause damage after they have penetrated well into deeper tissues. These corrosives are far more serious. They will migrate into tissues and cause deep, serious burns. The corrosives that cause delayed effects tend to be most damaging. If a corrosive is spilled on the skin, the burning sensation from tissue damage may be delayed. Never wait to determine whether or not the exposure "burns" before taking action. Inhalation of corrosive vapors or ingestion of corrosives causes severe edema (swelling) and extensive burning of the respiratory tract or mouth and throat. [9]

Most people do not intentionally harm themselves with corrosives. These events occur accidentally and catch the victim by surprise. Sudden pain and shock contribute to the panic that causes disorientation, and the victim may entirely forget the location of or to use eyewash fountains or body showers. Someone else must force the corrosives victim to wash the corrosive away thoroughly. In the case of eye burns, this may require holding the victim's eye open in order to irrigate properly the affected eye. If the skin (or eye) is burned with a corrosive, immediately irrigate with a continuous flow of water for a minimum of 15 minutes to prevent or reduce potential damage. Do not apply chemical neutralizers to the skin. Seek medical assistance immediately. Laboratory protocols require that at least two people work in the chemical laboratory at one time. If you work alone and you are injured, you will have no help in the event of an accident. [10]

Label all containers of corrosive acids or bases with both a CORROSIVE and DANGER label. Always wear protective equipment including the proper gloves and goggles when working with this class of chemicals. Wear a chemical splash shield as well as goggles when pouring or transferring corrosives. **Corrosives should not be placed above eye level.** Place corrosives in a tray (such as a plastic photo tray) or container large enough to contain the contents in case of an accident. A working eyewash fountain (Figure 4-2) and body safety shower (Figure 4-3) are a must in the laboratory or processing area. These are required by law. A fume hood, as well as other adequate ventilation, is necessary to reduce the buildup of vapors. Acids such as glacial acetic acid will volatilize (evaporate) into the ambient atmosphere and produce very irritating vapors to anyone in the breathing zone. Use a commercial spill kit with chemical neutralizers for cleanup of a corrosives spill.

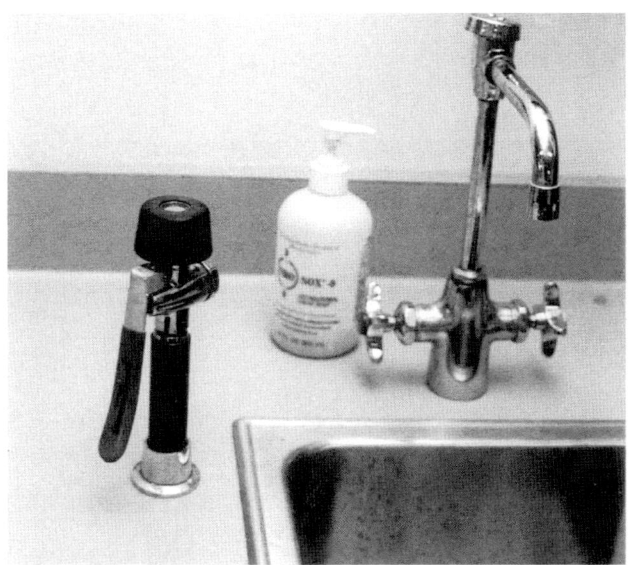

Figure 4-2: Eye wash station located at laboratory sink.

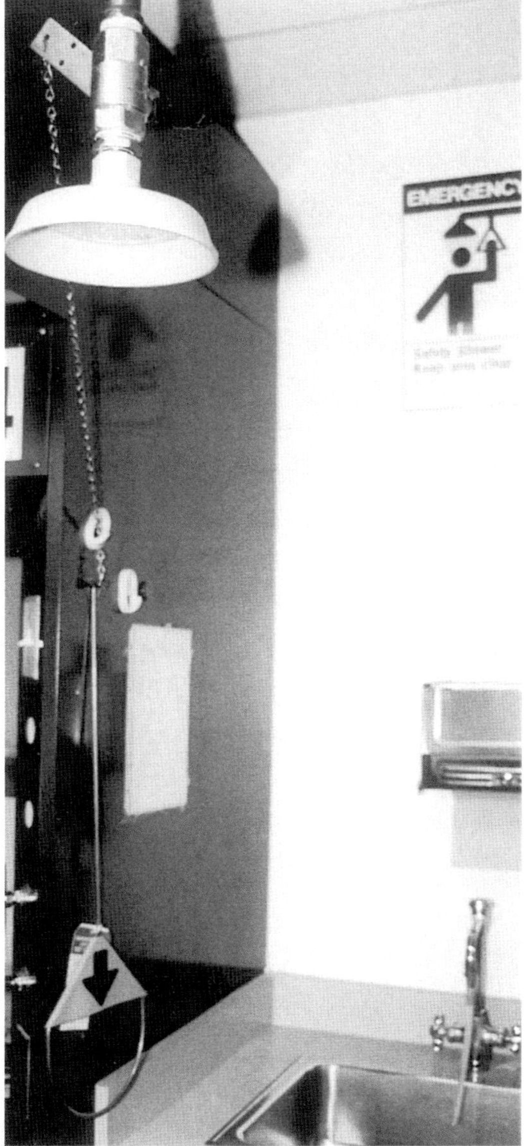

Figure 4-3: Full body safety shower installed in chemistry laboratory for use in the event of an incident.

Among the corrosives that may be encountered in the forensic identification laboratory are liquids such as organic acids (acetic and hydrochloric acid and acids used by questioned document examiners to analyze inks), organic solvents, and solids. What solid corrosive do we use in our profession? Iodine. This material is extremely corrosive. There are many more corrosives which will be encountered in the chemical laboratory, but most are not used in forensic identification work.

Toxic Substances

Toxic substances are also called poisons. They can, in relatively small quantities, cause illness or death when ingested (lead, mercury), inhaled (fumes, gases, vapors such as sulfur dioxide, hydrogen cyanide), or absorbed through the skin (mercury, methanol). Are all chemicals toxic? Is a particular substance toxic? The answer is "Yes, certainly." All substances are toxic at some level (although not necessarily every substance to every species). [11] Even water can be toxic; humans cannot survive in it as a pure medium. Oxygen can be toxic. All chemicals should be considered toxic until you receive further information about the substance.

The numerous toxic chemicals used in the laboratory are toxic only in their free or chemically available forms. The toxicity of these chemicals in the body depends on their absorption and distribution (protein binding, transformation, storage, excretion), tolerance and rate of metabolism. Toxic effects may be categorized as *local* or *systemic* (as in bioaccumulative such as with carcinogens), *acute* or *chronic*. [12] Exposures usually termed *acute* or *chronic*, mean that the effects are immediately manifested or occur again and again over time and may intensify with time.

Maximum allowable safe-exposure limits to toxic materials have been developed from the best available data reflecting the human health effects of these toxic materials. They are called *threshold limit values* (TLV's). These values, being averages, do not reflect individual sensitivities. The federal government uses TLV's to set a safe-exposure level for most workers exposed to toxic materials. (TLV's are recommended by the American Conference of Governmental Industrial Hygienists. They are not enforceable by law unless no other legal standard exists.) Regular measurement and monitoring of the contaminant level in the workplace reduces the likelihood that employees will be exposed in excess of the TLV. *Permissible exposure limit* (PEL) is a term closely related to TLV. OSHA standards use PEL to describe the level and duration of allowable employee exposures to the OSHA-regulated toxic chemicals (over an eight hour period). [13]

Containers of toxic substances should be labeled DANGER and TOXIC. Always handle toxic chemicals under the fume hood. Again, these materials may pose other hazards such as flammable or corrosive. For instance, methanol is extremely toxic but is also flammable. Whenever possible, substitute less hazardous materials for toxic ones. For example, many departments have substituted ethanol for methanol in their formulations of Rhodamine 6G. Get medical help or advice if prolonged or unexpected contact with a toxic substance occurs. Thorough washing after the use of toxic chemicals is mandatory, as is medical surveillance at regular intervals. [14] Always use personal protective equipment such as laboratory coats, aprons, goggles, gloves, shoe covers and/or chemical splash shields when working with toxic materials. And it bears repeating: "Wash your hands before leaving the laboratory."

The forensic identification specialist should approach the use of chemicals with the same sense of professionalism which s/he applies to other aspects of the field. Always read the labels on chemical containers. Labels contain information on the type of hazard posed by the chemical contents. They will often also recommend the proper personal protective equipment. Consult the MSDS for information on the properties of the substance, for the proper protective clothing, storage conditions, any incompatible chemicals, and any other safety information when handling any chemical for the first few times. The MSDS's are one of the best sources of information available on any chemical substance and should be reviewed periodically the same as any other technical literature.

5
Biological Hazards

"Biological hazards are any virus, bacteria, fungus, parasite, or any living organism that can cause disease in human beings." [1] These hazards can be transmitted by animals or by exposure to contaminated water, insects or infected people. Federal legislation has been enacted which dictates the handling of pathogenic materials. 29 CFR 1910.1030, the Bloodborne Pathogens Standard. The requirements under this standard are very specific to biological materials. All employers are required to develop safety policies in line with the regulation.

Some protocols for handling biological materials are much the same as those for chemical substances. However, chemical hazards and biological hazards are very different and pose different risks. A few statements need to be repeated. **Always employ universal precautions by handling all biological materials as though they were infectious.** [2] For the forensic identification specialist, this includes the fingers and hands of deceased individuals. Handle these materials in a manner which will introduce a minimum of dried particulate into the air. Additionally, if you are required to attend autopsies, demand that you be provided complete personal protective equipment. You should be equipped <u>at least</u> as well as the pathologist. Unfortunately, a minority of pathologists see themselves as being made of some kind of metal that can not be infected! I know a man who refuses to use gowns, gloves, or masks and expects the same of the identification specialists. He insists that these individuals get their camera right into the body cavity for the photography and belittles them if they show reluctance or concern. You do <u>not</u> have to work under these circumstances, <u>ever</u>! You are entitled to protective equipment. If the equipment hinders your ability to perform the job, then develop procedures to perform the task using the protective equipment.

The hazards of working with and around biological materials come from the danger of contacting and receiving an infectious exposure from bacteria, fungi, viruses, or parasites. Some of these can be found in dead tissues and some in biological fluids. Most people have a serious concern regarding Hepatitis B and Acquired Immunodeficiency Syndrome (AIDS). This section will discuss these two diseases in detail and recommend strategies for coping with possible exposures. Many specialists have heard of these infections but may not have a very in-depth understanding of what they are or how they affect the body. Both these viruses are found in blood or other serous body fluids, in the greatest quantities in blood. Therefore, federal and state legislation addresses them under the category of bloodborne pathogens.

Bloodborne Pathogens

Hepatitis Viruses

We have all heard of hepatitis, but what is it? Hepatitis refers to "inflammation of the liver". Hepatitis can be caused by chemicals, autoimmune disease and frequently, by biological agents. In the United States, four types of viral hepatitis are considered important. Hepatitis A (HAV) which used to be called "infectious hepatitis," is spread by fecal contamination. This is the type of hepatitis most often contracted through children or restaurants and catering services when food preparers have not followed good hygiene after using the toilet. It can affect anyone and in the U.S., it can occur in situations ranging from periodic cases to epidemics. Hepatitis B (HBV), which used to be called "serum hepatitis," poses one of the greatest risks to the forensic identification specialist. An effective vaccination is available for this virus. Delta Hepatitis (HDV) affects persons who have already been infected with HBV and can increase the severity of acute and chronic liver disease. It is a defective virus that is dependent upon the existence of Hepatitis B to stay alive. HDV is covered by the HBV vaccination. Non-A, Non-B (HCV) hepatitis is the name once given to a group of diseases caused by viral agents. These viral agents are now recognized as the causative factor in Hepatitis C. A bloodborne virus that is efficiently transmitted by blood transfusions and by needle sharing among intravenous drug users causes the "post transfusion" type of HCV. [3] Hepatitis C now poses as serious a risk to the forensic identification specialist as Hepatitis B. Hepatitis E (HEV) is transmitted in the same manner as Hepatitis A. Fortunately, it does not often occur in the United States. There is no vaccination for Hepatitis E.

Hepatitis B Virus (HBV)

So what if you do become infected with HBV? What is likely to happen to you and what symptoms will you possibly experience? Results of infection will take two possible outcomes. The first is self-limited acute hepatitis B. The body destroys many liver cells in a valiant effort to rid itself of the infection, producing antibodies (these antibodies are to both the core and surface particles of the virus), eliminating the virus from the body, and creating a life-time immunity to re-infection. Almost a third of these cases of acute infections produce no symptoms. Another third experience a relatively mild reaction with flu-like symptoms. The remaining third of cases are much more severe. They can result in jaundice (a yellowing of the eyes and skin), dark urine, extreme fatigue, anorexia (loss of appetite), nausea, abdominal pain, and sometimes joint pain, rash, and fever. Several weeks to months of time off work is necessary to recover, if not hospitalization. Fulminant hepatitis (or rapid and at full intensity) is about 85% fatal even with advanced medical care and occurs in about 1 - 2% of cases. [4]

The second possible outcome is development of chronic hepatitis B, with far more severe consequences. Approximately 6 - 10% of infected adults are unable to flush the virus from their liver cells and become chronic HBV carriers. HBV carriers are at high risk of developing chronic persistent hepatitis, chronic active hepatitis, cirrhosis of the liver, and primary liver cancer. One fourth of carriers develop the relatively mild, non-progressive chronic persistent hepatitis. Another fourth develop the chronic active hepatitis which is progressive, debilitating and often leads to cirrhosis of the liver in 5 to 10 years. This condition can result in death. Survivors develop terminal liver cancer in 20 to 60 years. [5]

There are vaccinations available for HBV. These vaccines can be taken as a means of prevention before or after exposure to the hepatitis virus. The HBV vaccine taken for prevention of infection before exposures occur are 100% effective for recipients who develop antibodies. Studies reveal that more than 90% of recipients will develop the necessary antibodies. The first series of vaccinations consists of three shots. Over a six month period, if this serum does not result in antibody protection, people at high risk for exposure should consider a second series. The second series is estimated to develop antibodies in 30 to 50% of the recipients. [6] The period of time of vaccine effectiveness is as yet unknown. Until U. S. Public Health Services comes out with specific direction for booster shots, individuals should seek advice through their physicians.

Hepatitis B Immune Globulin (HBIG) can be given in two shots one month apart to an individual who has been exposed. This vaccine is about 70 to 88% effective in preventing infection if administered within seven days of exposure. The addition of HB vaccine may "substantially increase" the post-exposure treatment effectiveness over that of HBIG alone and will also provide long term protection because the activities of the body's own immune system. This combined treatment is over 90% effective in preventing infection. [7]

In planning an approach to a vaccination program, consider the following comments found in the California Department of Justice's Hazard Communication Program for Infectious Biologicals:

> While benefit of pre-exposure prevention over post-exposure prevention is not quantifiable, the employee who is vaccinated can reasonably expect to avoid medically prescribed HBIG treatment after an exposure incident. There are definite benefits to the employee who has antibody protection at the time of exposure. Even with an initial weak immune response to an exposure, the body's immune system "remembers" what the hepatitis B virus looks like and can rapidly produce antibodies to mount a defense against the intruding virus. Whether or not pre-exposure vaccination ever provides antibody protection from HBV, the continuing use of "universal precautions" is required along with a medical evaluation subsequent to an exposure incident. For emphasis, ...safe work practices......cannot be reduced because an employee chooses to take advantage of vaccination against HBV.

Transmission of Hepatitis B

While the modes of transmission for Human Immunodeficiency Virus (HIV) are similar to those of HBV, the <u>much</u> higher concentration of HBV than HIV in infected persons increases the potential for HBV transmission. For an exposure where a source of blood is known to be infected with HBV and HIV, the likelihood of infection is approximately 100 times greater for HBV than HIV because HBV is approximately 100,000 times more concentrated than HIV. [8] According to a large body of experience relating to controlling the transmission of HBV in the workplace, the general practices employed to prevent the transmission of HBV will prevent HIV also. Additionally, blood-borne transmission of other pathogens will be avoided by adhering to the same precautions taken to avoid transmission of HBV and HIV. Even with control measures for HBV and HIV, adhere to general infection control principles and general hygiene measures, such as hand washing, to prevent transmission of other infectious diseases. [9]

Potential for HBV transmission in the workplace setting is greater than for HIV; however, modes of transmission for viruses are similar. Both viruses have been transmitted in occupational settings only by inoculation through the skin; or skin with an open wound such as chapped, abraded, weeping, or inflamed skin; or mucous membranes to blood, blood contaminated body fluids, or concentrated virus. **Blood is the single most important source of HBV and HIV in the workplace setting.** Protective measures against these viruses should focus primarily on preventing these types of exposures to blood. Additional considerations should be given to HBV vaccination as described above.

The risk of developing a hepatitis B infection following a needle stick or open cut type exposure to blood is directly proportional to the probability that the blood is infected with HBV. Other factors include an individual's immunity status and the means of transmission of the virus into a person's system.

Calculations of the probability of transmitting an infection were determined from hundreds of different individuals who had experienced needlestick type injuries in health care settings. [10] Statistics on the frequency of HBV carriers in the general population were published by the Department of Labor, in 1989, as follows: whites 2/1000; blacks 7/1000; foreign born Asians up to 130/1000.

Health care settings have been the focus of exposure case studies because they provide some of the best documentation, and therefore the most reliable information about HBV and HIV infections. The studies capture information on specific exposure incidents and the medical status and history of both the donor of the blood and health care worker. Results show that the most efficient means of disease transmission is by direct injection of the infected blood (by needlestick or another sharp object) into a worker's bloodstream. The Center for Disease Control's (CDC) researchers report that the probability of being infected with

HBV after a needlestick type injury involving direct bloodstream exposure is approximately 60 - 300 per 1000. A range for HBV infections is reported because there are two different infectious particles or antigens. [11] In fact, the virus has an inner core which contains DNA, enzymes, and various proteins and an outer shell (or surface) comprising a lipoprotein called hepatitis B surface antigen. The surface antigen in blood indicates that an individual is currently infected with the HBV and is potentially infectious to others. [12]

The second most common route of disease transmission is the infected blood directly contaminating the non-intact skin of an individual. Transmission of the virus onto mucous membranes such as found in the eyes, nose and mouth is the least likely method of infection. [13]

To give perspective to the statistical likelihood of becoming infected, calculations have been made of the number of injuries one person would have to experience before an infection occurs.

Probability of Blood Source Being Infected	HBV Status	Needlesticks
1(patient)	Infected	5.5
0.130 (foreign born Asians)	Unknown	42.7
0.002 (white gen. population)	Unknown	27,777

These calculations are based on 180 infections per 1,000 needlesticks. Be cautioned that "while the information above tries to put the probability of becoming infected from an exposure incident into perspective, every exposure incident must be assumed to have the potential for disease transmission requiring prompt first aid and medical attention!" [14]

Hepatitis C Virus (HCV)

The hepatitis virus is tenacious. It has mutated over the years and will no doubt continue to do so. This has resulted in a serious rise in cases of Hepatitis C Virus (HCV). There are currently approximately four million people infected with HCV. First identified in 1988, HCV was once referred to as Non-A, Non-B hepatitis. It is now the most chronic bloodborne viral infection in the United States. Available information indicates it is more difficult to contract and yet continues to be more prevalent in the general population. This reality has puzzled the research community. Four times more people are infected with HCV than HIV. Some people are unfortunately infected with both viruses.

Hepatitis C is often referred to as “the silent virus” because it lays inactive in the liver and may not express itself for decades. Many infected individuals do not know they are infected and have no clinical illness. However, the consequences of their chronic liver disease will become apparent in 10 to 20 years after infection. Perhaps five percent (5%) of individuals know that they are infected. Of those people infected, 15% - 25% with acute HCV will fight the disease off through their immune response. About 60% - 70% will become chronically sick with liver problems. Ten (10) percent to twenty percent who have chronic hepatitis C over a period of 20 – 30 years develop cirrhosis of the liver. One (1) to five (5) percent of infected individuals die of cirrhosis of the liver or liver cancer. Statistics on the prevalence of HCV are conservative because the survey made in the early 1990’s did not include incarcerated and homeless persons. These groups of people generally have a high occurrence of HCV.

Hepatitis C virus is contracted in the same ways as HIV and HBV. Sources of infection are 60% in drug (injecting) users who share needles, 15% through sexual contact, 10% resulting from blood transfusion prior to blood screening in the 1980’s, 5% from other causes such as hemodialysis, health care work and perinatal, and 10% have no recognized source for their infection. Once infected, 60 – 70% of individuals have no discernable symptoms. Jaundice may be apparent in 20 – 30%. The remaining 10 – 30% might have non-specific symptoms such as anorexia, malaise (a general poor feeling) and/or abdominal pain.

It is possible for HCV to be transmitted from any percutaneous (direct passage of blood through the skin) exposure to blood. However, exposures through activities such as tattooing, body piercing or acupuncture have not been shown to create an increased risk for infection. The risk of percutaneous exposure is high for individuals working in law enforcement who process crime scenes or handle physical evidence. While the incidence of occupation exposure resulting in HCV is low, all preventative measures should be taken. Once infected with HCV, the results can be devastating.

While rumors persist to the contrary, there is currently no vaccine for HCV. The HCV mutation occurs during the course of infection. Anti-HCV antibodies and HCV can exist in the blood simultaneously. Because the antibodies are not protective in the same manner as HBV, an effective vaccine will be very difficult to produce. So, the only action that can be taken other than prevention, is antiviral therapy after infection. The efficacy of the therapy is dependent upon a number of factors. A study of HCV reveals there are at least six different genotypes and at least 90 subtypes. Unfortunately, 70% of the infected U.S. population has genotype 1. Past therapies have resulted in substantially less success with people who are genotype 1. Additionally, the therapy requires total commitment of the infected individual to take all medications as directed. Unfortunately, 10 to 20 percent of people in treatment do not complete therapy because of unpleasant significant side effects. Persons with chronic hepatitis C who continue to abuse alcohol are at risk for ongoing liver injury. Any antiviral therapy may prove ineffective. The CDC reports that interferon therapy can be associated with relapse in people with a history of alcohol abuse. During therapy, an individual must be willing to abstain from all alcohol. This may require a person being given support through an alcohol treatment program while undergoing antiviral therapy. Some patients may have conditions such as severe cirrhosis that prohibits treatment. Additionally, persons who suffer from serious depression may not be good candidates for therapy. (Enduring the therapy can really take you down!) Without antiviral therapy, if the disease progresses to the worst condition, the only possibly life-saving action is a liver transplant.

The therapy regimen has been improved over the years. Initially, the most effective therapy consisted of a combination of alpha-interferon and ribavirin. These drugs achieved the sustained elimination of HCV infection for at least 6 months in 30 to 40 percent of patients. In November of 2000, *U.S. News and World Reports* reported on two new drugs, Pegasys and Pegintron. These drugs use a "shield molecule" called PEG to prevent interferon from breaking down quickly. As result, a person need only have one weekly injection instead of three, which in turn reduces negative side effects. About 50 percent of patients given either of these two new drugs along with a standard antiviral drug were essentially virus free after six months.

Now, let me put the above detailed information into perspective with a case history that strikes close to home. My brother was diagnosed with non-specific (non-A, non-B) hepatitis in 1975. He was counseled to eat healthy, get plenty of bed rest and avoid alcoholic beverages (which he did). During the years from 1977 to 1997, he had a physical examination every 2 years. His reading on liver function was a "little out of range" but he felt pretty good and was very active. However, in 2001, everything in his life changed. He felt tired to the point of inactivity (general malaise) and experienced abdominal pain in the region of his liver. Ultimately, he came under the care of a Hepatologist (a specialist in diseases of the liver). He had a liver biopsy that revealed he had developed a "fatty" liver (which may correct itself if therapy is successful). He also had a genotype test and learned he was a genotype 3. This was encouraging because unlike genotype 1, good results are often experienced with this genotype. His blood test revealed that he had 99 million viral particles per titer! This was the highest count his physician had ever seen or been aware of in any reported case. He did not suffer from chronic depression and so opted to try the antiviral therapy because he was so miserable. His therapy consisted of an alpha-interferon injection approximately every other day (3 times a week) and an oral dosing of ribavirin (2 pills three times a day). Then the real misery began. He felt sick with flu like symptoms and headachy for the first 3 – 4 weeks (antiviral therapy is a form of chemotherapy). After these initial reactions, he was occasionally a little feverish and experienced "hot flashes". He generally felt fine except for muscular weakness and had almost no endurance (tired very easily). Strength and energy to mow the lawn became a major effort. The therapy lasted for six months. Four (4) months after the onset of therapy, his viral count had dropped to 12,000 particles. Fourteen (14) months after onset of therapy, his viral count was 0. Is this a cure? No physician or researcher is really willing to call it as such. My brother was informed that if he was still clean after 6 months, there is a less than 2% chance of recurrence of the HCV. So why is this not considered a cure? Because it is too new a therapy with too few documented results to make such a proclamation. We know that hepatitis has a nasty habit of hiding out in the liver only to rear its ugly head years later. Until more HCV infected people undergo the newer therapies and remain "healthy" for a number of years, the verdict will be undeclared.

Further information on HCV can be obtained from the Centers for Disease Control. They have an excellent web site.

Human Immunodeficiency Virus (HIV)

In the years 1983 and 1984, French and American scientists isolated a human virus associated with Acquired Immunodeficiency Syndrome (AIDS). In 1980 the disease was generally unknown until doctors in Los Angeles and New York City began to encounter cases of a rare type of pneumonia called *Pneumo-*

cystis carinii, and a normally slow-growing cancer known as Kaposi's sarcoma. People infected with the AIDS virus may develop certain types of cancers such as Kaposi's sarcoma (which causes lesions on the skin and then at other sites). All victims were either young male homosexuals or drug abusers. Doctors called their symptoms "the immunologic consequences of some unknown process". Dr. Ward Cates, of the CDC, stated that the disease had a potential "much worse than anything mankind has seen before." By 1985, infectious-disease expert Dr. John Seale concurred when he wrote in the *Journal of the Royal Society of Medicine* that AIDS was capable of producing "a lethal pandemic throughout the crowded cities and villages of the Third World of a magnitude unparalleled in human history". [15] In June of 1987, *Reader's Digest* noted that "the epidemic is so wide spread and so lethal that experts are comparing it to the Black Death that killed a quarter of Europe's population in the fourteenth century". [16] By 1988, United Nation's Secretary-General Javier Perez de Cuellar referred to the AIDS epidemic as a "global conflict" that "threatens us with all the consequences of war". [17]

Again, in 1990 *Awake* noted: "At a conference in Marseilles, France, Dr. Jonathan Mann, director of the World Health Organization's Global Programme on AIDS, warned of a huge global spread of AIDS in the 1990's. As many as ten million may now be infected with the virus in 152 countries around the world. By the year 2000, AIDS may kill six million people. The report in the *Times* of London notes that Africa is hardest hit. In Dar es Salaam, Tanzania, 42 percent of women working in bars and restaurants reportedly carry the virus. In Cote d'Ivoire three out of ten adults were said to be infected. Of the crisis in the United States, the Hudson Institute warns that "a catastrophe is sweeping over America." It forecasts that the AIDS virus will infect some 14.5 million Americans by 2002 and kill more Americans in the 1990's than all the wars in the nation's history." [18]

We live in an international community where people travel from one side of the planet to another in a matter of hours or days. Coupled with the above-mentioned concerns and predictions by the medical community, we all have cause to feel anxious about AIDS. This fear has led to a good deal of misunderstanding and misinformation. The foundation of prevention is education and then adherence to established protocols.

What is the virus and how does it function in the body? First, let me clarify terms. Back in 1984, the French and American teams learned that the virus attacks a subgroup of white blood cells called T-4 lymphocytes. Human bone marrow produces about a million white blood cells every second. These are the "big guns" of our immune system. T-cells are a type of white blood cells in our bloodstream. There are three types of T-cells: helper, suppressor, and killer cells. These cells are involved in the biological warfare of the body and are among the most indispensable armed forces of the immune system. The AIDS virus singles out for attack these helper T-cells. Helper T-cells can be thought of as the *chiefs of operations* of the immune system, identifying enemies and stimulating the production of other warriors of the immune system, rallying them to join battle with the invaders. Once helper T-cells are immobilized, the immune system is rendered virtually helpless, leaving AIDS victims vulnerable to all sorts of diseases. [19]

Because lymphocytes were the focus of attack by the virus, the French called it (the virus) lymphadenopathy-associated virus (LAV). (Lymphadenopathy is a big medical word which means "disease of the lymph nodes"!) [20] The Americans, on the other hand, called it human T-cell lymphotropic virus-III (HTLV-III). Eventually, experts decided upon a universally accepted term of human immunodeficiency virus type 1 (HIV-1), shortened to HIV in most documents. Interestingly, HIV-2 has since been discovered in Africa.

The HIV is a member of a group of viruses known as human retroviruses. Its genetic material is ribonucleic acid (RNA) rather than deoxyribonucleic acid (DNA - the genetic material found in most living organisms). RNA is an acid that controls the combination of proteins in all living cells. In other words, RNA takes the place of DNA in these viruses. The HIV has a core which contains the RNA and some enzymes and an outer covering of lipids (fat or fat-type substance) and proteins. Because viruses, by definition, have no genetic material to reproduce on their own, they must find a host cell to reproduce. This is where the helper T-cells come into play. The HIV bind to the surface of the helper T-cells and release their RNA. The RNA is then copied by the attending enzymes into double-stranded DNA that is incorporated into the DNA of the host cell. In this way, the host cell is "tricked" into producing more virus particles from the viral DNA. As HIV gradually depletes the number of cells essential for host immune function, the infected person becomes more susceptible to opportunistic infections. [21] Once the immune system is destroyed, other germs (bacteria, protozoa, fungi and other viruses) and cancers that ordinarily would never get a foothold cause the "opportunistic diseases". These diseases are called as such because they use the opportunity of lowered resistance to infect and destroy. Some of the most common of these diseases are *Pneumocystis carinii* pneumonia and tuberculosis. Evidence also indicates that HIV may also travel to and attack the nervous system (via white blood cells), resulting in brain damage. [22]

Once a person is infected with HIV, the infection can take one of several directions. Some people remain well but can infect other people. Others develop less disabling conditions than AIDS. In some people, the virus destroys the protective immune system, and these people will have classic AIDS.

Signs and symptoms include loss of appetite, weight loss, fever, night sweats, skin rashes, diarrhea, fatigue, lack of resistance to infection, and swollen lymph nodes. <u>Consult a physician for diagnosis</u>, since these are also signs and symptoms of many other diseases. [23]

There is no vaccination for AIDS for purposes of prevention or post exposure control of the disease.

Transmission of Human Immunodeficiency Virus

HIV has been isolated from human blood, semen, breast milk, vaginal secretions, saliva, tears, urine, cerebro spinal fluid (the fluid around the brain and spinal cord), and amniotic fluid (the fluid in the womb surrounding a human fetus). However, studies implicate only blood, semen, vaginal secretions and breast milk in the transmission of the virus. [24]

HIV is not transmitted by casual contact with infected persons. Studies of persons living unknowingly with people infected with AIDS (i.e., they took no precautions) reveal no evidence of transmission by hand shaking; talking; food sharing or sharing of utensils, plates, or drinking glasses; or by sharing of the house or household facilities. Nor did personal interactions including hugging or kissing involving the exchange of saliva transmit the virus. You can't get AIDS from coughing, sneezing, or using swimming pools, or hot tubs, toilets, door knobs, or telephones. Other studies have shown that mosquitoes or other animals do **not** transmit HIV. [25] Even with reliable study results, people tend to panic and shy away from HIV infected people. This isn't the first time people have misunderstood the mode of transmission of a disease. At one time, people believed that epidemics were caused by bad air (hence the disease named malaria). They had no scientific knowledge (understanding) of microbes. A great deal of scientific investigation has documented HIV's modes of transmission. HIV is contracted by engaging in sexual intercourse with an HIV-infected person; using needles contaminated with HIV; by inoculation, mucous membrane or non-intact skin contact with HIV-infected blood, blood components or blood products; by receiving transplants of HIV-infected organs and tissues including bone, or transfusions of HIV-infected blood; and by transmission from a mother to her child around the time of birth. [26]

Your occupational concern is the risk from an HIV-infected needle (stick) or other sharp. An exposure incident is defined as a specific situation where any amount of a substance requiring "universal precautions" is deposited on: 1) damaged skin, 2) mucous membranes, or 3) by "percutaneous" (through the skin) puncture (e.g., contaminated needle stick, contaminated knife wound, bite from a bloodied mouth, etc.). So what are the risks of infection? In 1988, the Centers for Disease Control (CDC) estimated the number of HIV carriers in the U.S. population to be from 4/1000 to 6/1000. However, one high risk group (i.e. prostitute intravenous drug users) in one state was found to be infected at a rate of 500/1000. [27]

Again, as with HBV, exposure case studies from health-care settings provide the best and most reliable information regarding infections. Hundreds of needlestick or sharp object injuries occur daily in the United States. CDC researchers report the probability of being infected and becoming ill after a needlestick type injury involving direct bloodstream access is approximately 5 per 1000. [28] As with HBV, statistical calculations have been made from individuals in health-care settings who have received one or more needlestick type injuries. The following is a calculation of the number of injuries that one person would have to receive before the statistical data predicts an infection.

Probability of Blood Source Being Infected	HBV Status	Needlesticks
1 (patient)	Infected	344
0.5 (prostitute + IV drug)	Unknown	688
0.006 (general population)	Unknown	57,777 [29]

All the statistical projections in the world don't really provide comfort. The best approach to decrease the risk of infections is to follow "universal precautions" and all other protocols. These will be discussed later.

Other Bloodborne Pathogens

There are other infectious diseases which are characterized by a phase in which the agent causing infection may circulate in blood for a prolonged period of time. With the exception of syphilis and malaria, these diseases are rare in the United States. [30] This translates to a very low risk factor to health care workers or public safety workers. However, with an increase in world travel, including refugees and immigrants, it behooves each of us to be aware of these other diseases.

Syphilis

Syphilis is a sexually transmitted infectious disease that is on the increase in the United States. The disease is caused by infection with *Treponema pallidum*, a spirochete. [31] (Spirochetes are an order of slender spiral micro-organisms.) [32] A single lesion or wound that will heal without treatment appears in the first stage of infection. Within weeks or months, a second stage occurs, marked by rash, fever, and the spreading of the spirochetes into the blood and lymph system. There may be a long latency period before the third stage involves the skin, bones, central nervous system and cardio-vascular system. There is a high death rate associated with syphilis. A couple of infamous characters who died of this disease were Al Capone and King Henry VIII. There are documented cases of transmission by needlestick. Treatment with antibiotics after exposure may prevent infection. [33]

Malaria

Malaria is a potentially fatal mosquito-borne parasitic infection of the blood cells. Its symptoms are noted as sudden, periodic attack or recurrence of fever, chills, sweats, and anemia. This disease is an important health risk to immigrants from many malaria-ridden areas of the world and Americans who travel to these areas. Transmission by mosquito has been documented in the United States. It has also been transmitted by needlestick. Malaria is caused by the red blood cells becoming infected by a protozoan parasite of the *Plasmodium*. (Most protozoa are one-celled animals.) Treatment involves drug therapy but recurrences are common. [34]

Babesiosis

Babesiosis is a tick-borne, parasitic disease similar to malaria. The *Babesia microti* parasite attacks the red blood cells and causes an often severe and sometimes fatal disease. The disease occurs mostly in the northeastern United States, especially in certain islands off the northeastern coast. The symptoms include fever, chills, drenching sweats, tenderness or pain in the muscles and joints, nausea and vomiting, and anemia. The parasite can be transmitted by transfusion of fresh blood. Treatment involves drug therapy. [35]

Brucellosis

Brucellosis is a fever-type illness caused by members of the bacteria genus *Brucella*. The disease is also called Malta Fever or undulant fever, and is typically associated with occupational exposure to livestock (principally cattle, swine, and goats) or with ingestion of unpasturized dairy products. The symptoms include fever and weakness, sweats, and pain in the joints. Transmission by blood transfusion has been reported. [36]

Leptospirosis

Leptospirosis is a prolonged illness characterized by fever, rash, and occasionally jaundice. It is caused by strains of thin, spiral, and hook-ended spirochetes (micro-organisms) called *Leptospira interrogans*. The phase in which the organism is found in the blood lasts only 1 or 2 weeks. The disease is typically acquired by contact with urine of infected animals, including cattle, swine, dogs, and rats. As of May 1989, there were no reported cases of transmission by blood in a hospital setting. [37]

Arboviral Infections

Arboviruses include a large group of viruses that multiply in both vertebrates and arthropods such as mosquitoes and ticks. These viruses are known to cause diseases such as yellow fever and viral encephalitis (inflammation of the brain). [38]

OSHA reports that "arboviral infections generally do not lead to high or sustained levels of viremia (presence of viruses in the blood) in humans, therefore, there is little potential for person-to-person transmission of these infections through blood products or needlestick exposure". However, the document goes on to note that the exception is Colorado tick fever (CTF) caused by a tick-borne virus which infects red blood cells. Symptoms include fever, chills, headache, muscle and back ache. Transmission by blood transfusion has been documented. [39]

Relapsing Fever

Relapsing fever is considered a rare disease, caused by spirochetes of the genus *Borrelia*, transmitted by head lice, body lice, or ticks. This infectious disease is marked by intermittent attacks of high fever. In the U.S., a few cases of tick-borne relapsing feces are reported in localized geographic areas (western United States). Although cases of occupational transmission have been very rare, there have been documented instances of such transmission as result of patient care practices. Treatment for this disease involves antibiotic drug therapy. [40]

Creutzfeldt-Jakob Disease

Creutfeldt-Jakob disease, a rare disease with worldwide distribution, is a degenerative (causes deterioration or impairment) disease of the brain caused by a virus. It is believed to be transmitted by ingestion of, or inoculation with, infectious material, primarily tissue of the nervous system. No cases of transmission by blood in a hospital have been reported. There have been rare instances of transmission secondary to implants of the membrane tissue which surrounds the spinal cord and brain, in the receipt of human growth hormone, and insertion of unsterilized electrodes which had been inserted into the brains of Creutzfeldt-Jakob disease patents and then used on others. [41]

Human T-lymphotropic Virus Type I

Human T-lymphotropic Virus Type I (HTLV-I), the first human retrovirus to be identified, is very common in southern Japan, the Caribbean, and in some parts of Africa. It is also found in the U.S., mainly in intravenous drug users. The virus can be transmitted by transfusions of cellular compounds of blood (whole blood, red blood cells, platelets). HTLV-I has been associated with a malignancy of the blood and blood forming tissues known as adult-T-cell leukemia/lymphoma. It has also been associated with a disease of the nervous system in which there is some evidence that it may be associated as well with blood transfusions. As of May 1989, there were no reports of occupational acquisition of HTLV-I. [42]

Universal Precautions

The use of universal precautions is based upon the fact that you can not tell by just looking at a person whether they carry HIV or HBV or any other bloodborne pathogen. Neither can you detect pathogens simply by looking at blood or other human body fluids. So how do you deal with the dilemma of working with these biological materials posing an unknown exposure risk? Applying "universal blood and body fluid precautions." This has been described as a preventive exposure strategy developed in 1985, in response to the threat posed by the transmission of the human immunodeficiency virus (HIV), the causative agent of acquired immunodeficiency syndrome (AIDS), for health care and clinical laboratory personnel. Specific precautions include an array of work practices (i.e., use of personal protective equipment and basic hygiene) and engineering controls (methods of containment). The term "universal" means that every patient and blood sample is assumed to be infected and should be handled accordingly. Therefore, every arrestee and blood sample submitted for analysis is to be considered infectious for HIV or other bloodborne pathogens. [43]

For the forensic identification specialist, this means that all blood, human tissue and other body fluids which contain visible blood must be treated *as though it is* infected. If lighting is poor and there is a chance that tissue or body fluids may contain blood, then apply universal precautions. By following universal precautions, you prevent contamination from routine handling of the biological materials. Assuming infection can save your life!

If you have the responsibility of collecting clothing/bedding or other items from a crime scene which may be biologically contaminated, or receiving them into evidence at the laboratory, handle them as though they are infectious. If you have to lay them out to dry, protect the surface of the counter or table top with butcher paper or plastic. Wear protective clothing and nitrile gloves (latex will do if that is all you have available). Think ahead before gloving your hands. Inspect your skin for breaks, soundness and intactness. If you have any breaks, cover them with an adhesive bandage. If you are working with materials which have gross blood contamination, then wear double nitrile gloves. This will allow you to remove contaminated protective equipment with a clean pair of gloves. In addition to protective clothing and gloves, wear a surgical particulate mask and eye goggles (or face shield). Any time you handle these items, wear this protective equipment to protect your personal clothing, skin, and mucous membranes. Upon completion of drying, properly package the items, apply hazard warning labels to outside of the packaging, and decontaminate the drying surfaces by removing and disposing of cover materials and cleaning the surfaces. Clean all surfaces with a dilution of common household bleach (sodium hypochlorite). Make this dilution with 1 part of liquid bleach added to 9 parts of water. [44] In fact, routinely decontaminate all potentially contaminated surfaces.

Limit access to laboratory areas where potentially infectious materials are handled to those employees with case work responsibilities. Always remove lab coats when leaving the laboratory and never wear them into other areas. Never eat, drink, store food, or apply cosmetics in the laboratory. And make it a standard habit to wash your hands with soap and water after handling evidence, before you leave the laboratory, and before and after using the lavatory.

If you process the fingers or hands of deceased individuals for prints, always apply universal precautions. Wear a laboratory coat and nitrile gloves (latex will do if that is all you have available). Again, think ahead before gloving your hands. Inspect your skin for breaks, soundness and intactness. If you have any breaks, cover them with an adhesive bandage. If you are working with materials which have gross blood contamination, then wear double nitrile gloves. This will allow you to remove contaminated protective equipment with a clean pair of gloves. In addition to protective clothing and gloves, wear a surgical particulate mask and eye goggles or face shield. Upon completion of processing, seal fingerprint cards in a heat sealable bag, apply a hazard warning label, and decontaminate the area. Detailed information on these procedures are found in Section 12.

Employer Responsibilities

Employers do have a responsibility for developing programs to protect workers. Based upon reviews of the pertinent data, 29 CFR Part 1910 states that certain employees face a significant health risk as the result of occupational exposure to blood and other potentially infectious materials because they may contain bloodborne pathogens, including hepatitis B virus which causes Hepatitis B, a serious liver disease, and human immuno-deficiency virus, which causes Acquired Immunodeficiency Syndrome (AIDS). The Agency preliminarily concludes that this significant health risk can be minimized or eliminated using a combination of engineering and work practice controls, personal protective clothing and equipment, training, medical follow-up of exposure incidents, vaccination (where applicable), and other provisions.

Another CDC document recommends that employers, in developing programs to protect workers, should follow a series of steps: 1) classify work activity, 2) develop standard operating procedures (SOPs), 3) provide training and education, 4) develop procedures to ensure and monitor compliance, and 5) redesign the workplace. [45]

In classifying work activities, the employer should evaluate all tasks their forensic personnel perform and determine which activities risk exposures. Essentially, three categories can be established as follows: 1) activity routinely has contact with blood or other body fluids, 2) activity usually performed without blood exposure but exposure may occur in an emergency, and 3) activity does not involve predictable or unpredictable exposure to blood. Employers should provide personal protective equipment to all employees engaged in activities in the first two categories and ensure and enforce the use of personal protective equipment by all employees involved in activities in the first category.

Secondly, the employer must develop a detailed work practices program which includes SOPs for all tasks having the potential for exposure. (Writing and implementing the work practices program for all laboratory and crime scene processing as an integral part of the chemical hygiene plan). Once SOPs are set forth, the worker must be educated in a formal program to familiarize workers with the necessary work practices to avoid potential exposures. Employees should not engage in work activities which pose a risk of potential exposure until such a time as they have received training on the SOPs, work practices and the necessary personal protective equipment.

It is imperative that employers monitor employee compliance with SOPs, required work practice observance, and proper use of personal protective equipment. These standards go right back to the initial discussion of laboratory responsibilities.

Whenever possible, make changes in the work environment that correct problem areas of potential exposures. Use devices or engineering controls (physical or mechanical systems which eliminate hazards at their source, such as biological safety cabinets, fume hoods, and glove boxes). An additional engineering control may be the use of specifically marked plastic bags for collection of waste materials contaminated with biohazards. Another control required by law is the use of puncture resistant sharps containers. (Usually a plastic, metal or hard cardboard tube.) These containers eliminate the need for employees to transport sharp items, such as broken glass, scalpels, and needles while looking for a place to dispose of them. (Figure 5-1) A sharps container should be present in every laboratory. Never over-fill the container! You can receive a serious cut or stick trying to dispose of a sharp into a full container.

Changes in the approach to a task could also have beneficial results. For instance, there is a serious health risk of needle sticks when packaging and transporting syringes at crime scenes. Rather than packaging in paper bags, place all syringes in puncture-resistant sharps containers. When sealing bags of evidence, use evidence tape rather than staples. Develop policies to eliminate this type of hazard. The supervisor may set policy which dictates that no needles or syringes with the needle attached will be accepted by the laboratory for latent print processing without his/her approval. Clearly mark the outside of any submitted evidence containing needles.

In addition to all the previously mentioned responsibilities, the employer must also provide a program of medical management to reduce risk of infection by HBV, including vaccinations if there is a risk that employees may come into contact with blood or other potentially infectious material as the result of their work assignment. Additionally, the program provides medical testing after a confirmed exposure incident

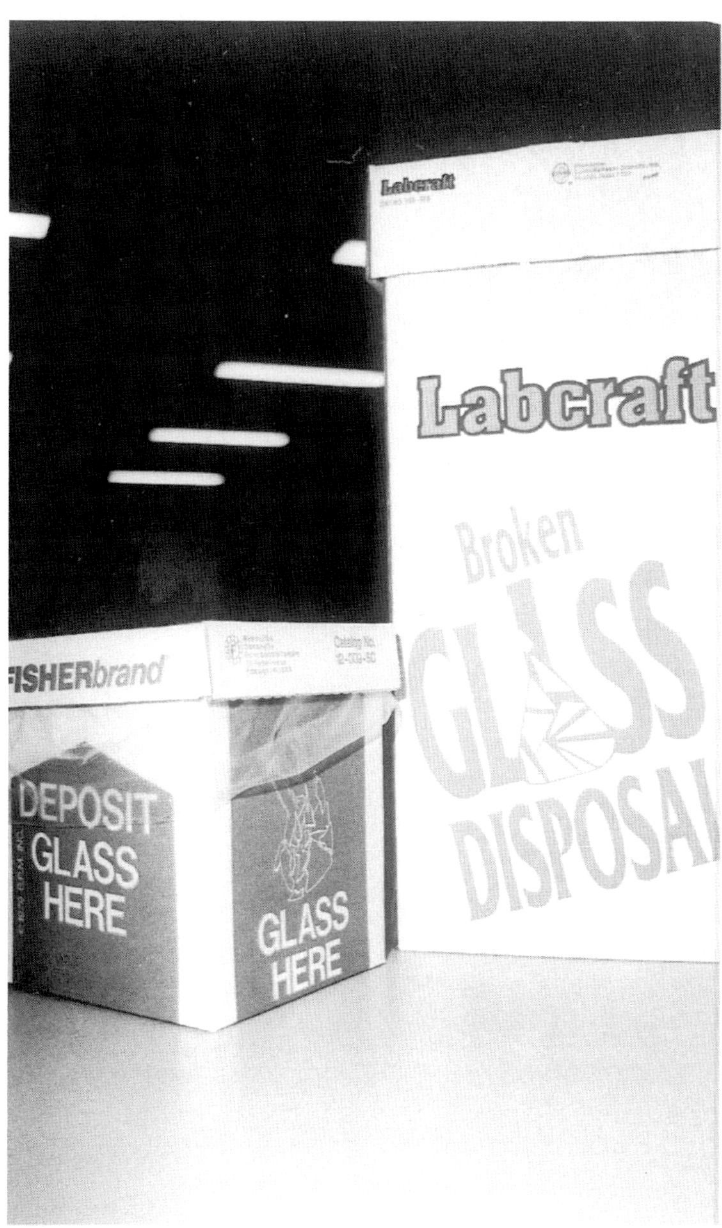

Figure 5-1: Commercially available "sharps" containers used for disposal of broken glass, scalpels, and needles.

and counseling concerning HIV and HBV. A licensed health professional should provide these services. [46] The licensed health care professional should be a physician. If exposure of an individual worker occurs, medical management consisting of collection of pertinent medical and occupational history, provision for treatment, and counseling regarding future work and personal behaviors may reduce risk of developing disease as result of the exposure. [47] Following work, decontamination and disinfection of the work environment, devices, equipment, and clothing or other forms of personal protective equipment can reduce subsequent risk of exposures. Clean up after a spill, after work, or daily. Proper disposal of contaminated waste has similar benefits. [48]

To summarize, biological hazards can pose a serious (and possibly deadly) threat to the forensic identification specialist. However, with comprehensive written policies and protocols and with conscientious work practices, the potential for exposure incidents can be limited. It bears repeating one more time: **Always employ universal precautions by handling all biological materials as though they were infectious.**

6
Routes of Exposure

Chemicals can harm (or cause injury) in several ways. Forensic identification specialists must always be alert to potentially harmful situations that generally occur through the misuse or improper handling of chemicals in the workplace. All chemicals can cause harm if misused or handled improperly. The danger from a chemical depends on three aspects of exposure: *1) dose*, or how much, *2) duration* and *frequency*, or how long and how often, and *3) route*, or how the person is exposed. [1]

The quantity of the chemical received is the critical factor. Generally speaking, the larger the dose, the shorter the time it takes for harm to occur. Smaller doses require more time to injure someone. As the dose increases, so does the degree of harm or severity of the injury. At some point, the quantity will cause death. Very small doses may not result in any immediate injury but can create long-term problems. Threshold is "the dose at which a chemical begins to be harmful. A chemical may have, for example, a toxicity threshold of 6 gm such that drinking < 6 gm is not harmful but > 6 gm causes severe nausea." [2]

The duration of a chemical exposure directly affects the severity of the injury. An acid spilled onto the skin will do less damage when you wash it off quickly. The longer you leave this substance on the skin, the more serious the burn. Quickly removing a substance from the skin reduces any resulting illness because the chemical has less time to penetrate.

The frequency with which a person is exposed to a chemical can directly affect the type, time of onset, extent, and severity of the toxic effect. One exposure (acute toxicity) to some chemicals can cause an immediate injury, while other chemicals won't injure until exposure (chronic toxicity) is repeated over time. The determining factor is how the body eliminates a particular substance. Some chemicals are easily eliminated while others build up in the body until they reach a harmful level. [3]

Harmful agents can take different routes to gain entry to the body. Chemical or biological hazards must come in contact with cells and enter the body. [4] These exposures occur in four ways: by dermal absorption, inhalation, ingestion, or injection. [5] The employee must be alert to the possible route of exposure to any harmful agent s/he may be using. Material Safety Data Sheets provide such information. The section labeled "Health Hazard Information" will note the primary route of entry (i.e., inhalation), target organs, acute effects, chronic effects, and first aid measures.

Absorption

A common route of entry is absorption of substances through the skin or mucous membranes such as exist in eyes, nose and mouth. Usually, skin absorption is a slow process. Cuts or abrasions on the skin shorten the time. Although intact skin does provide a natural barrier to some chemicals, many other compounds can be absorbed through intact skin. [6] Chemicals can be absorbed through the skin when clothing, shoes or a laboratory coat are contaminated with chemicals.

Entering through the eyes, chemicals can be rapidly absorbed into the bloodstream. Because of open passages between the eyes, nose and mouth, chemical in the eyes and/or nose can be swallowed. These exposures happen when splashing chemical liquids or powders in the face or rubbing the eyes. Gases, mists, fumes and dusts can also enter through the eyes. [7]

To avoid chemical exposures, use personal protective equipment during every laboratory procedure. This equipment includes laboratory coats or smocks, dust masks, chemical goggles and/or face shield, and the appropriate gloves for the chemicals being handled. Latex gloves will not provide protection from organic solvents. (Such organic solvents are the alcohols and any petroleum products. These include acetone, methanol, ethanol, propanol, petroleum ether, hexane, heptane, and Freon.) Only a rubber glove such as neoprene assures adequate protection. The equipment provides a protective barrier between the wearer and the substance being handled.

Absorption or dermal exposures produce skin irritations, rashes, burns, or various forms of dermatitis. An exposure to mucous membranes will probably result in a burning sensation of the mucosal surfaces. Laboratories need readily available quantities of water. Eye exposures require a water flushing for at least

15 minutes. In addition to eye washes, drenching body showers and sinks must be provided for flushing of other body areas. [8]

Inhalation

Inhalation is the major route of entry for hazardous chemicals. [9] These exposures occur commonly through the inhalation of air contaminated with gases, vapors, dusts, mists or fumes [10], as well as sprays, aerosols and smoke. (Most solid materials do not evaporate rapidly enough to create vapors. These vapors and gases are generated by volatile liquids.) Normal breathing brings airborne contaminants from the nose and mouth into the lungs. From the absorption into the lungs, chemicals pass into the bloodstream and reach the brain. [11] This route provides the most rapid entry into the body and the most rapid harmful effects. [12]

Apply chemicals in the safest manner possible to avoid inhaling them. Work in well-ventilated areas and use the fume hood when working with volatile chemicals, sprays or mists. Never spray Ninhydrin, or any other amino acid reactive reagent. [13] Spraying these reagents, especially the commercially prepared formulations that contain a lacquer, creates an aerosol which may be too heavy to be drawn up and out by a standard fume hood. (Fume hoods are engineered to draw fumes and vapors — not aerosols.) Sprayed Ninhydrin will bounce on the backboard of the hood and out the front. I routinely experienced this problem in the laboratory. Co-workers constantly complained that the hood was not drawing up to standard, even though it did pull at more than 100 lfm. After spraying the Ninhydrin formulation, latent print analysts could smell the chemicals and would react with coughing, sneezing, dry throat and stinging eyes. Changing the procedure of application eliminated this problem. (In fact, all published research literature recommends the dipping or brushing of Ninhydrin. Access to commercially prepared formulations led to spraying for convenience.)

Understanding nasal functions gives insight. One explanation says:

> Odors enter the nasal passages when you breathe in. First, though, odorous air has to make it past the "guards." Lining the nostrils are the trigeminal nerves, which trigger sneezing when they sense stinging or irritating chemicals. These nerves also give pleasure by reacting to the pungency of some flavors. Next, odorous molecules are pushed upward by eddies that form when air currents swirl around three bony, scroll-

> like protrusions called turbinates. The airstream, moistened and warmed along the way, carries the molecules to the epithelium, the primary reception area. Situated in a narrow channel high up in the nose, this thumbnail-size patch of tissue is packed with some ten million sensory neurons, each tipped with numerous hairlike projections, called cilia, bathed in a thin layer of mucus. So sensitive is the epithelium that it can detect 1/1,300,000,000 ounce of certain odorants in a single whiff of air.
>
> But exactly how odors are detected is still shrouded in mystery. Humans can distinguish as many as 10,000 odors. And there are more than 400,000 odorous substances in our environment, with chemists constantly creating new ones. So how does our nose make sense of all this olfactory hubbub? Well over 20 different theories attempt to explain the mystery. Some evidence was found in 1991 that there are tiny proteins, called olfactory receptors, woven through the cell membranes in the celia. Apparently such receptors bind differently to differing types of odorous molecules, thus giving each odor a distinctive fingerprint. [14]

How does all of this relate to our smelling chemicals in the laboratory? Have you ever noticed that you could detect the smell of some pervasive odor that seemed to fade away with time? Well, the olfactory bulbs in the nose, informed by the brain, bring about these changes. They may be assisted by the receptor cells on the cilia, which are said to fatigue easily. [15] This may be a helpful feature in the face of potent foul odors (such as putrid flesh. You never really get used to it.), but it can pose a hazard in the laboratory. One chemical which affects the nose in this way is ozone. The Material Safety Data Sheet states that, "Olfactory fatigue develops rapidly, so do not use odor as a preventative warning device." [16] Herein lies the hazard of relying only on your nose to detect an unsafe chemical condition. You never want to do so. Do not ever get into the habit of opening chemical containers and "whiffing" the vapors in order to identify the material inside. This is an excellent way to dose yourself with very dangerous chemicals.

Inhalation exposures can be detected by one simple test: if you can smell the chemical, then you have received an exposure. This does not necessarily mean, however, that the exposure was excessive or health threatening. Few people smelling gasoline vapors at the pump run to the hospital for treatment. You expect to smell chemical odors in the chemistry laboratory where chemicals are used. Whether an exposure is dangerous or debilitating will depend upon the individual's sensitivities and the permissible exposure limits established for the substance.

Certainly, if you can or have smelled something and then experience an inappropriate or debilitating reaction (nausea, light-headedness, dizziness, or loss of consciousness), medical aid is justified and warranted.

Also consider the risk of exposure while photographing dried, chemically developed evidence prints under high-intensity light. Fume-sensitive specialists reacting with tears, coughs, or labored breathing to reheated, dried Ninhydrin deposits have worn air-purifying respirators equipped with high-efficiency particulate (HEPA) cartridges to trap the airborne contaminate. [17]

Ingestion

Ingestion is another common and obvious route of exposure. People can unknowingly eat or drink harmful chemicals, so do not eat, drink, smoke, or apply cosmetics in the laboratory or any area where chemicals are stored or used. Never store food or drinks for personal consumption in a laboratory refrigerator used for chemical, biological, or evidence storage. Food stuffs absorb vapors from other materials in the refrigerator. Avoid touching your face or placing pens or pencils in your mouth. This precaution is very difficult to remember, because most of this kind of touching occurs at a subconscious level. It is an unspoken law that as soon as you don your gloves, your nose will itch. It is a natural reflex to scratch it with a swipe of your glove, sleeve or arm. Resist the urge. Frequent hand washing is the best preventative measure to avoid transferring contaminants to the skin or mouth. Wash your hands every time you complete a procedure and before leaving the laboratory. Your best protection from ingestion is to become fanatical about hand washing. Wash, wash, wash.

Injection

Injection hazards present themselves in the handling of sharp or pointed items. Develop protocols for the receiving, handling and disposing of any "sharps," especially when dealing with possible biological hazards. Prevent injection accidents. Pick up broken glass, etc., with tongs or other grasping material. Bring the sharps container to the area of breakage, rather than carrying broken material to the sharps container. Always use care when placing sharps into a "sharps" container. Do not overfill containers with sharps or broken materials. Others may be punctured or cut trying to place additional items into the container. All laboratories should have a supply of these inexpensive "sharps" containers. They are usually made of cardboard lined with plastic.

Make a report to your supervisor about any exposure that causes concern or requires medical attention, including simple first aid. Your supervisor needs to be apprised immediately of any incident. Both verbal and written reports are important. Do not assume that a written report has been completed. Write one yourself or ask to see the completed report to ensure its accuracy. These reports become a part of your medical records and are kept for thirty years after you leave the department.

7
Ventilation Systems

Proper ventilation in the laboratory is a major concern for both safety and comfort. Adequate ventilation reduces chemical odors and heat generated by electronic equipment as well as the presence of hazardous flammable and toxic substances in the air. For this reason, the general dilution ventilation system should provide 4 to 12 room air changes per hour, providing that adequate outside air is available to dilute any contaminants. Laboratory air contains a variety of potential hazards that require the air pressure in the laboratory to be less than the adjoining corridors and the rest of the building, so laboratory air is drawn out through the laboratory exhaust vents rather than into the building.

Any persons working with hazardous materials must be provided adequate ventilation. The laboratory ventilation systems are often poorly maintained or poorly designed. Additionally, the systems may be improperly used, such as in the spraying of aerosols in fume hoods (see Section 9 on spraying of chemicals). Ventilation systems commonly used by the forensic identification specialist are chemical fume hoods as well as other miscellaneous or specially exhausted enclosures.

It is especially important that forensic document examiners who work with the Electrostatic Detection Apparatus be provided a well-ventilated area or room. The Corona Wand generates ozone, a severe respiratory hazard with a threshold limit value of 0.1 parts per million (ppm) in an 8 hour period. [1] Even though ozone has a characteristic odor often associated with electrical sparks or lightning in concentrations of less than 2 ppm, the MSDS for ozone warns that olfactory fatigue develops rapidly. In other words, do not rely on your nose. General and local exhaust ventilation must be provided to meet the exposure values. Ventilation should dilute and disperse small amounts of ozone into the outside atmosphere. Ozone is highly irritating, and properly maintained engineering ventilation systems are crucial to a safe work environment. (Additionally, the MSDS provided by Genium Publishing describes ozone as highly toxic.)

Good laboratory ventilation, though essential, is not sufficient to protect workers from toxic and flammable vapors. Any procedures involving hazardous or volatile chemical manipulations require the use of a fume hood; therefore, most chemical processing of physical evidence in the laboratory will be performed in the chemical fume hood. Use the hood to draw any hazardous material (specifically vapors, fumes, dusts, and mists) away from the breathing zone of the user. The hood has a sash to minimize the front opening during use. Remember, the hood should make it possible to enclose as much of the process or operation as possible. When the hood is not in use, keep the sash closed, especially if any chemicals are being stored in the back.

Store chemicals in vented safety storage cabinets rather than in the fume hood. (See Section 16 on storage of chemicals.) If material is stored in the hood and the hood is turned off, vapors can build up to a dangerous or toxic level. Leave only minimum amounts of chemicals in the hood, and only those you use regularly. Never place these chemicals in a position which blocks the air flows necessary for adequate ventilation.

Laboratory hoods are safety devices made especially to prevent toxic, flammable, or noxious vapors from entering the laboratory atmosphere, to provide a physical barrier from unexpected and undesired chemical reaction, and to contain accidental chemical spills. The hoods are enclosed, except for the openings which provide for exhaust, on three sides and are designed to draw air inward by means of mechanical ventilation.

Fume hoods are one of the most important aspects of worker safety and, therefore, require certain essential maintenance and operating procedures. However, this equipment is only a mechanical safety device and is secondary in nature to safety protocols. A fume hood can never substitute for safe working practices or chemical disposal.

A schedule of evaluation and maintenance is essential. Always evaluate fume hoods before use to assure adequate face velocity. Mechanical ventilation must remain in operation at all times when the fume hood is in use and for a sufficient time afterward to clear the fume hood of any airborne hazardous substances.

Fume hoods are manufactured in various shapes and sizes. A fume hood which is permanently installed, or wired-in, should meet certain basic requirements. It should be placed away from laboratory traffic patterns. People walking past the fume hood disrupt the flow patterns and cause eddies of air to move in and out of the fume hood front. When your co-workers are using the fume hood, try not to pass back and forth behind them and decrease the efficiency of the air flow. Install the fume hood away from doors, windows, or other air diffusers which can create cross-drafts at the face of the fume hood.

Design the duct connections to the fume hood to avoid sharp angles or introduction of other branches to within six duct diameters of the fume hood and reduce turbulent air patterns inside the system. Locate the fan for the fume hood outside the building on the roof to maintain negative pressure in the duct carrying contaminated air from the fume hood to the fan. Locate air-cleaning equipment ahead of the fan to reduce deterioration of fan parts caused by the action of contaminants. Never vent fume hoods into the main air ducts for other areas of the building. Place exhaust stacks above the roof line and away from air supply equipment. [2] The design and installation of ventilation systems are technically complex. A registered professional engineer or a certified industrial hygienist should

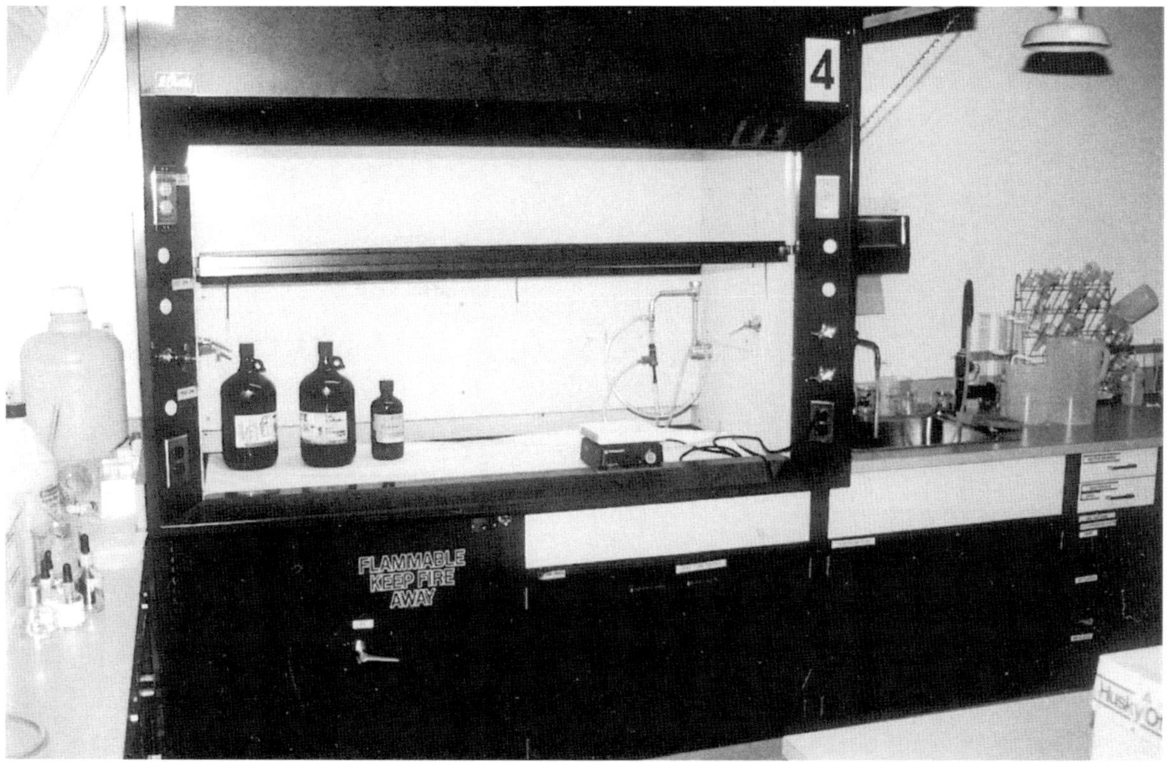

Figure 7-1: Permanently installed fume hood next to sink and full-body safety shower.

approve any designs. Most state OSHA departments have specific regulations for ventilation systems. Those states that do not have their own OSHA come under the auspices of federal OSHA. All regulations can be found in 29 CFR 1910.1450.

Standard laboratory fume hoods can be viewed in Figures 7-1 and 7-2. These fume hoods are large enough for two people to work at the same time. If a fume hood is to be used by more than one person at a time, it must provide 2.5 linear feet per person to allow adequate space and ventilation. Federal standards allow for a minimum velocity of 60 linear feet per minute (lfm) [3]. I recommend a higher standard to provide a more adequate airflow. In California, the governing standard is an average face velocity of at least 100 lfm with a minimum of 70 lfm at any point in the fume hood. Fume hoods measured at any less velocity are considered deficient. [4]

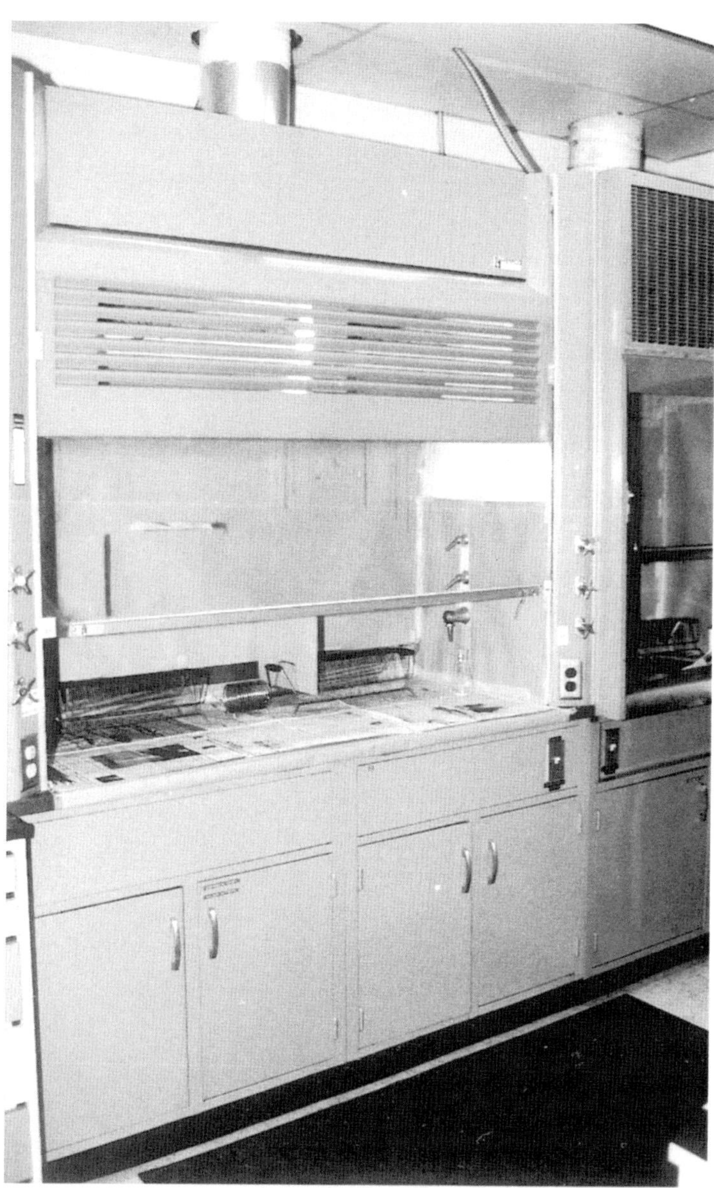

Figure 7-2: Two fume hoods installed side by side. Note the nonslip mat on the floor in front of the hoods.

If a fume hood cannot be built into the laboratory setting, purchase a portable fume hood. These fume hoods are available in different shapes and sizes. Some are designed and manufactured to set on a counter top, and some are located on movable carts with wheels. Figures 7-3 and 7-4 are examples of portable fume hoods. Portable fume hoods are equipped with a carbon (charcoal) filter system and require an electrical outlet for the power plug. Portable fume hoods are very efficient if maintained and are adequate for most types of chemical processing.

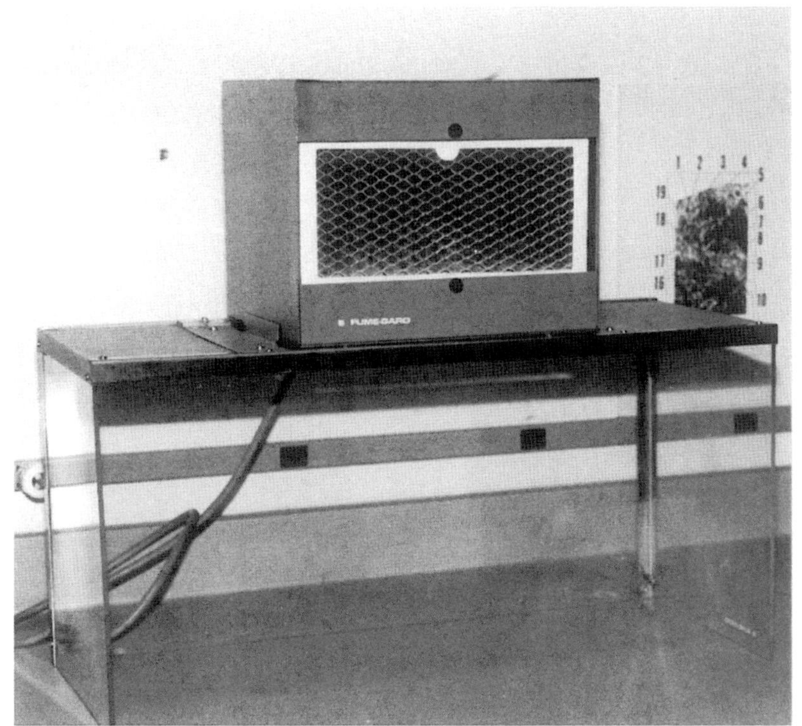

Figure 7-3: Portable fume hood with carbon filter. Fume hood is designed to sit on a counter top.

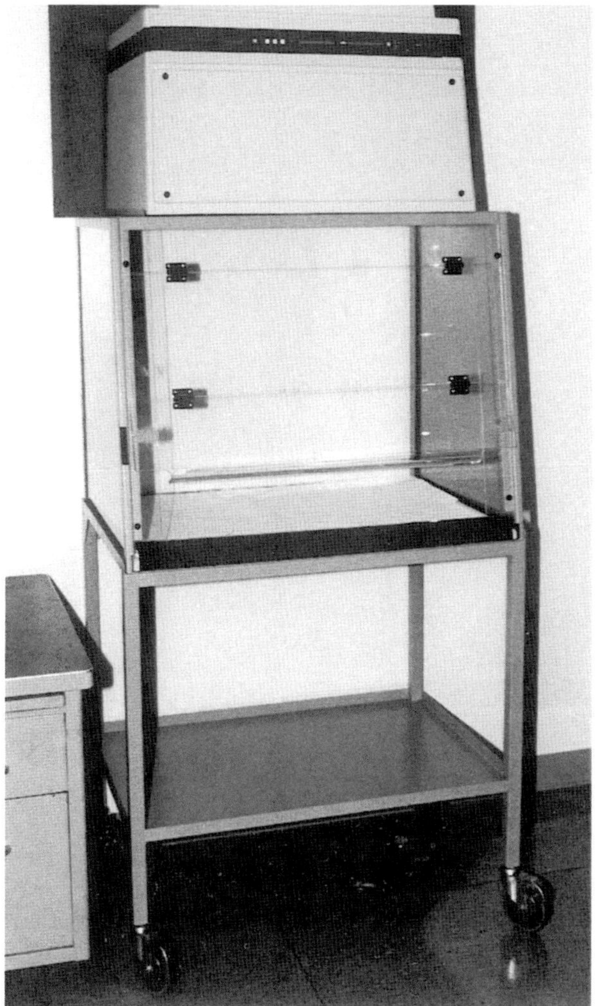

Figure 7-4: Portable fume hood with carbon filter installed on a movable cart.

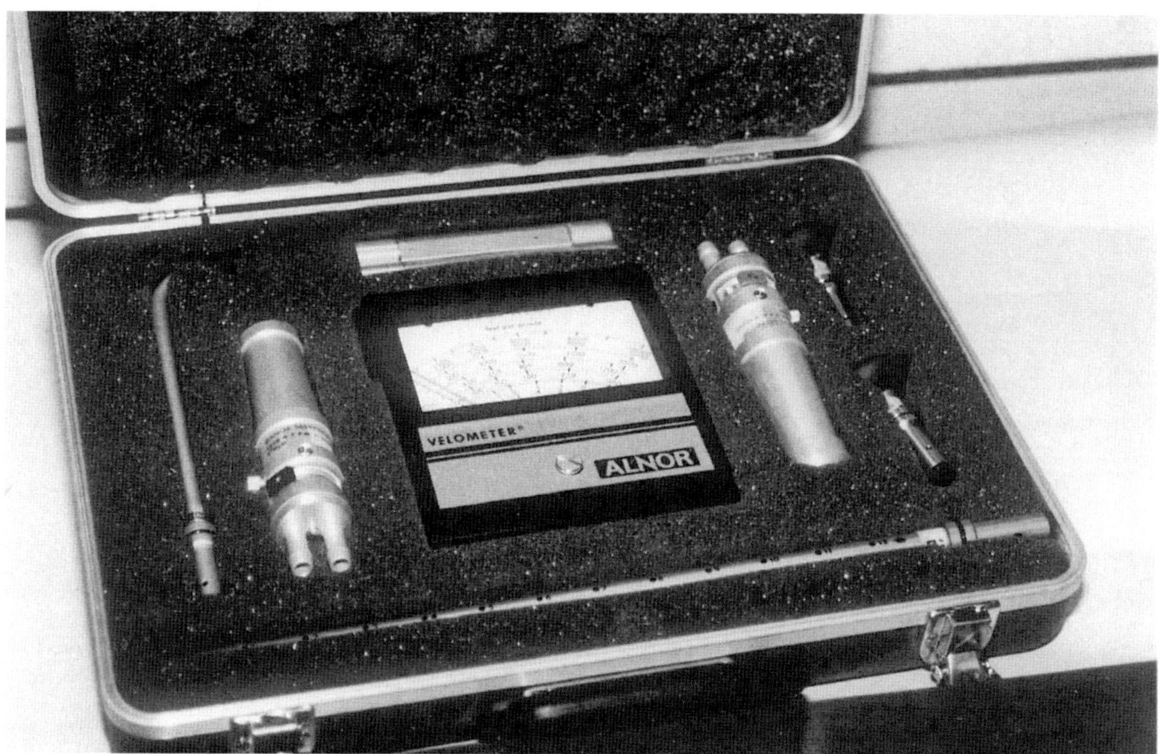

Figure 7-5: Velometer. This instrument is a direct reading instrument for measuring air velocities inside ventilating ducts, or in open areas, such as fume hoods. It may also be used for measuring duct static pressure.

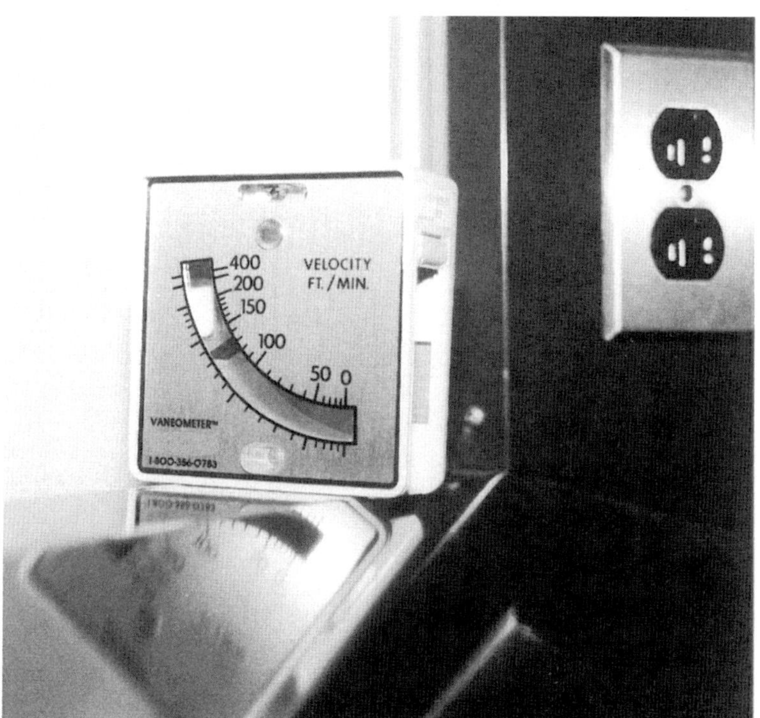

Figure 7-6: Vaneometer placed on the edge of fume hood. Reading indicates fume hood is drawing at 135 linear feet per minute.

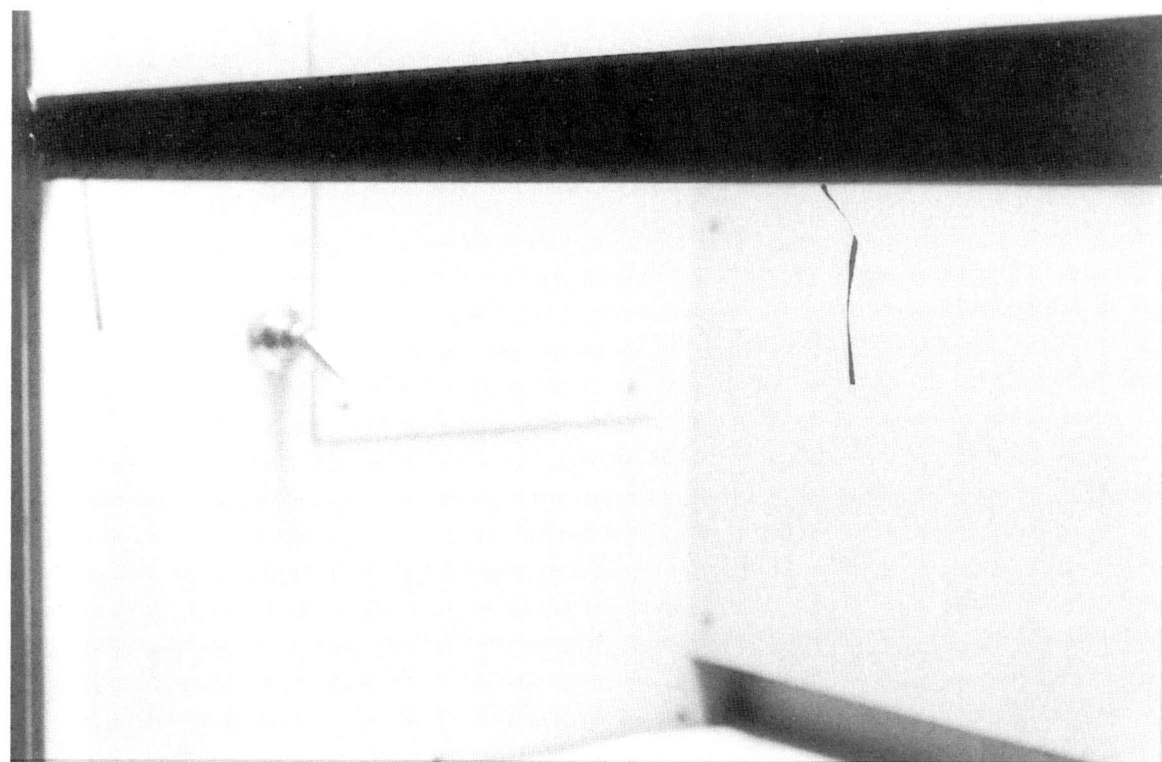

Figure 7-7: "Tail" of tape attached to the sash of a fume hood. The position of the tape indicates the fume hood is turned "off."

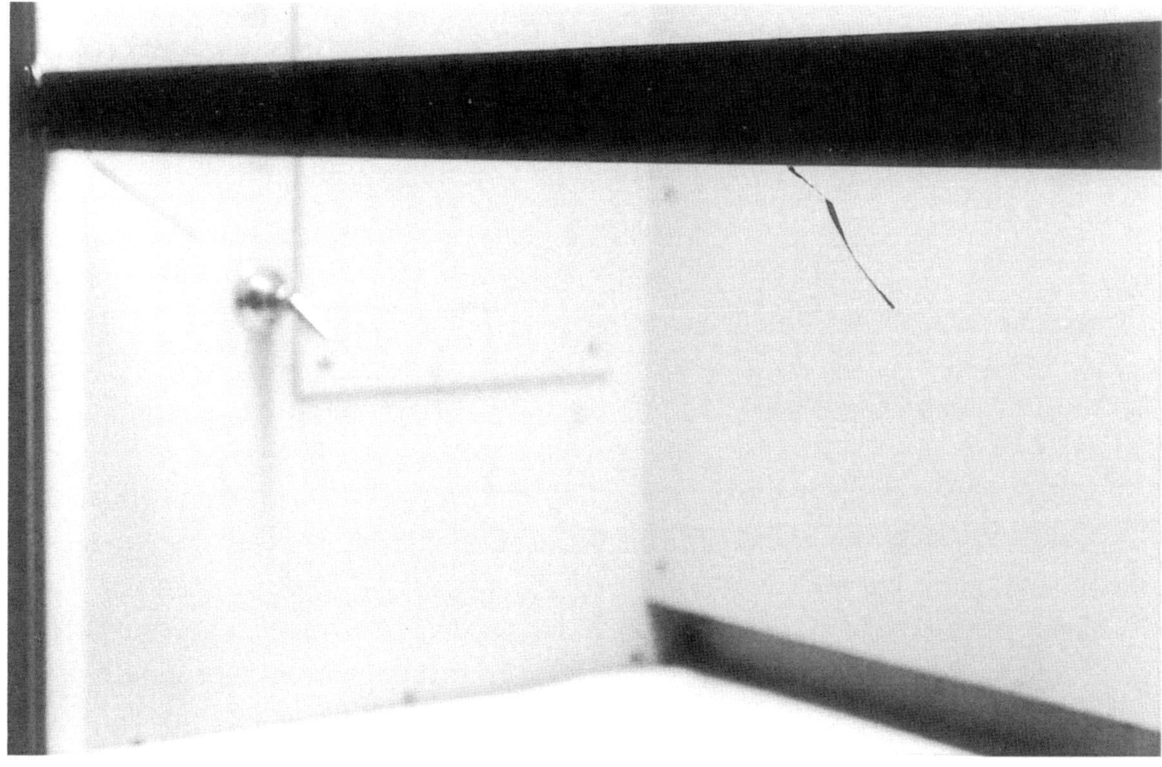

Figure 7-8: "Tail" of tape indicating the that fume hood is "on," drawing air in, up and to the back of the fume hood.

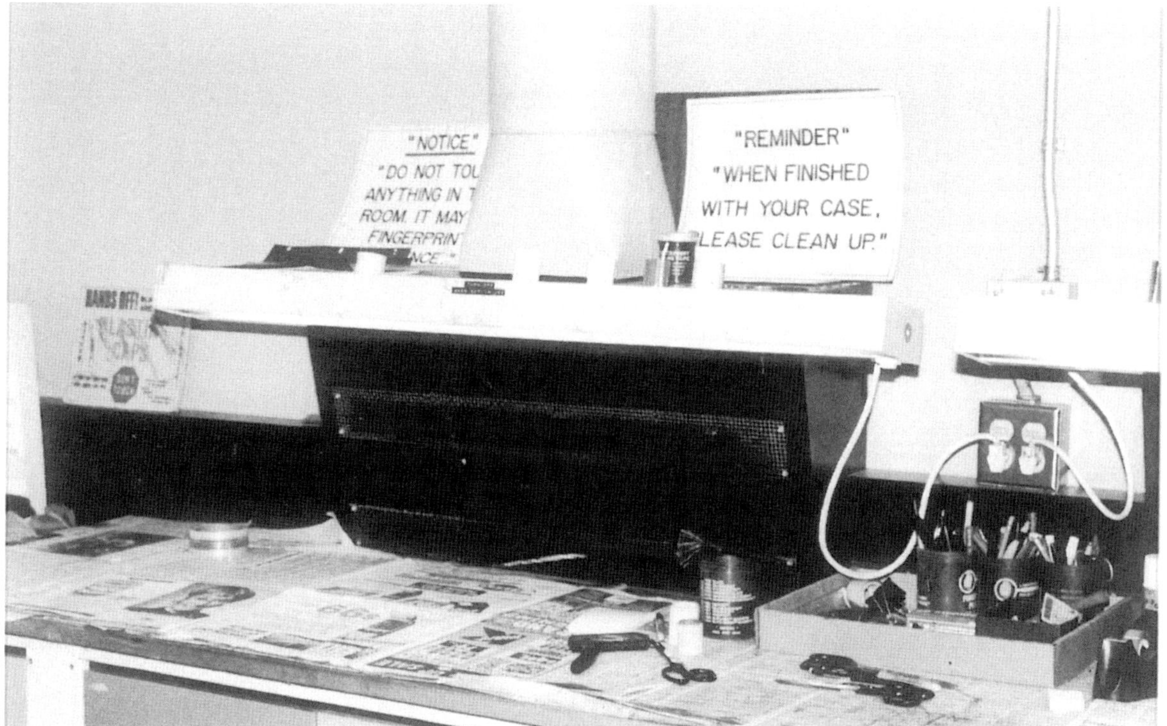

Figure 7-9: Slot fume hood designed to draw fingerprint powders across the surface of the bench top and out the ducting.

Regardless of which type of fume hood you use, establish and mark the sash position. Set a velometer (Figure 7-5) or vaneometer (Figure 7-6) on the outer edge of the face of the hood. Raise or lower the sash until you determine the minimum and maximum air flows. Mark these points on the sash and/or jamb of the fume hood with arrows or velometer readings to show the maximum opening to meet the fume hood velocity requirement. Attach a "tail" to the bottom of the sash to confirm air is being pulled up and out the back of the hood when the system is turned on. Use pieces of tape like that used in cassette tapes (Figures 7-7 and 7-8). If a tape tail falls off, or is somehow removed, replace it immediately. These tape pieces need only be 4 or 5 inches long. Permanent stops should restrict closure of the sash so that during work with flammables enough air flow is maintained to prevent explosions.

A type of specialty exhaust system useful to the forensic identification specialist is a laminar flow or "slot" hood. This type of system is seen in Figure 7-9. The purpose of the fume hood is to pull airborne particulate from the surface of the bench top to the rear of the work area and up the ventilation ducting. This system is excellent when using fingerprint powders. The powders are very fine and easily airborne. If slot fume hoods are not available, the specialist must wear a particulate or dust mask when processing evidence with powders. With the fume hood installed, not only do you not need a mask (although you can still wear one if you wish), but you keep to a minimum powder particulate accumulation on surfaces in the laboratory.

Always use proper ventilation, including a fume hood, for chemical processing. The efficiency of a fume hood depends upon its design and subsequent maintenance. Measure the ventilation rates of all fume hoods, record the data, and keep the measurements for reference. Routinely monitor the entire laboratory ventilation system to assure its efficiency for the safety of both the laboratory and the other areas of the building.

The law requires ventilation systems wherever hazardous, toxic or flammable chemicals are in use. The forensic identification specialist is within his or her rights to refuse to perform any tasks related to such chemistry without adequate mechanical or engineering controls. Ventilation systems are only one aspect of safety and can never be substituted for sound work practices.

never liked to wear
safety glasses.
Now she doesn't
have to.

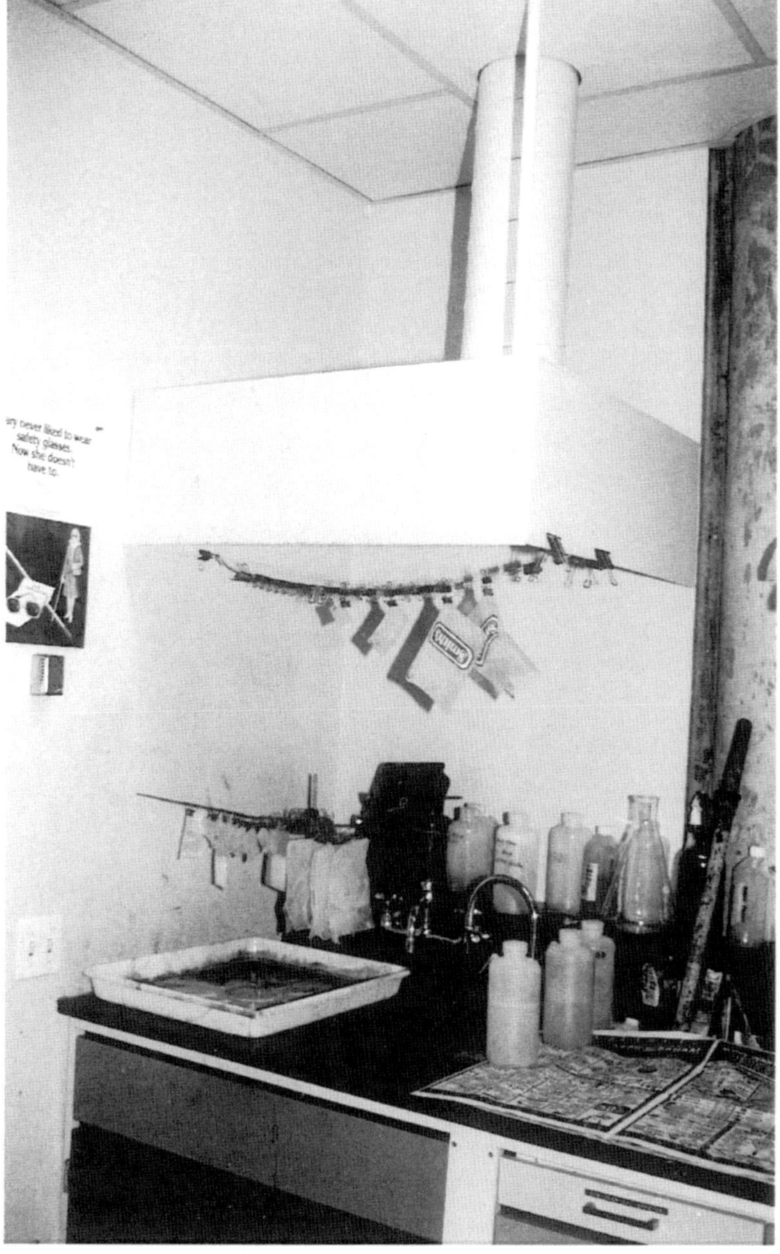

Figure 7-10: Ventilation system built over a sink area used for processing with fluorescent dye stains.

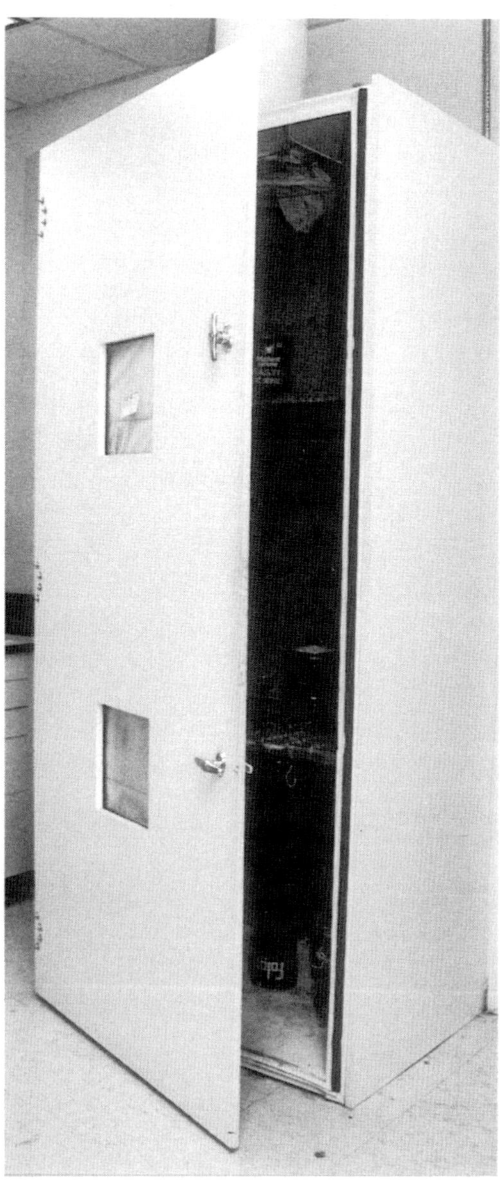

Figure 7-11: Ventilated cabinet for processing oversized items with cyanoacrylate esters.

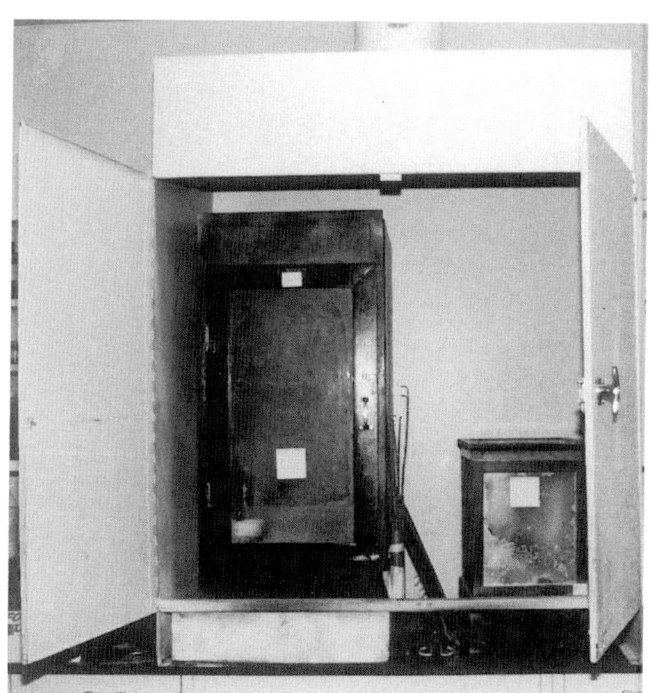

Figure 7-12: Ventilated enclosure for containment of small fuming cabinets.

8
Personal Protective Equipment

Many people consider personal protective equipment to be the first line of defense against hazards in the laboratory. In fact, it is the last line of defense. All engineering controls should be in place, i.e., fume hoods, ventilation systems, sharps containers, laboratory design, substitution of less toxic materials, etc. Your personal protective equipment is the final barrier to protect you from the hazards in the laboratory. These hazards could be noise, vapors, flying glass from a shattered beaker, or wet chemistry. Protective equipment does not replace engineering controls. Conversely, engineering controls do not replace personal protective equipment. One goes hand-in-hand with the other. Personal precautions include using all protective equipment and then following of all laboratory protocols. You may need to insist that the equipment be made available and the protocols be written. The forensic identification specialist must be willing to educate her or his management on the elements of a safe laboratory and the mandates of the OSHA act.

The law reads: "Protective equipment, including personal protection for eyes, face, head, and extremities, protective clothing, respiratory devices, and protective shields and barriers, shall be provided, used, and maintained in a sanitary and reliable condition wherever it is necessary by reason of hazards of processes or environment, chemical hazards, radiological hazards, or mechanical irritants encountered in a manner capable of causing injury or impairment in the function of any part of the body through absorption, inhalation or physical contact." [1] Let there be no doubt in your mind that this covers the processing of physical evidence. Whether you work in the laboratory performing forensic document examination, latent print development or photography, this standard applies to you.

A general discussion of the various types of personal protective equipment is intended to give you a basic understanding of the types of equipment and their uses. There are numerous brands and manufacturers of equipment. They will all make great claims to being "the best" and/or the most innovative. If you are going to purchase a number of pieces of any type of equipment, first buy only one of the items and test it out in your laboratory under working conditions to determine its quality and fulfillment of your safety needs. Cost is not always an indicator of quality. Many middle-priced pieces of equipment work as well as expensive equipment. Always give consideration to the type of material used to manufacture the item and the design of the item. However, the old adage, "You get what you pay for," is also true. Inferior products are inferior no matter what the window dressing. If there is a great price discrepancy between pieces of equipment of the same general description, ask probing questions of the vendor. Consider any information on protective materials and make the best selection for the situation. There are always exceptions to the rule. Where one material may usually be the best selection, in another given situation it may be the worst choice. When in doubt, research your options.

Respiratory Protection

There are a variety of respiratory protective devices ranging from the simple soft felt mask used to filter nuisance levels of dusts and particulates to the self-contained, positive-pressure, encapsulating suit which can offer total body and respiratory protection from toxic substances and oxygen-deficient environments. You would not generally use the latter as a forensic identification specialist though it may be appropriate to investigate clandestine drug laboratories. Preferably, this type of initial investigation should be performed by a criminalist or chemist. (See Figure 8-1.)

If the laboratory is properly designed and operated with adequate ventilation systems and efficient fume hoods or other types of vent systems, you will not need additional respiratory protection for most procedures. The exceptions are accidents or procedures which cannot be performed in the fume hood. Any specialist who may ever, for any reason, need to wear a respirator must be included in the respiratory protection program. This includes the use of "dust" masks when powder-processing evidence in the field. Yes, a dust mask may be classified as a respirator (by some industrial hygienists). Any of us who have worn a dust mask can attest to the fact that they impede your ability to breathe freely.

According to requirements of the OSHA respiratory standard, 29 CFR Part 1910.134 (b)(10), any individual who is to wear the respirator must be capable of wearing it under working conditions. This means that s/he must be physically able

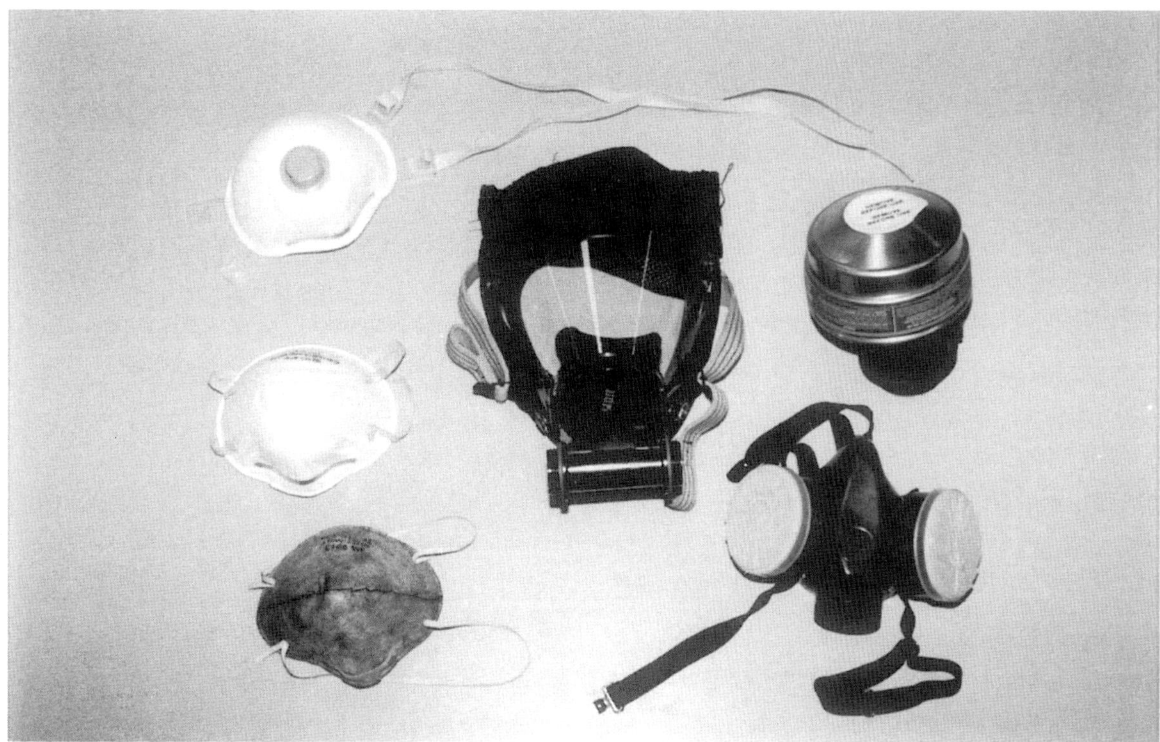

Figure 8-1: Respiratory protection (from center, clockwise): Full-face mask and air-purifying canister, half-face respirator, nuisance odor mask impregnated with charcoal, particulate/ dust mask, and particulate/dusk mask with exhalation valve.

to perform her or his work and use the equipment. A physician must determine if the worker's medical condition permits wearing a respirator. This examination will include a pulmonary function or spirometer test. Anyone with poor respiratory function should not be asked or permitted to wear any respirators which require breathing through a protective filter or cartridge. This can prove to be an interesting situation. In one state agency, a latent analyst who had suffered from severe bronchial problems since childhood was tested and failed the spirometer test. He had been assisting in the investigation of clandestine drug laboratories, but with the advent of a safety program, respirators became required personal protective equipment. Management informed this individual that he could no longer respond to clandestine labs. He felt quite "put out" at this determination, insisting that there was no problem, he could do the work, and he would even waive his rights should there be any adverse effects. In fact, he was an avid jogger and was probably in better physical condition than most of the other analysts. Over the years, his lungs had compensated for his decreased breathing capacity. However, since he did not successfully pass the spirometer test, he was removed from the response team for this type of crime scene.

The health of the respirator user should be checked on a regular basis. A number of medical conditions preclude the wearing of a respirator: emphysema, asthma, reduced pulmonary function (variety of causes other than the preceding two), severe hypertension, coronary artery disease, cerebral blood vessel disease, epilepsy, claustrophobia (brought on by wearing the unit), or other relevant conditions as determined by the examining physician. [2] Since the intent of the respiratory device is to protect the health of the user, the forensic specialist should participate in an ongoing and complete medical surveillance program to establish a baseline as well as to periodically check the users health. The employer maintains these records for the duration of employment plus thirty years after separation from service with the department.

A number of factors affect the selection of the proper respiratory device. The most important consideration is the properties of the chemical or material for which the protection is needed. What is the permissible exposure-limit (PEL) or threshold level value (TLV) of the material? Is there a skin absorption potential? Is it immediately dangerous to life and health (IDLH)? What type of material is it, i.e., acid, solvent, dust, carcinogen, etc? Will air or oxygen need to be supplied? What levels of material are expected to be present? Does the material provide an adequate warning of its presence by an odor or by irritation of the respiratory system or the eyes? Any devices selected must comply with the specifications of ANSI (American National Standards Institute) Z88.2, bear an appropriate NIOSH (National Institute of Safety and Health) or MSHA (Mine Safety and Health Administration) approval number, and provide the degree of protection needed under the existing working standards. [3]

Another extremely important aspect is proper fit. A proper fit means that there is a protective seal between the device and the face which will prevent any air or vapors from entering into the interior of the unit. The respirator must fit to each user individually. Facial hair, such as sideburns or a beard, will interfere with the exhalation valve and seal. Remove any such hair. In fact, some men who have a heavy beard growth are able to obtain a proper fit in the morning but not in the evening. Some skin conditions may obstruct a proper fit. Facial structure may pose problems, especially in fitting a half-face respirator. Some women are difficult to fit because of the small size of their faces. A narrow face with a prominent nose bridge or high cheek bones challenges the fit. Respirator manufacturers are constantly designing new devices to overcome these problems. It is totally unacceptable to maintain respirators in the laboratory for common use. Every individual must be assigned his or her own personal respirator. Such assignment carries responsibility for proper maintenance of the device.

Every user must be trained to use the respirator, to fit test the device and to maintain the device in good working condition. A knowledgeable person must administer a qualitative fit test. This person is usually with the safety or medical department; however, if you have no such person, consider approaching your local fire department for assistance. Firefighters routinely use self-contained breathing apparatus and have usually had excellent training or access to a trainer in respiratory protection. To perform the test, the trainer usually uses a particulate irritant such as a nontoxic smoke or an organic solvent which generates a distinctive odor. The most familiar of these is *isoamyl acetate*, which smells distinctly like banana. The user dons the respirator and then the trainer wafts the smoke or solvent around the respirator to challenge the seal. If the user detects any smell or irritant, the seal is inadequate.

Any training program should include, as a minimum, (1) how to care for the device, including how to inspect it for proper functioning as well as normal care, (2) how to put the respirator on and check to see that it is performing its function, (3) the function and limitations of the device, (4) proper cartridge selection, and (5) the health risks associated with either not using the protection or failing to use it properly. Give refresher training every year. [4]

Prepare written procedures covering safe use of respirators in dangerous atmospheres that users might encounter in normal operations or in emergencies. [5] These written protocols should additionally include all information on respirator and cartridge selection, fit testing, maintenance, function and limitation of devices, and health risks.

The most common respiratory protective device used by the forensic identification specialist is the dust mask. The term "dust" mask is a little bit misleading, as this mask can also be used as protection against paint fumes, moderate levels of organics, and acid fumes. My experience is that commercial masks marketed for painters are usually inadequate for use with fingerprint powders. 3M manufactures a good mask for training and latent case work; however, there are many other masks on the market. A dust mask is the simplest form of an air-purifying respirator. Do not use dust masks for hazardous dusts but for exposures to inert or nuisance dust levels below 15 mg/M^3. [6] People who wear glasses often have problems using these masks. Glasses fog over quickly making it frustrating to try to see. A mask of different design has an exhalation valve which directs exhaled breath down and out. This style of mask also seems to decrease the level of warmth that builds up in the mask during use. Other special design features include molded bridge pieces and small sections of metal over the nose bridge that can be pinched for a closer fit to the nose and cheeks. Some masks have a chemical absorbent built into the felt material to absorb some fumes and gases. One such mask, a nuisance organic vapor mask, has charcoal impregnated into it. Pathologists use it when working autopsies to filter some of the smell of decomposed flesh. The somewhat inexpensive dust mask is meant to be worn for relatively low levels of air pollutants and then discarded. Do not wear this disposable equipment more than once or by two different people. Generally speaking, dust masks have a lifetime of eight hours.

Never wear these masks in an environment with less than 19.5% oxygen. Sensations of oxygen deprivation are insufficient warning signals for this hazard. At oxygen concentrations of 10 to 16%, you can function for short intervals, but the lack of oxygen to the brain will significantly impair your judgment. At levels below 6%, death occurs in only a few minutes. It is quite likely that more persons have died from lack of oxygen while wearing air-purifying respirators than have died from the direct effects of toxic materials. Air-purifying respirators, such as the dust mask or cartridge style, are not approved for use in atmospheres which are immediately dangerous to life and health. [7]

There is an ongoing controversy whether the dust mask is a respirator. NIOSH and MSHA tested and approved many dust masks that have been classified as respirators. Some industrial hygienists will hang to the letter of the law and consider the masks as respirators. Dust masks are difficult to fit and to fit test. If the mask does not fit snug to the face and is only pinched across the nose, air and contaminants will take the path of least resistance and enter around the edges of the mask. Respirators are used in environments having a measurable concentration of contaminant that exhibits warning properties. Nuisance dusts do not quite fall into these categories. While a dust mask is a good device for nuisance dusts or fingerprint powders, heavy concentrations of powders or other contaminants may require the use of a half-face respirator equipped with a high-efficiency particulate air (HEPA) filter. Remember that respirators require the wearer to have a medical evaluation and fit testing. If dust masks are classified as respirators, the users have extra burdens.

The half-face cartridge respirator is the type most often used in an ambient environment where there is no concern about irritation or absorption of material through the skin. This style of respirator is molded of a flexible plastic or silicone rubber which covers the nose, cheeks and mouth. It provides a seal to the skin of the face. The face piece is provided with receptacles for two sets of cartridges and/or filters. Since these respirators are certified as complete units, the face piece of one manufacturer's device cannot be equipped with the cartridges of another manufacturer. Mixing them will invalidate any guarantees of safety. Many devices are also manufactured with non-removable and non-interchangeable cartridges. These must be discarded after breakthrough. One advantage of the air-purifying, cartridge/filter style respirator is that a series of filters and cartridge can be "stacked" to provide protection against a large variety of contaminants. This type of respirator has a greater capacity and wider application than the dust mask. The normal protection factor provided by a half-face respirator accepted by OSHA is either 10 times the PEL or the cartridge limit, whichever is lower.

Besides fit testing, the other most important factor of using cartridge respirators is cartridge selection. Every cartridge is color-coded and marked for the contaminant it filters, i.e., organic vapors; ammonia or methylamine; organic vapors, chlorine, hydrogen chloride or sulfur dioxide; etc. The cartridge is adequate to filter out only the contaminant for which it is certified. For example, a cartridge certified for organic vapors will not offer protection against methylamine (commonly found in clandestine drug laboratories). This important concept is the key to proper protection. If you are unsure of which cartridge to select, consult a criminalist or chemist. The forensic identification specialist will normally need either the organic vapor or methylamine cartridge.

Keep in mind that it requires effort to breath through the filters. Even though there are check valves to aid the exhalation cycle, inhalation still requires air to pass through the cartridges. There are power-assisted air-purifying respirators (PAPR) manufactured with a small battery-operated pump through which the air is fed into the face piece. The cartridges are located on the pump instead of the face piece. The pump, including the battery, is usually attached to the belt and is relatively light weight. This arrangement increases flexibility. The usual nickel-cadmium batteries are designed to provide 8 hours of continuous operation if properly maintained. This style of device is more expensive than a non-powered unit.

A power-assisted air-purifying respirator is a positive-pressure system. This means that the air inside the face piece is at a higher pressure than the air outside the face piece. A positive-pressure system provides more protection than the ordinary half-face respirator, because it is very difficult for contaminants to enter around the seal on the face. Additionally, even if the pump fails, the user can continue to breath through the filters until he or she can exit the hazardous environment. Under ANSI Z88.2 standard, this type of respirator can be used in an immediately dangerous-to-life-and-health (IDLH) atmosphere as long as at least one standby person with the proper equipment for entry and rescue is present outside the affected area. Communications between the worker within the area and the standby person may require the use of throat microphones connected to amplifiers or radios. [8]

To guard against chemicals splashing, you can wear chemical splash goggles and/or a face shield in addition to the half-face respirator. One caution bears mentioning. Goggles with ports or other openings to circulate air and decrease fogging will not protect your eyes from vapors and gases. Some respirators and goggles are simply incompatible in fit. Use a full-face respirator in an environment known to present chemical gas/vapor hazards to the eyes.

Full-face respirators resemble the half-face device except that they provide a shield which covers the upper part of the face and the eyes. This respirator has the advantage of being easier to fit to the face, so the current ANSI Z88.2 standard and OSHA allow a higher protection factor, generally by a factor of five or less, depending upon the contaminant. [9] One of the major drawbacks of full-face respirators is their difficulty for persons who wear glasses. An adapter can attach corrective lenses to the face piece, but constant movement requires periodic adjustment. Some workers remove the temple pieces of their glasses and tape them to the bridge of their nose. Either of these arrangements is a poor compromise. By OSHA standards, contact lenses cannot be worn in a full-face respirator. Another drawback to these units is the problem of fogging. Warm air exhaled inside the face piece may cause the face shield to fog up. Anti-fogging coatings and/or the installation of nose cups to direct warm, exhaled air through the exhalation valve may eliminate this problem. At very low temperatures (below -32 degrees Celsius or -25 degrees Fahrenheit), your warm, moisture-laden breath can create ice to jam the exhalation valve open or closed, or the moisture may freeze and block the free flow of air through the valve. [10] As with the half-face respirator, power-assisted air-purifying full-face units are available. This style of device is more expensive than a non-powered unit. The full-face unit, in turn, is more expensive than a half-face unit by a factor of four or more.

The full-face respirator will not protect you in an environment which is oxygen deficient (contains less than 19.5% oxygen). Cartridges simply filter various contaminants from the air; they do not provide oxygen where it does not exist.

Claustrophobia is an additional consideration in wearing the full-face respirator. A person who can show medical documentation showing he or she suffers from this condition cannot be forced to wear such a respiratory device.

Never ask or require any individual who cannot smell odors (such as with a head cold) or who has no sense of smell to wear an air-purifying respirator. When these devices become saturated in a contaminated environment, the user begins to "smell something," exits the scene and replaces the cartridge with a new one. Any person with an impaired sense of smell cannot determine when the cartridge is no longer providing protection.

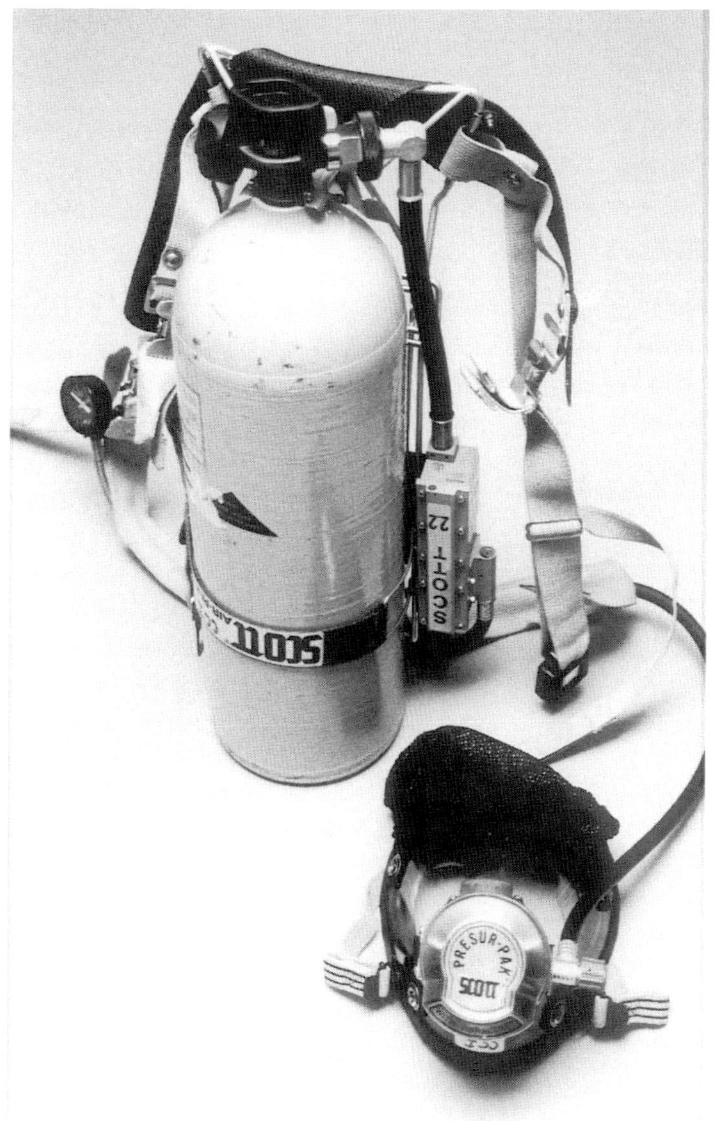

Figure 8-2: Self-contained breathing apparatus consisting of full-face mask, air tank with supporting frame and straps, and regulator.

Once cartridges have been opened from their protective wrapping and placed on the respirator, do not reuse them. Neither should you place used cartridges in sealable plastic bags to use at a later time. The safest practice is to use new cartridges for each event.

The last type of respirator is the air-supplied respirator. This device provides a source of breathable air to the wearer independent of the ambient environment. This is the only respirator to wear in an oxygen-deficient atmosphere. Some designs are approved for IDLH environments. There are two basic designs. One supplies air from a source outside the area of contamination, while the other provides a supply of air carried by the wearer. (Figure 8-2) Each of these two designs has two types of units: "demand" and "pressure-demand." "Demand" means that the demand valve allows a flow of air only during the inhalation phase, resulting in negative pressure inside the face piece the rest of the time (less pressure on the inside). That means the seal of the face piece can leak as the contaminated air outside tries to equal pressure inside the face piece. "Pressure-demand" means that a positive pressure is maintained inside the face piece at all times so that outside air is unlikely to leak into the respirator. This makes the pressure-demand unit far more desirable, more often purchased, and the only type approved for IDLH environments.

Supplied-air devices receive air from a source outside the area of contamination, connected to cylinders or air compressors by a hose. The supplied air must be of high purity. There are some hazards and concerns. The cylinders may contain oxygen rather than compressed air. Compressed air may contain some low concentrations of oil. It is not permissible to use oxygen with supplied-air devices which have previously used compressed air because contact of high-pressure oxygen with oil may result in a fire or explosion. Compressors used to supply breathing air must be equipped with a high-temperature alarm, or carbon monoxide alarm, or both if the compressor is lubricated with oil. The air provided by the compressor must be passed through an absorbent filter to insure a pure air supply. Regulations permit hoses up to 300 feet long. [11]

The weak link in this type of system is the hose. The hose can restrict movement, can be kinked or damaged, and requires a retracing of steps when exiting the area. To assure escape in the event of pump or hose failure, the user must carry an auxiliary tank of air connected to the respirator. The major advantage of this system is the unlimited supply of breathable, high purity air when unlimited numbers of cylinders are available or a compressor is used.

Respirators that are self-contained breathing apparatus (SCBA) come in two styles. Those designed for the user to carry the air supply have the limitation that they only provide the amount of air which the user can carry. Most of these devices are matched to a full-face piece, but other styles are available. The air supply is carried in a tank on the user's back and the air flow is controlled by regulators and valves. The tanks holding ordinary air have a 30-minute air supply that really may last only 15 minutes when a user performs strenuously. This supply limits the amount of productive time for the user. These respirators are heavy and can be unwieldy. Latent print analysts with one state agency decided they could not process clandestine lab evidence effectively while wearing these respirators. The latent print personnel developed protocols that they would never "suit up" in any respirator (at these scenes) of a higher level of protection than the full-face air-purifying type. Pressure-demand versions of the SCBA are the preferred style and are acceptable for IDLH atmospheres if some other type of egress pack (respirator) is also worn by the user.

The other style of SCBA uses pure compressed oxygen. After air pressure is reduced in the cylinder, the air exhaled by the wearer passes through a chemical pack that removes the carbon dioxide and returns the pure air to supplement the oxygen from the portable canister. These systems are often much smaller and lighter than the device that incorporates an air tank. As a result of appropriate sizing of the oxygen tank and air-purifying chemical, these systems can last a fixed time, typically an hour, although some will last considerably longer. This system provides the user with more productive time, but the system poses a significant hazard if a fire is involved. [12] These type of systems, if pressure-demand and equipped with a full-face piece, are approved for IDLH environments.

Maintenance of your respirator is essential. Contaminants can cause damage to the face seal material as well as to the valves. Even though the device has been cleaned and properly stored, chemicals may have permeated the materials used to construct it. Always inspect your unit before you wear it and have a routine schedule of inspection regardless of usage. Keep and maintain records of inspection, cleaning and repairs.

The use of any type of respirator in most types of interior laboratories should be the exception rather than the rule. Laboratories should have engineering controls in place to maintain a safe atmosphere for workers who follow safe laboratory practices. Respirators are worn most often in the field. Often the specialist is working under adverse conditions such as heat. Respirators are not especially comfortable, and even the dust mask adds to the heat. Do not give in to the temptation to remove your respirator and take your chances. Do not let anyone cajole you into believing your respirator is not necessary. Especially, do not let someone's making fun of you discourage you from using a respirator. The level of contamination in an environment is not always obvious. Encourage your management to be safety minded, to provide necessary safety programs, to enforce safety requirements, and to promote a positive safety attitude.

Eye Protection

Eye protection is essential in the laboratory environment. Interestingly, in private industries such as chemical manufacturing, an employee who forgets to wear his or her safety glasses would be counseled for the first oversight. The second oversight would result in separation. I cannot stress enough the importance of this type of personal protective equipment. Every time you enter the laboratory, your eye protection should be on your face.

The OSHA standard governing the requirement for eye protection is 29 CFR Part 1910.133. It is based on ANSI standard Z87.1-1968. There are later revisions of this standard, and more revisions will probably continue to be issued. No doubt more protective measures will be required. There are many commercial products available which meet the current requirements. (See Figure 8-3.)

The hazards posing the greatest threat to your eyes are from impact and splashing chemicals. Always wear eye protection while working with chemicals in the laboratory or in the field. Provide visitors to the laboratory with temporary eye protection. Such inexpensive, disposable safety goggles are commercially available.

While safety glasses (which look like prescription eye wear) provide protection from impact, they offer little or no protection from chemicals running

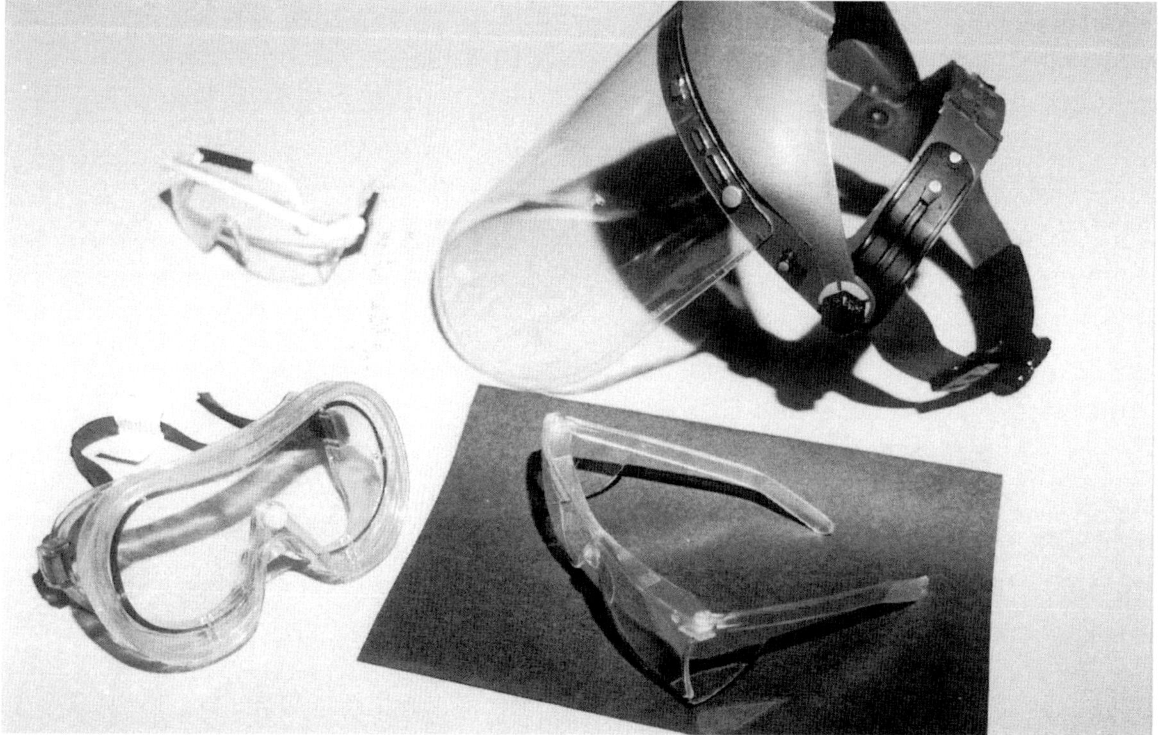

Figure 8-3: Eye protection (clockwise, top): Chemical face shield, safety glasses with side shields, chemical splash goggles, and safety glasses.

down the forehead and into the eyes because of their loose fit. Safety glasses, especially a style which provides side shields, do protect you from flying glass. The open structure of safety glasses causes no more problems with heating or fogging than regular prescription glasses.

Some people want to believe that contact lenses provide eye protection, but they provide no physical or chemical protection for the eye and actually pose serious hazards. If chemical(s) should be splashed into your eye(s), your contact lenses will trap the contaminant underneath them. You substantially reduce or eliminate the effectiveness of flushing the eyes with water. An additional problem is that capillary attraction (an effect of surface tension) may increase the amount of chemical trapped on the surface of the eye that otherwise might have been removed by tearing. The trapped chemicals are burning away and doing their damage in the meanwhile. Most people wear contact lenses for cosmetic and/or convenience reasons. When an individual must wear contact lenses for special eye conditions, the wearer should also always wear chemical splash goggles at all times while in the laboratory. Otherwise, do not wear contacts in the laboratory.

Chemical splash goggles provide the best eye protection. Most meet the standard in ANSI Z87.1 for laboratory eye protection. A wide variety of goggles are available on the market for the different tolerances people have for fit and design. This type of eye wear should fit snugly and comfortably around the eyes and should provide good peripheral vision. If possible, try to select a goggle which is compatible with your respirator and/or which can be worn over your prescription eye glasses. Select an easy-to-clean style so you can keep your goggles clean in order to maintain clear vision while performing tasks. Goggles should be designed with ports or openings around the edges of the lens to allow for their breathing and to help prevent fogging. You should not overheat and perspire from wearing them. Some people feel the design which incorporates openings around the lens (as opposed to ports on the sides) prevent fogging more efficiently because the movement of your head assists the passage of air flow directly over the interior of the lens and removes heat. Additionally, you can apply anti-fogging coatings to the lens; however, these coatings often prove ineffective.

The lenses of most safety goggles (and safety glasses) are made of polycarbonate. This material is typically 0.060 inches (1.52mm) thick. It is the material of choice, being lightweight, tough, and resistant to impacts and scratches. Some models coated with silicone are resistant to a number of chemicals. [13] Since a strap secures goggles to the head and creates a snug facial fit, they are more stable in lateral impacts which would probably dislodge safety glasses.

The quality of splash goggles is as varied as the styles. Test prospective goggles under actual working conditions before purchasing such an important piece of protective equipment. Again, there are many models and as many prices. Price may not be an indicator of quality. If great claims are made about performance, test them in the laboratory before buying. Be sure that you are happy and comfortable with your selection because in the laboratory, you should live in them.

Chemical face shields supplement protection to the face. They can be worn with safety glasses or goggles, but should never be worn as a substitute for such eye protection. The face shield protects the areas of the face not covered by your eye protection, as well as the throat. Wear a face shield over safety goggles when transferring or pouring chemicals. Shields are also constructed of polycarbonate. Store your face shields in an accessible place near the fume hood and keep them clean.

Chemical Protective Clothing

Use chemical protective clothing to provide a barrier to protect you from hazardous substances in the laboratory. You want to prevent chemicals from reaching your skin by permeating the material of which your clothing is made, or by entering through penetrations in the clothing. [14] Gloves are a type of protective clothing. Much of the material presented in this section also applies to other types of clothing, i.e., coveralls, laboratory coats, jump suits, encapsulating suits, and aprons. (See Figure 8-4) The publication *Guidelines to the Selection of Chemical Protective Clothing* will provide necessary information on the materials used to manufacture this type of protective equipment. The primary drawback to the manufacturer's rating system is that the evaluations are subjective, i.e., the material is given "excellent," "good," "fair" or "poor" protection based on visible degradation of the product. *Guidelines* points out that, "it has been found that chemicals can permeate a material without there being any visible sign of problems." [15] Also consider the information not contained in the data, such as the temperature at which the tests were performed on the various materials. Permeation depends significantly on the temperature. Additionally, the thicknesses of the materials also are frequently not given. [16] Obviously the thickness of a material will have some effect on the amount of time it takes for a contaminant to penetrate to the other side.

Chemicals may diffuse through the barrier material, or they may chemically

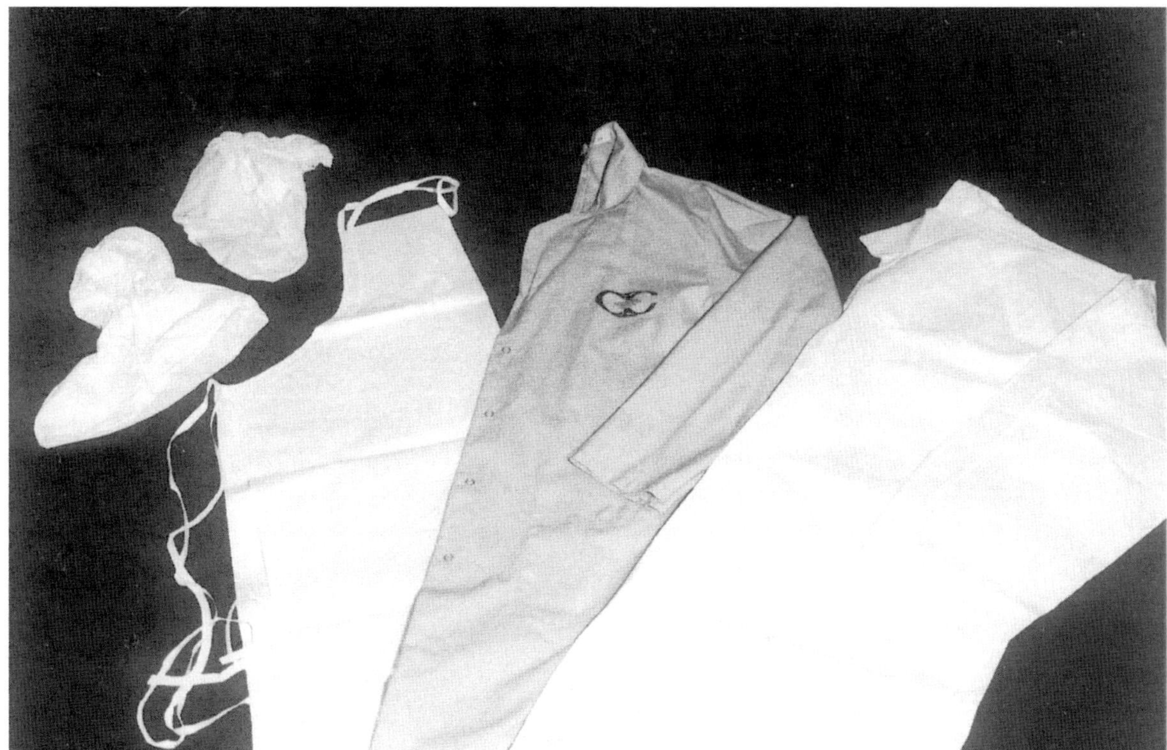

Figure 8-4: Chemical protective clothing (left to right): Tyvek® shoe covers, disposable Tyvek® apron, cotton laboratory coat, and disposable Tyvek ® laboratory coat.

react and degrade the performance of the material. Chemical reactions change the chemical properties or leach out some components of the barrier material. You want a barrier material to be a poor absorber of the challenging chemical and to have a slow rate of permeation. [17] Because a barrier material can continue to absorb chemicals for a long period of time after wear (in storage), discard or launder any protective clothing which has received a challenging exposure. Generally speaking, if you are wearing a Tyvek laboratory coat, you may use it on more than one occasion, but the coat is meant to be disposable and discarded after use. For this reason, most specialists will wear a laboratory coat made of fabric and supplement it with a rubber apron when pouring or mixing chemicals. Routinely launder your cloth laboratory coats every one or two weeks if you have worn them in the laboratory.

Most all protective clothing has seams that may have been chemically or heat welded, but they are still susceptible to tearing or splitting under stress. This type of clothing is more likely worn at crime scenes when working with biological materials or at clandestine drug laboratories. Unwelded or unsealed seams still have pinholes where chemicals can penetrate. Most clothing will have normal openings for zippers, pressure-locking lips or buttons. Protective clothing should have some type of overlapping flaps over these openings to prevent chemical penetration. Duct tape can be used to secure the overlapping flaps and to tape areas around the wrists and ankles. However, duct tape does not protect against exposure to chemicals. Use it to close openings.

It is important to develop an understanding of the materials used in protective clothing. Materials such as Tyvek or paper can protect against particulate contaminants and other nuisances but really offer little or no protection against hazardous contaminants. Use them as an outer covering over the primary protective gear, such as fully encapsulating suits to limit the amount of direct contamination on the primary surface. Then discard them. [18]

Another type of material, called elastomers (a natural or synthetic elastic substance, such as rubber or neoprene) provide better protection against chemical degradation, permeation, and penetration from toxic and corrosive liquids or gases. This is why rubber aprons and neoprene gloves provide such adequate protection in the laboratory when working with wet chemistry. Elastomers are sometimes combined with a flame-resistant fabric called Nomex to enhance durability and protection. [19]

Abilities of elastomers to resist degradation and permeation range from poor to excellent. The selection of a particular material should be based on its resistance to chemical degradation as well as on its ability to resist permeation and other performance characteristics. Other factors to be considered include:

- **Temperature of service** – Higher temperatures increase the effects of all chemicals on elastomers. The effect varies with the material and chemical. A material quite suitable at room temperature could fail at elevated temperatures.

- **Conditions of service** – A material which swells upon contact with the chemical may function well in a test situation but fail in actual use.

- **Grade of the elastomer** – Elastomers are manufactured in different grades, each providing different degrees of protection. Process changes, curing times, and overall quality control cause grades to vary from lot to lot. [20]

Following are some of the materials used to manufacture protective clothing:

- **Butyl rubber** – Resists degradation by many contaminants, except halogenated hydrocarbons and petroleum compounds, a common deficiency of most protective materials. Especially resistant to permeation by toxic vapors and gases. Expensive material used in boots, gloves, splash suits, aprons, and fully encapsulating suits.

- **Chlorinated polyethylene** – Also referred to as CPE. ILC Dover product. Used in splash suits and fully encapsulating suits. No data on permeability. Considered to be a good all-around protective material.

- **Natural rubber** – This is also a synthetic latex. Resists degradation by alcohols and caustics. Used in boots and gloves.

- **Neoprene** – Resists degradation by caustics, acids, and alcohols. Used in boots, gloves, and respirator facepieces and breathing hoses. Commonly available and inexpensive.

- **Nomex** – Product of Dupont. Aromatic polyamide fiber. Noncombustible and flame resistant up to 200°C, thus providing good thermal protection. Very durable and acid resistant. Used in fire fighters' turnout gear and some fully encapsulating suits as a base for the rubber.

- **Polyethylene** – Used as a coating on polyolefin material such as Tyvek, increasing resistance to acids, bases, and salts.

- **PVA** – Polyvinyl alcohol. Resists degradation and permeation by aromatic and chlorinated hydrocarbons and petroleum compounds. Major drawback is its solubility in water. Used in gloves.

- **PVC** – Polyvinyl chloride. Resists degradation by acids and caustics. Used in boots, gloves, aprons, splashsuits, and fully encapsulating suits.

- **Saranex** – Made of Saran, a Dow product. Coated on Tyvek. Very good general purpose disposable material. Material of choice for suits worn at clandestine drug laboratories. The major drawback is that wearing Saranex is like wrapping your body in Saran Wrap. Heat stress is a serious problem. Take frequent breaks to open the suit and the let the body breathe. Replace fluids with electrolytes because of sweating and dehydration.

- **Tyvek** – Product of Dupont. Spun-bonded nonwoven polyethylene fibers. Has reasonable tear, puncture, and abrasion resistance. Provides excellent protection against particulate contaminants. Inexpensive and suitable for disposable garments.

- **Viton** – Product of Dupont. Fluoroelastomer similar to Teflon. Excellent resistance to degradation and permeation by aromatic and chlorinated hydrocarbons and petroleum compounds. Very resistant to oxidizers. Extremely expensive material used in gloves and fully encapsulating suits. [21]

With all the possible barrier materials available, what are the types of protective clothing which should be worn in the laboratory?

Gloves

Gloves are another vital piece of protective equipment. Some specialists are unaware of the different types of gloves or ignore the use of them altogether. We all know peace officers who handle evidence without benefit of gloves, but a number of forensic specialists do the same. One philosophy is: "If I don't use gloves, I'll be more aware of the evidence and be less likely to over-handle it and leave my prints or destroy prints of evidentiary value." While there may be some logic to this statement, there is also a fallacy. If the specialist gets into the habit of wearing gloves all the time when handling evidence, s/he is more likely to remember to wear gloves when working with chemicals. Your safety depends on building work habits which promote personal protection.

Ignorance of the functions of different glove materials can cause another problem. For instance, many specialists are in the habit of wearing latex gloves for all processing. There is nothing wrong with this material if you are working with deceased or latent print powders. However, a latex glove provides no protection when working with solvents such as acetone, methanol or petroleum ether. Organic solvents will penetrate the latex material and the skin of your hands as though bare. Match your gloves to the chemicals (hazardous materials) you handle. (See Figure 8-5.)

Most manufacturers will provide qualitative descriptions of the effectiveness of their gloves that can be very subjective (Excellent, Good, Fair, and Poor). Some firms will provide technical support data on request. Still, the Permeation-

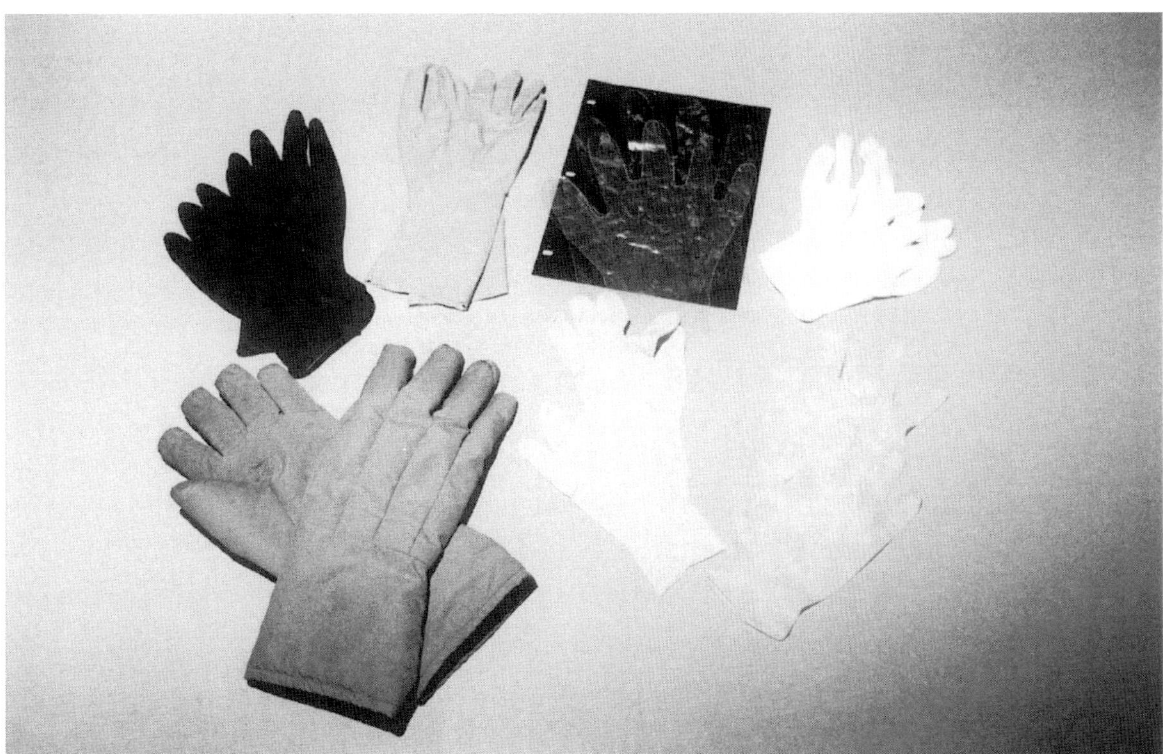

Figure 8-5: Gloves (clockwise, top): Polyvinyl, cotton, latex, nitrile, low temperature (Cryo), black neoprene, and green neoprene.

Degradation charts supplied by manufacturers are better than nothing in terms of guidance for selection. You must realize that a material may resist degradation by a contaminant but still be very permeable to it. [22] The third edition of *Guidelines for the Selection of Chemical Protective Clothing*, a two-volume work, was sponsored by the U.S. Environmental Protection Agency and the U.S. Coast Guard. The first volume contains an overview of the general topic of chemical protective clothing and tables which can be used to select and use this clothing properly. Twelve major clothing materials are evaluated in the context of about 500 different chemicals and permeation data, including 25 multiple-component organic solutions. Volume 2 is a technical support base for Volume 1. [23]

The forensic identification specialist will probably use three or four types of gloves depending upon the processing being performed. **Cotton** gloves provide the least protection, but are wonderful for applying latent print powders or for the questioned document examiner endeavoring to not leave latent prints on porous surfaces. The gloves will not provide protection from any chemicals and should not be used with evidence which has been chemically treated. You can wear the gloves repeatedly.

Polyvinyl gloves are quite thin and appear as a clear plastic. These gloves are adequate for working with latent print powders, but you can "leak" your fingerprint through this material onto the surface of the evidence. They provide no protection against organic solvents or acids. Discard these **disposable** gloves after use.

Many specialists think **latex** gloves provide adequate protection for all processes. Latex is quite good for using latent print powders and working with deceased or other biological materials (double them for this event). These gloves, however, will not protect you adequately from most wet chemistry. Many people experience an allergic reaction to latex. If you develop any type of dermatitis after wearing a latex material, you should consider pursuing this possibility. Discard these **disposable** gloves after use.

Nitrile gloves (also called Buna-N, milled nitrile, nitrile latex, NBR, or acrylonitrile) provide better protection than plain latex and have some resistance to petroleum compounds, alcohols, acids and caustics. These gloves are readily available, inexpensive and thin, allowing for a sense of dexterity when handling materials. Discard these **disposable** gloves after use.

Neoprene gloves provide the best all-around protection for working with caustics, acids and alcohols. They are readily available and moderate in cost. These gloves are made of a heavier material than nitrile and can be purchased with an embossed surface to assist in gripping. They are available in sizes from 7 to 11 to fit women as well as men. These gloves can be washed with any laboratory soap after use and will last for some time before requiring replacement. They are really the glove of choice when working with most wet chemistry.

Always give consideration to glove thickness and cuff length. The longer and thicker the glove, the greater the protection. Jacket cuffs can be worn over the cuff of the glove to prevent any liquid from spilling into the gloves. Rolling the cuff of the glove will accomplish much the same purpose.

Whichever glove you decide to purchase, ask to see some data on permeation rates (the amount of time before any given contaminant will penetrate through the glove material) and degradation rates (amount of time before any given contaminant will cause a breakdown or decomposition of the glove material). These tables are usually provided at no cost by various safety supply companies.

Laboratory Coats/Aprons

You must wear linen or Tyvek laboratory coats any time you are in the lab. When mixing, pouring or transferring chemicals, wear a chemical apron over your laboratory coat.

Foot Protection

Wear shoe covers to protect your footwear from splashes or spills. (NEVER wear sandals or canvas shoes in the laboratory.) Wear shoe covers at crime scenes where biological fluids may be present. Wear rubber boots that meet the specifications of ANSI Z41.1-1969 to process clandestine drug laboratory sites. These boots should be made of PVC, neoprene, butyl rubber or some other elastomer if you expect them to protect you against liquid hazardous chemicals. [24] You may also wear boots with steel toes for added protection.

Hearing Protection

Most laboratory environments will not require the use of hearing protection unless that particular facility is undergoing a hearing conservation program. The laboratory should make every attempt to decrease excessive noise levels. OSHA has adopted a comprehensive hearing conservation program in 29 CFR Part 1910.95. However, this standard applies to an employee exposed to an 8-hour, time-weighted average of 85 dB (decibels) as properly measured on specially calibrated instrumentation. [25] This standard will not apply to most forensic identification specialists. Forensic latent print specialists who also conduct firearms examinations must protect their hearing when test firing firearms. (See Figure 8-6.)

There is a wide variety of hearing protection devices on the market. The most basic and least expensive is the simple ear plug placed in the ear. Ear plugs are manufactured of a soft foam, silicone or PVC material which conforms to the ear canal and effectively reduces noise levels, especially at higher frequencies. Many of these plugs can be washed and reused. Ear plugs, however, are not

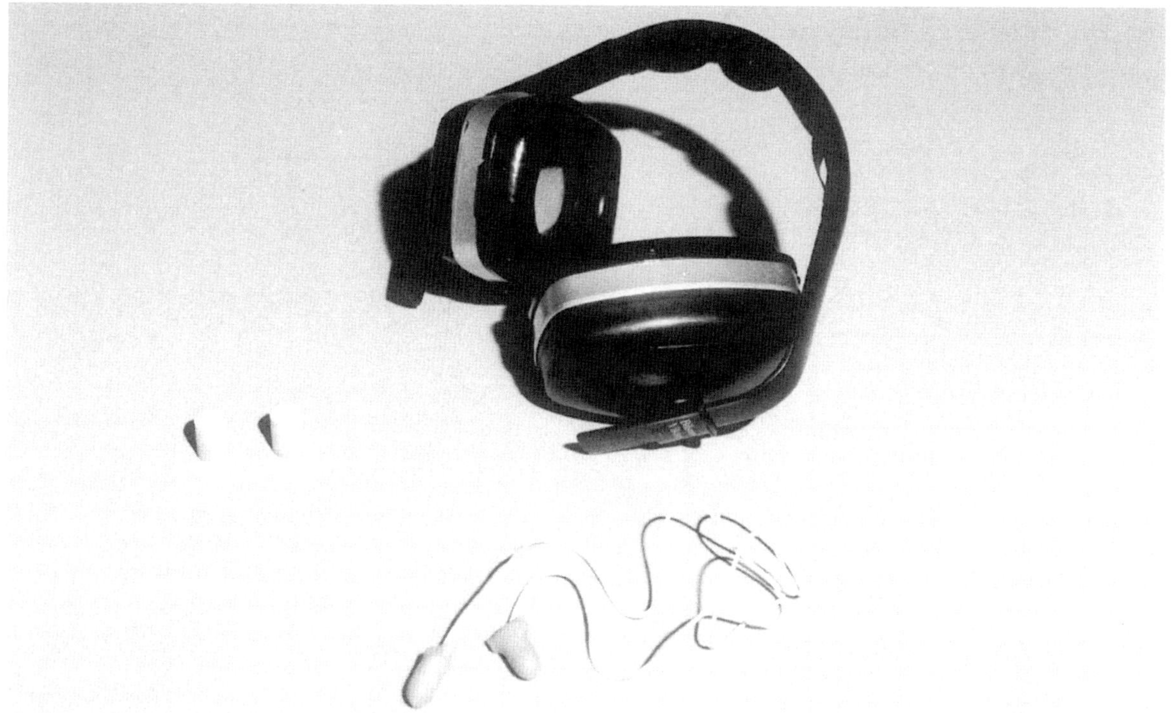

Figure 8-6: Hearing protection: Hearing protectors, ear plugs with cords, and ear plugs without cords.

sufficient for firing of weapons (high caliber and/or short barreled). Combine the ear plug with hearing protectors for better protection. Hearing protectors have cups that cover the ear completely and seal from noise. They are not very expensive compared to the disposable ear plugs and will pay for themselves in time. Hearing protectors will reduce the intensity of sounds by 20 to 30dB. Attenuation of hearing protection devices varies with frequency. [26] These devices should meet the ANSI standard S3.19-1974.

The user who wears glasses has one problem using hearing protectors. The temples of the glasses will actually break the seal of the hearing protector around the ears, reducing the hearing protectors effectiveness by 5 to 10dB. The specially designed hearing protectors made to eliminate this problem may be expensive. The better solution to this problem is to combine ear plugs with hearing protectors.

Choice of protective clothing will depend upon the severity of application. For exposure to severe abuse and if the environment is unusually hazardous, choose the most durable and protective material available. In many cases, less protective and/or durable, such as disposable, selections will be adequate. [27] Experience is your best guide. Expensive and/or well-known brands may high levels of failure or other problems, where less-known and moderately priced products may have a good record of performance. Document any problems you have with any protective clothing. Make decisions based upon needs, research, and experience — not solely on competitive pricing.

9
Spraying Chemicals

For many years, chemicals used in the development of latent impressions, such as Ninhydrin, have been sprayed. This method of applying chemicals to the surface of the evidence was used because spraying is convenient, quick and easy. Since commercially prepared cans or bottles of mixtures can be purchased, using spray containers eliminates having to mix a variety of chemical components. Forensic identification specialists have also mistakenly thought that spraying with a can or bottle could be performed out of doors, thus eliminating the need for a ventilation system. In reality, the chemicals used in latent print development should rarely be sprayed.

For optimum results, the recommended application for nearly all techniques is dipping or immersion into the solution. This allows full contact between the chemical and the latent residue. Spraying presents serious health and safety hazards. Spraying also wastes chemicals and does not promote good chemical reaction. The latent print analysts in one state bureau always sprayed their ninhydrin and felt that it gave great results. After they were ordered to cease spraying and began dipping the evidence, they approved the more numerous developed latent prints the change in procedure produced.

There are two basic rules to follow: 1) Never spray a formula which contains any chemicals that react with amino acids (proteins), because the chemical will react with your exposed human tissue, and 2) Never spray a formula that contains any organic solvents or [1] chemicals that contain carbon compounds. [2] Such organic solvents are the alcohols and any petroleum products, including acetone, methanol, ethanol, propanol, petroleum ether, hexane, heptane, and Freon. Organic solvents pose serious health hazards to human tissues. Solvents such as acetone and methanol are known to attack the liver and central nervous system. Methanol is especially known for its propensity to attack the optic nerve.

The real problem with spraying formulations is that the chemicals become an aerosol (a fine suspension of solid or liquid particles) that a fume hood cannot remove adequately. Handle and apply all chemicals in a regulation fume hood. Aerosols sprayed in the fume hood inevitably travel to the back of the hood, hit the backboard and bounce back out the front. This is why people often complain that when spraying Ninhydrin, they can smell the chemicals and experience coughing and sneezing and irritation to their throats. Often times, people will mistakenly believe that the fume hood is not functioning up to standard, when the hood would probably have to be capable of a face velocity around 400+ linear feet per minute to pull aerosols. [3] When you must spray chemicals, such as at a crime scene, use a self-contained breathing apparatus (air supplied). Dust or particulate masks are only adequate for use during dusting with fingerprint powders, affording inadequate protection against chemical fumes or vapors.

If spraying is a "must," do it in the fume hood while you wear an air-purifying respirator equipped with an organic vapor cartridge. The cartridge is marked on the side with information on which chemical vapors it is designed to filter. However, forensic specialists should never use any respiratory equipment without medical certification. [4] Respirators impede the individual's ability to breathe. The law also requires an individual to be trained in the use of respirators before actual use. [5]

The only latent print development techniques recommended for spraying are Small Particle Reagent (Molybdenum disulfide in detergent and water), Zinc Chloride, and "Liquid Iodine" (Iodine in Freon or cyclohexane). Use proper respiratory equipment to apply these chemicals: a fume hood and/or air-purifying respirator with an organic vapor cartridge, or at crime scenes, a self-contained breathing apparatus. Small Particle Reagent is the only formulation that can be applied at the scene while using a dust mask. It contains no amino acid reactive chemicals or organic solvents but do not breathe the dry Molybdenum particulate. Apply all other formulations, including Ninhydrin, DFO (1,8-Diazafluoren-9-one), Amido Black, Silver Nitrate, Gentian Violet, and Sudan Black, by dipping or immersion, and all dye stains, such as RAM, MBD and Rhodamine 6G, by wash bottle.

In addition to using a fume hood and/or respirator while working with chemicals, other personal protective equipment is also a necessity. Always wear a laboratory coat, apron or coverall. Rubber or neoprene gloves are required for protection against acids and organic solvents. A chemical splash shield will protect the face from splashed or spattered chemicals. If a chemical shield is not available, chemical goggles or laboratory safety glasses will protect the eyes.

Remember, you use protective equipment to provide a barrier between you and the chemicals being handled. The greatest hazard in performing forensic identification work today is neglecting to learn and apply safety protocols. Safety is not quick, easy and convenient. Do not be lulled into the lax attitude that safety is not important. Ignorance and indifference are deadly.

10
Laboratory First Aid Kit

Every chemical laboratory should be equipped with a basic first aid kit. This kit should be intended for immediate treatment of most minor injuries or burns. It should not be equipped to function as a substitute for the home medicine cabinet. Most laboratory accidents involve only one individual so the kit need not be large or stocked with a large number of items. In the event of a serious accident, call emergency medical personnel immediately. Never attempt to treat a serious injury in the laboratory.

The kit should be well marked and easily accessible to all laboratory personnel. Generally, this entails mounting the kit on a wall at a level that is reachable to all possible users. Such a kit should contain the following items:

Adhesive bandages, various sizes
Sterile pads, various sizes
Sterile sponges
Bulk gauze
Eye pads
Adhesive tape
First aid booklet
Antiseptic wipes
Cold packs
Burn cream
Antiseptic cream
Absorbent cotton
Scissors
Tweezers

The first aid kit should not contain tourniquets, aspirin (or other medications taken internally), iodine, or Merthiolate. You could add to the kit other items like Ipecac, used to induce vomiting, and activated charcoal to help absorb poisons internally. [1] If these items are included in the kit, have employees at the site who have specific training in how to use them properly. [2] Do not include any other items for internal application in the kit. Rather, it is better to have people formally trained in first aid and CPR in the laboratory. The safety officer or some other designated individual should inspect and maintain the first aid kit.

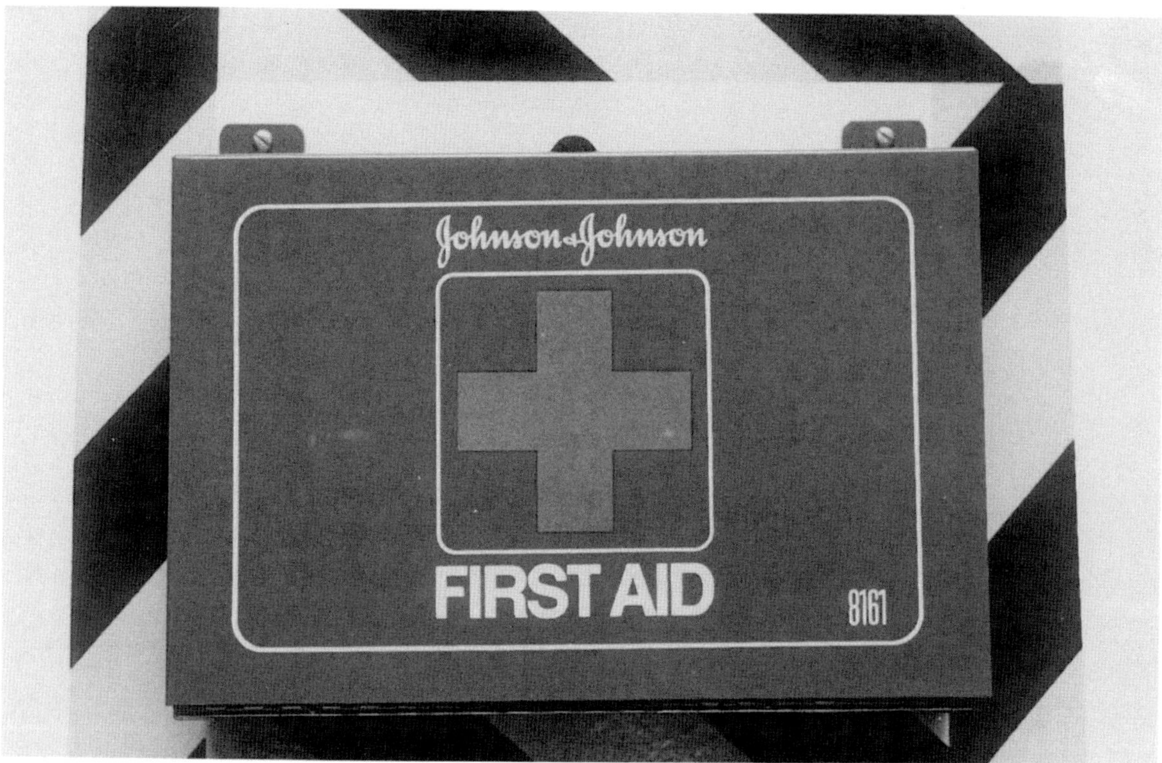

Figure 10-1: Commercially available First Aid kit mounted to laboratory wall.

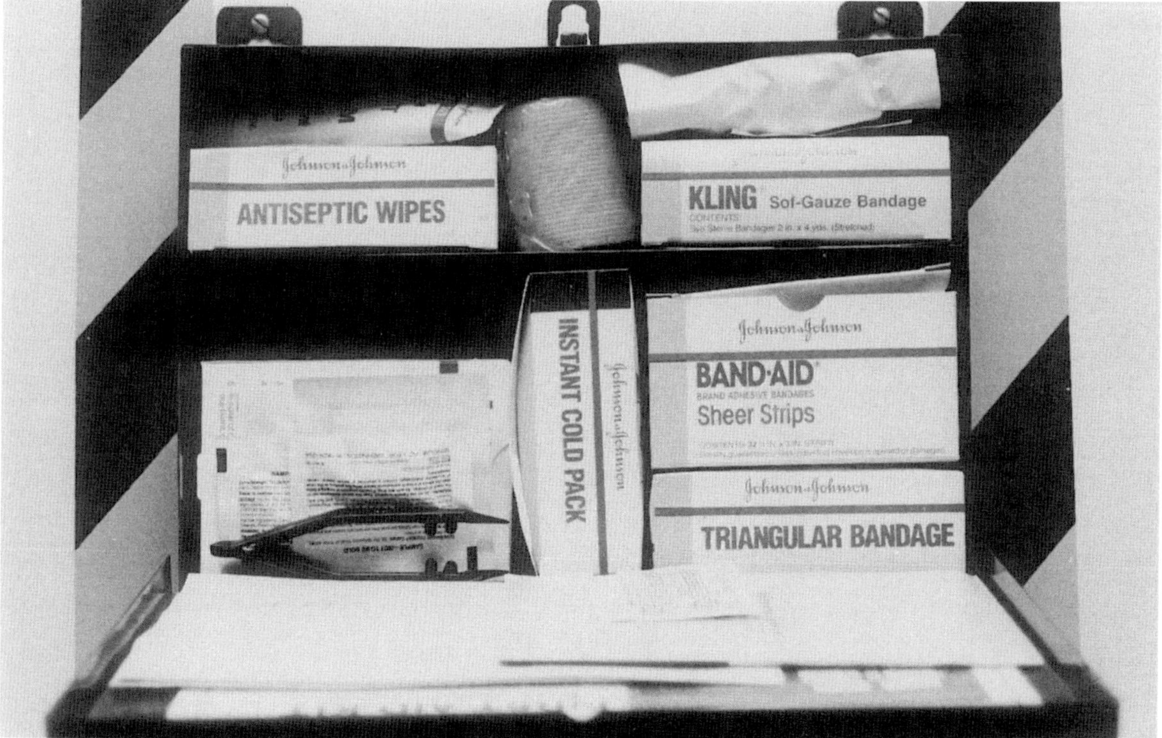

Figure 10-2: Contents of standard laboratory First Aid kit.

Nancy Masters

11
Mixing Chemicals

When working in the chemical laboratory, you must observe personal precautions. These precautions include the use of all protective equipment and the adherence to all laboratory protocols. The forensic identification specialist may need to insist that management make the equipment available and write the protocols. Each individual must be willing to educate his or her management on the elements of a safe laboratory and the mandates of the OSHA Act.

Before beginning the mixing process, review the written formulation. Refresh your memory on what the procedures are and which chemicals are to be used. Gather together all the necessary equipment, glassware and chemicals you will need to complete the formulation. Always select clean glassware which is marked for a larger volume than you will be mixing (i.e., use a 20 ml beaker to mix 10 ml of product). It is unwise to mix an amount of chemical equal to the size of the mixing container. The action of the stirring bar in the liquid (which creates a vortex) may cause the level of the liquid to move up and over the lip of the container.

Another recommendation is that you line the surface of your fume hood before proceeding with mixing. This will catch any spilled chemical and make cleanup much easier. Some departments require this procedure before any chemical preparation. [1] This lining can be replaced as it becomes evident that it is chemically contaminated.

When preparing reagents, use a few basic rules to prevent accidents. Always read the label on any container before using the contents. Every container should have a label which will indicate the name of the chemical, the company which manufactured or imported the chemical and the chemical's physical and health hazards. The label might include instructions on storage and handling, protective clothing and equipment to be worn and suggested safety practices. Always familiarize yourself with the properties of any chemical by reviewing the Material

Safety Data Sheet before actually handling the container. Problems arise when previously emptied bottles are filled with newly mixed preparations and the label not replaced, or when secondary containers are filled and not labeled. Any label on a secondary container should indicate the type of preparation contained within, the initials of the preparer and the date of preparation.

Be sure you know what material is in the container. There are a couple of "truisms" in chemistry. One is that acids taste sour, e.g., vinegar is a dilute solution of acetic acid. Another is that bases have a slippery texture or feel slimy. These are good things to know, but this does not mean that you should touch or taste chemicals to determine their nature. Treat all chemicals with respect. Do not let them make contact with your skin, mucous membranes or respiratory system. Know what you are handling and do not take risks. If you have any doubts, ask questions of a chemist or others who have access to the laboratory.

I have a special comment for forensic identification specialists who mix their own photographic chemicals. While it is true that most photographic chemicals are biodegradable, that does not mean that they pose no health risk. If you are mixing gallons of solutions in holding tanks, avoid breathing the dusts or vapors. Wear a dust/mist respirator and safety goggles. Some technicians have developed headaches after mixing large batches of these chemicals.

Do not risk contamination of the contents of the original container. Discard any excess chemicals which have come into contact with other chemicals. If you pour out or extract an excess amount of chemical from the stock container, discard it rather than return it to the stock contents. Do not risk contaminating the stock container. Do not lay container stoppers down to pick up contaminants that might be introduced back into the stock bottles. Use plastic, disposable pipettes, an eye dropper, or an auto-pipette to reduce pouring out excessive chemicals (Figure 11-1). Plastic, disposable pipettes or eye droppers allow you to extract small amounts of liquid (1 ml or less). Auto-pipettes allow you to set the amount you wish to extract and withdraw that amount only (usually up to 25 ml). They come with disposable tips you can discard after use. Use of the auto-pipette also eliminates the need to lift and tip large, heavy and/or full containers of chemicals.

When pouring chemicals from one container into another which has a narrow mouth, whether a bottle or graduated cylinder, use a funnel. This will help avoid spillage and the unnecessary release of chemical vapors or fumes. Always handle chemicals with the greatest of care.

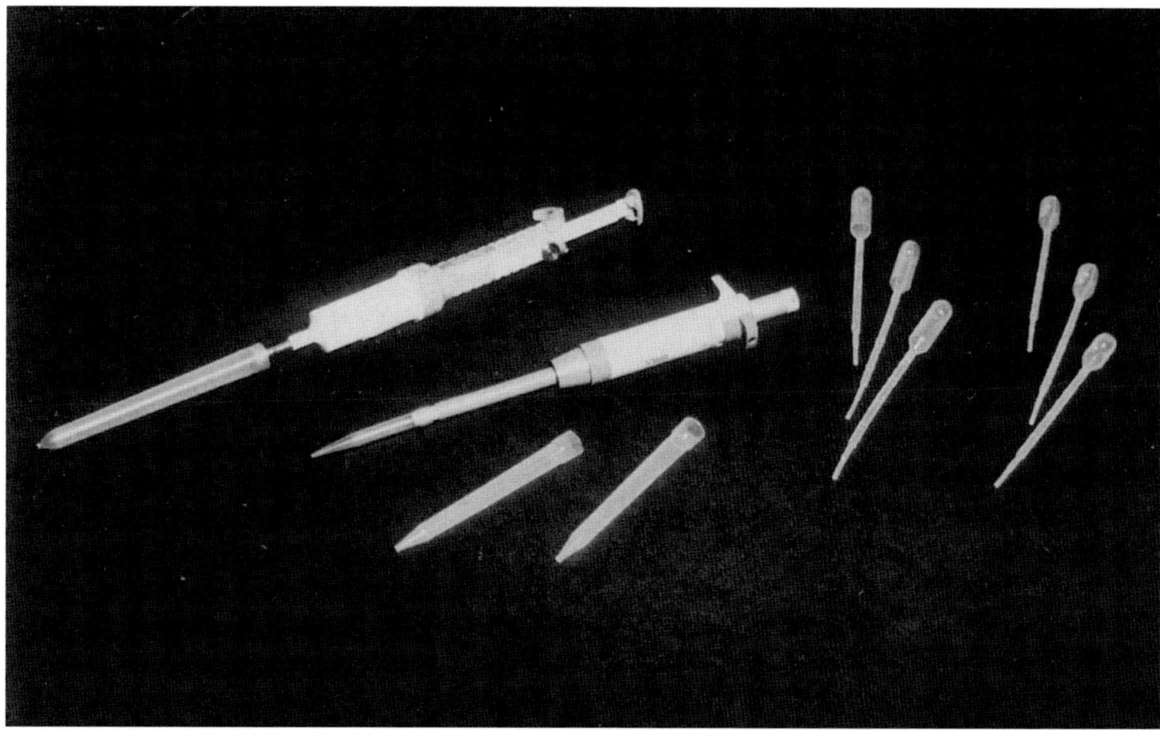

Figure 11-1: Auto-pipettes with disposable tips and plastic disposable pipettes.

When chemicals are placed in a secondary container (such as when you mix Ninhydrin), always apply a label identifying the contents and warning of hazards to the outside of the container. Consider color-coding your secondary labels to indicate the type of chemical hazard. Color coding should be in compliance with National Fire Protection Association (NFPA) guidelines. A blue label or bar indicates a health hazard, red–fire hazard, yellow–reactivity hazard, and white–special hazard or protective equipment required.

You seek a reagent when you mix a formula, e.g., Ninhydrin, Rhodamine 6G, Zinc Chloride. The carrier material (often called the solvent) is the material into which you measure the reagent to complete the formulation. Example: Ninhydrin is the reagent and acetone (or Freon, methanol, petroleum ether, etc.) is the carrier or solvent.

When preparing reagents, always open chemical containers at arm's length and with the opening away from the face. Mix reagents or transfer chemicals from one container to another in a fume hood whenever possible. Never pipette chemicals by mouth. [2] Replace caps on chemical containers immediately after use and tighten them down. If a particular substance is especially hazardous, it is a good practice to seal the container with plastic tape at the cap. [3] When picking up chemical containers, do not lift them by the cap. If someone has not properly closed the container, you may have a spill and/or broken container.

A properly equipped forensic identification laboratory should contain a series of different sized graduated cylinders for measuring chemicals. However, you can use a measuring cup when the cylinder is not available. To convert from metric to U. S. customary units or back the other direction, there are a couple of basic equivalents to remember:

1 cc = 1 ml; 30 ml = 30 cc = 1 fluid ounce

Therefore, if the only measuring device available is a Pyrex measuring cup, and the formula calls for 240 ml, use an 8 ounce cup. One liter (1,000 ml) converts to approximately 34 ounces. In most latent print formulations, being 1 ml off will not throw the formulation out of balance. A triple beam balance can also be used in lieu of an electronic balance.

When mixing chemicals, if the mixture layers out or separates (two liquid layers or solid in a liquid), you know they are not soluble. The mixture may work depending upon the application. Usually, though, it means that the reagent is not properly mixed and the chemical interaction is not taking place. Here are a couple of useful tips for mixing latent print formulations: 1) "Like dissolves like." Polar compounds, like salts, acids and bases, dissolve in polar solvents, like water or alcohols; alcohols and ketones (such as acetone) mix well. 2) "Do as you oughta, add acid to water." Water poured into strong acids can release a large amount of heat, resulting in a low-grade explosion or spattering of the acid out of the container.

Investment in an electric magnetic stirrer is well worthwhile. This device probably does a more thorough job of mixing than doing it by hand. Mixing reagents in a fume hood requires a magnetic stirrer be available at one end of the hood. After placing a magnetic stirring bar (a piece of plastic with a magnet in its center) in the bottom of the beaker, place your measured amount of liquid chemical into the beaker. Set the beaker on the stage of the magnetic stirrer and turn the stirrer "On" (Figure 11-2). Most magnetic stirrers are calibrated so you can set the speed of the stirring action. Depending upon the volume of chemicals you are mixing, you may wish to set the speed where it will create a vortex in the material. If the vortex is uneven (lopsided or to one side of the beaker), try centering the beaker on the stage or platform of the stirrer. Cover the top of the beaker with a square of clear plastic or glass to minimize splash or spatter and decrease the evaporation of solvents such as acetone or petroleum ether from the mixture. It is not usually necessary to mix the formulation beyond the point that any solid material has dissolved or that you would reasonably expect liquid components to have thoroughly intermixed. Upon completion of mixing, remove the magnetic stirring bar with a stirring bar rod, a long plastic rod with a magnet at one end to draw out the magnetic stirring bar.

Transfer the mixed formulation into a secondary container and label the container immediately. The label should document the name of the formulation, the initials of the preparer and the date of preparation. It should also contain any special health hazard information such as "poison" or "flammable."

Laboratory Cleaning

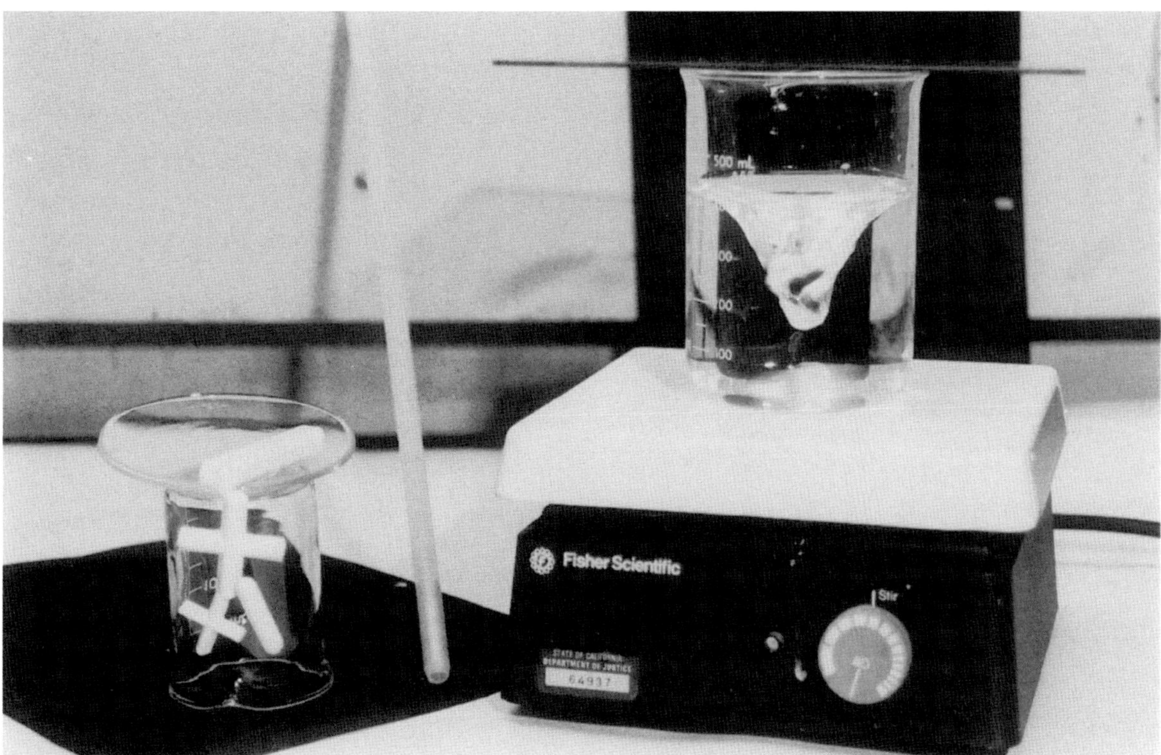

Figure 11-2: Beaker containing liquid on platform of operating magnetic stirrer. Note sheet of glass on the top of the beaker. Various shapes and sizes of stirring bars and magnetic stirring bar rod (for removal of stirring bars from mixture) appear to the left of the magnetic stirrer.

Immediately wash all equipment and glassware used in the preparation of formulas. Many commercial laboratory detergents are available on the market. Thorough washing will require a variety of sizes of brushes and sponges be available in the laboratory. Always wear some type of rubber gloves when washing equipment to protect you from any chemical residues remaining on the equipment and to provide some protection in the event of glassware breakage. If a particular formulation creates a residue which is difficult to remove, leave the piece of glassware with soapy water in it to soak for a day. Try not to develop the habit of leaving used, contaminated glassware standing in the chemical sink full of water or sitting around on the counters or in the fume hood. Every specialist should be held responsible for cleaning up his or her mess. Nothing creates more dissension that an individual who refuses to clean up the laboratory. Co-workers place signs that read, "Your mother doesn't work here. Clean up your mess!" Another tactic includes assigning one individual, to do *all* the laboratory cleanup on a rotating schedule. However, this tactic rarely works and may create even more hostility.

Line all counter tops with some type of heavy paper (such as butcher paper) to decrease the areas that must be physically washed down. Every couple of weeks or once a month, replace with clean paper. If a chemical spill occurs, immediately replace the paper. If you are not using paper to cover the counter tops, wash them down with a liquid cleanser containing an antimicrobial material as well as a viralcide and fungicide (of a type such as hospitals use). One caution: Avoid any cleansers which have heavy formulations of phenol. Phenol is toxic in large concentrations, and many cleansers are available without this component. Any time you process deceased casework or any evidence which may contain material of a biological nature, you must clean thoroughly.

There is another alternative to lining counter tops with paper. Paper can hold and "hide" biological material, acting as a reservoir and increasing exposure time to such hazards. A solution is to invest in stainless steel trays constructed with "lipped" edges, no sharp corners and smooth surfaces. They are easy to clean and serve as a secondary container in the event of a spill. They also cut down on waste which is generated in the laboratory. (This is an important consideration since good laboratory management will dictate the creation of the least amount of waste possible. Once generated, waste is a problem. The best approach is to prevent generating waste.) Possible disadvantages to the stainless steel tray system are the initial expenditure and the mechanics of handling the trays to wash them in the event of a spill. You must clean these trays daily.

The effort of everyone is needed for a positive health and safety program and an efficient laboratory. All personnel must be willing to follow all appropriate protocols and to do their share of the dirty work. Supervision should tolerate no less.

12
Deceased Casework

Section 5 dealt generally with Biohazards, and this section deals specifically with deceased casework, addressing procedures for processing hands and/or fingers of John and Jane Does.

The most important consideration in processing this type of casework is the confinement of the biological contaminants. The three most serious potential infectious agents are AIDS (HIV), Hepatitis, and tuberculosis.

HIV is not easily "caught." It doesn't survive for very long outside the body and needs a fluid environment. However, the virus may survive in the deceased in the morgue for many days. [1] HIV needs direct contact to enter the body via blood-to-blood contact (as does Hepatitis B and Hepatitis C). There must be an adequate amount of AIDS virus in the sample to infect you (for example, it may take more than one exposure if entry is made through a wound).

Hepatitis is a more serious concern. Its age (many years of existence) makes it very resilient. Hepatitis A is acquired only through infected fecal material entering the mouth. (This is the type of hepatitis infection people often contact through restaurant foods because employees do not wash their hands after using the toilet.) Hepatitis B (HBV) and Hepatitis C (HCV) enters the body via blood-to-blood contact, such as occurs in blood transfusions.

Tuberculosis is an infectious disease caused by the tubercle bacillus. [2] This bacillus is a spore and requires direct exposure to infect, such as through the sneeze of an infected individual. [3] Sputum containing the tubercle bacillus may be on a surface such as the floor of a crime scene. If the specialist is searching for trace evidence such as hairs and fibers and comes into contact with this infected expectorated material, wafts the material up and into the face, and inhales the tubercle bacillus, he or she could become infected with tuberculosis. [4] The only other likely tuberculosis exposure to the forensic identification specialist comes when photographing autopsies. Although tuberculosis most commonly affects the respiratory system, other parts of the body such as the lymph nodes, gastrointestinal and genitourinary tracts, *bones*, joints, nervous system, and skin may become infected. [5] During autopsy, a bone saw cuts the skull cap half, creating bone dust. One-third of the staff at the New York medical examiner's facility have acquired tuberculosis from inhaling infected bone particulate. (The spore is not an airborne hazard.) In Sacramento County, California, only limited autopsies are performed when a deceased is known to be tuberculosis infected, so the skull cap is not removed. Bone dust reveals some HIV and hepatitis contagion. [6] There is no known correlation between the bone dust and the infection of safety employees or health care workers. NIOSH has approved no particular respirator for working with such biohazards. Since the bone dust is a particulate, perhaps a half-faced respirator equipped with an asbestos filter may provide adequate protection. [7] The forensic identification specialist expected to photograph at an autopsy should be at least as well protected as any pathologist or pathologist's assistant. Demand at least a laboratory coat, eye goggles or full face shield, nitrile gloves and a dust/mist respirator. If the protective equipment hinders your ability to use your camera, then the pathologists should accommodate you.

You should be aware that infectious microbiological organisms will vary in hardiness outside the host. Direct and indirect exposures are possible at crime scenes. A crime scene is an uncontrolled environment. You must be vigilant on hygienic practices. Always apply universal precautions and use respiratory protection if you have the slightest doubt regarding the infectious potentials. Think of it this way: when in doubt or for peace of mind, use a respirator with a HEPA filter.

Designate a special area of the laboratory for deceased casework. That area should be equipped with a small refrigerator, a laboratory sink, cabinets and counter-top space adequate for processing, adequate lighting fixtures and a ventilation system separate from the main chemical laboratory. A small room is ideal for this purpose. It need not be any larger than will accommodate the necessary supplies and two individuals at a time. (See Figures 12-1 through 12-4.)

Store all necessary supplies in this area: paper for lining the counter top(s) or stainless steel trays, latex or nitrile gloves, safety goggles, organic nuisance dust/mist respirators, face shield, ridge building materials, scalpels and scissors,

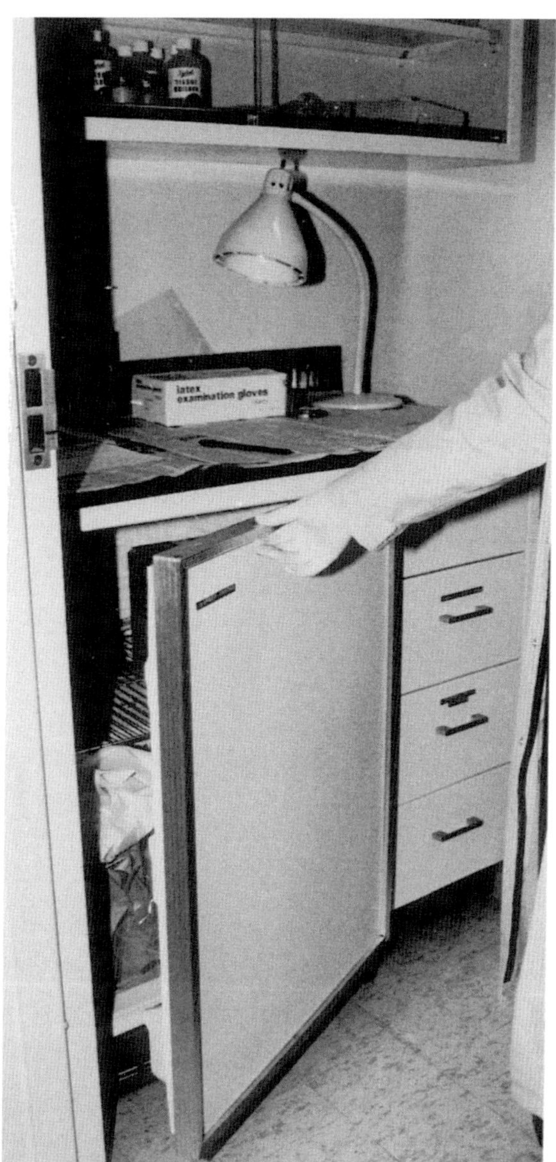

Figure 12-1: Deceased processing area: Laboratory refrigerator for storage of deceased fingers and hands.

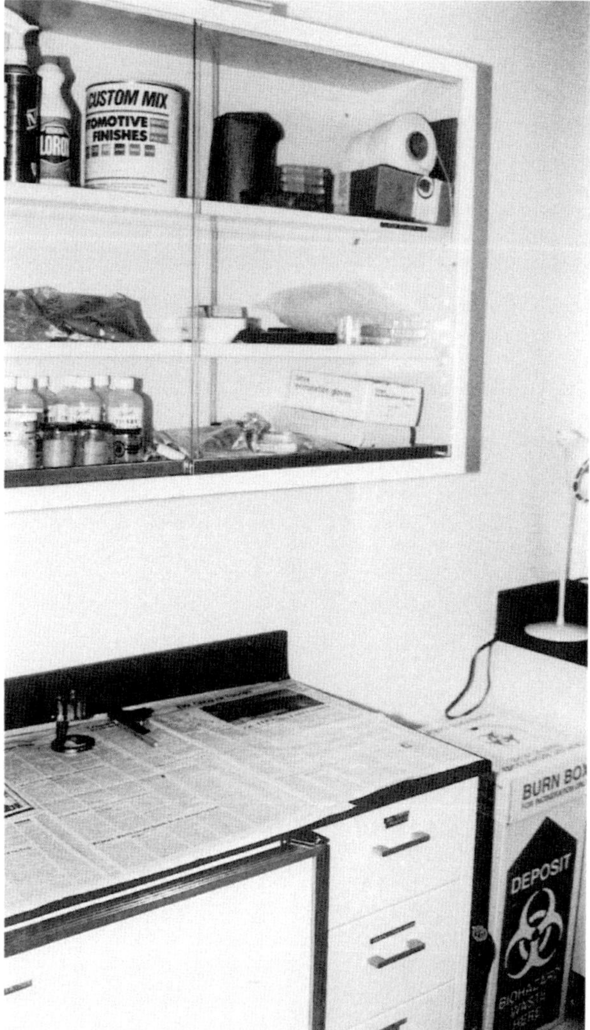

Figure 12-2: Deceased processing area: Storage cabinets for supplies needed to process deceased casework.

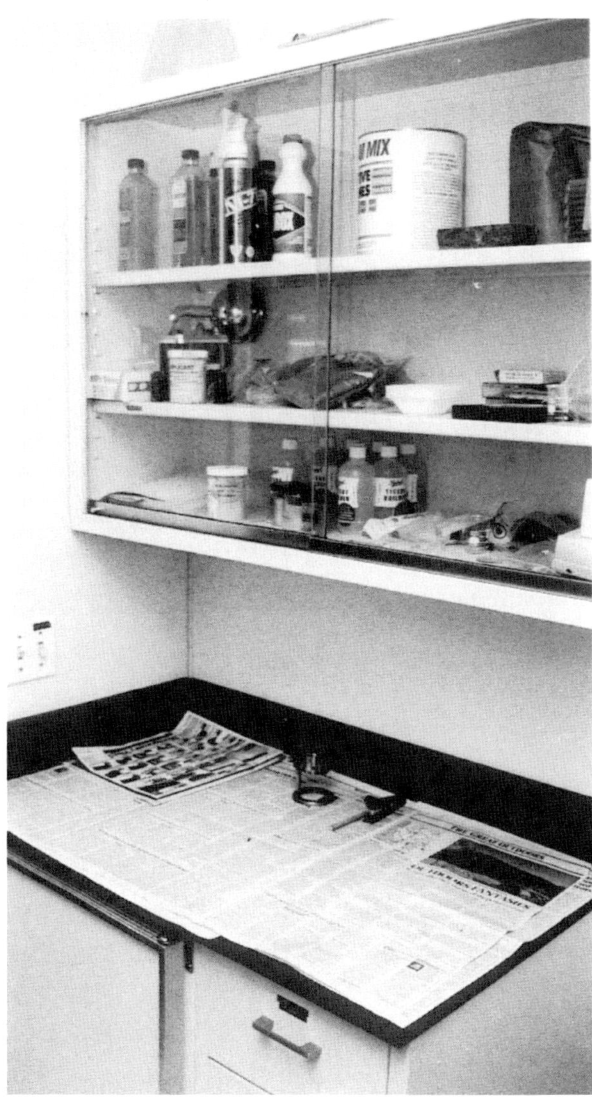

Figure 12-3: Deceased processing area: Additional view of storage area in deceased processing room.

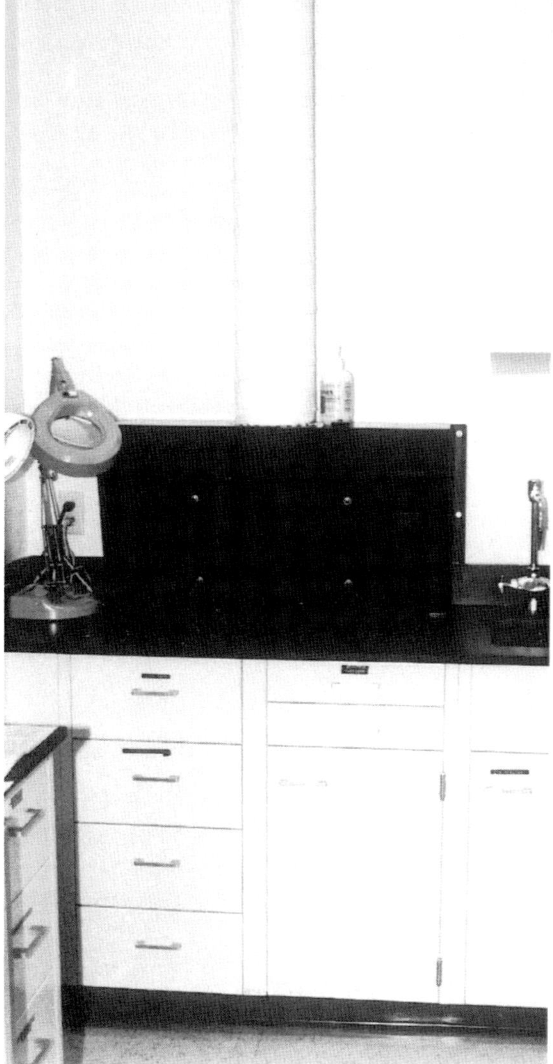

Figure 12-4: Deceased processing area: View of cabinets, counter top complete with installed wet sink, and slot hoods for ventilation of nuisance odors and fingerprint powders.

lift tapes and powders, inking supplies, fingerprint cards, pens or pencils, brushes for cleaning the friction ridges, trays, cleansers and brushes for cleaning processing equipment, biohazard bags for linen and biohazard or other plastic bags for disposable materials, waste containers, heat sealable bags and sealer, and hazard warning labels. Include other supplies your department deems necessary.

After you sign the deceased case into the forensic identification section and assign case number, place the container in the special refrigerator designated for deceased casework.

Under universal standards handle all deceased casework as though it is infectious. The forensic identification specialist should don a laboratory coat for protection of the forearms and personal clothing before processing the case. Use a dust/mist respirator (mask) to protect the nose and mouth from the entry of splashed or sloughed biological material. One analyst who chose not to use the mask had his hands slip and land a piece of deceased flesh on the corner of his mouth. Eye goggles or a face shield will prevent materials from being splashed or otherwise projected into the eyes.

Specialists traditionally wore double latex gloves, because latex is porous material and because the specialist could peel off the top (contaminated) pair if necessary without exposing the bare skin of the hands. Double gloving gives a false sense of security. Latex gloves are often flawed and reseal themselves after punctures. Another consideration is that latex causes dermatitis in some people. There are other glove materials with important qualities of being hypoallergenic, having good sheer strength, allowing dexterity, and giving evidence of flaws. Nitrile gloves, for instance, may be a better option than latex. Nitrile gloves, once punctured or otherwise flawed, literally tear or rip, alerting the wearer to use a new pair. For purposes of decontamination, double-gloving is still an option. A pair of latex gloves can be worn under the nitrile gloves for proper decontaminating or changing an outer flawed glove without exposing the wearer's bare skin.

When selecting personal protective equipment, think about your possible exposure(s) and the available materials. Make the best selection for the situation. Whether you decide on latex, nitrile, neoprene or vinyl, wear all protective equipment at all times while handling deceased materials.

If you have not already covered counter tops, first line them with disposable paper. Place all necessary processing equipment on the counter top to prevent unnecessary handling of cabinet and drawer handles during processing. You must decontaminate any areas you may have touched during processing.

Handle deceased material so as to propel into the air a minimum of particulate. Deal with any difficult ridge problems in some manner other than scalpels and/or syringes. Use bone snips or pruning snips rather than a scalpel for removal of fingers. Try soaking fingers or removed skin in ridge builder or other solutions. Attempt to place the skin between glass slides for photography. Consider using a laser or alternate light source to side-light the ridges for photography. Use a syringe as a last resort, because you risk sticking yourself with a contaminated needle. This does not seem likely, yet health-care workers report that they commonly stick themselves in the process of trying to "stick" other people. A good safety practice is to avoid situations that introduce hazards.

Try to avoid formaldehyde. Quite often fingers or hands are received in this solution because it functions as a preservative. While many dictionaries define formaldehyde as a disinfectant, it will not kill viruses. Do not use formaldehyde unless absolutely necessary and use only in a fume hood. The fumes irritate and corrode the mucous membranes. Lung disease, emphysema and malignant tumors may result from exposure. [8] It is carcinogenic in certain animals. [9] In the state of California, *Director's List of Hazardous Substances* names formaldehyde, based upon information developed (by the Director of the Department of Industrial Relations) from the International Agency for Research on Cancer (IARC), the Environmental Protection Agency-Federal Clean Water and Clean Air Acts, and the CAL-OSHA list of airborne chemical contaminants (GISO 5155). [10]

Formaldehyde will not work as a softening agent, because it hardens tissues and is so used in histology (study of tissues) for preservation. Hardened or dehydrated fingers/hands would soften better in ordinary tap water. [11] Soak hard or mummified fingers for 24 to 48 hours in a 1% solution of Eastman Kodak Photo Flo 200 for good results. [12] You could also use a set of solutions, Restorative and Metaflow, manufactured by Dodge Chemicals. Obtain these through Dodge Chemicals, 165 Cambridge Park Drive, Cambridge, Massachusetts 02140, (617) 661-0500.

Once you obtain all prints, place the fingerprint card into a heat-sealable bag and seal it. The print card and tape are contaminated. As forensic identification specialists, we know about biological hazards and can protect ourselves with barriers. However, other people are actually performing classification or searching procedures with the prints obtained from deceased. We have a moral obligation to protect those people from unnecessary exposures as well. Place a hazard warning label on the outside of the bag to indicate it contains a biological material that may pose a health risk and warn not to handle without gloves. Additionally, the print card will eventually go in your case file, where it will contaminate other materials in the file if the card is not heat sealed.

Upon completion of processing, immediately clean up the work area. Place hands/fingers and any pieces of skin/flesh back into the original container, seal it and place it in the refrigerator until an officer or shipping company picks it up. Place all lift tapes, papers, paper towels, butcher paper from counter tops, used gloves (wash your hands as soon as you remove both pairs of gloves), and dust/mist respirators inside and seal a red bag labeled "Biohazard" and/or "Infectious Waste." However, you may need a waste hauler to remove and dispose of the bag. Otherwise, use a durable plastic bag. This bag is then sealed at the top and left for removal by janitorial personnel who know that the bags contain biological material. Have the bags compacted as soon as possible. These materials will probably eventually end up in a landfill site. Once covered, the pressure from the dirt and resulting natural heat will effectively sterilize the contents in the plastic bag. [13] The red plastic bags marked "Infectious Waste" can be purchased through most hospital or cleaning supply companies. The bags are usually labeled in both English and Spanish.

Wash all equipment you used in the processing in a disinfectant detergent solution. A disinfectant containing phenol is corrosive and toxic, not needed for adequate disinfecting. A 70% alcohol solution will kill HIV in 7 (seven) minutes, but alcohol has no detergent or cleaning properties. Common household bleach (sodium hypochlorite) will kill everything, but it is corrosive, and people tend not to trust the weak smell and appearance of the solution. If you wish to use bleach, a 1:9 or 1:10 dilution is adequate. Mix about two cups of liquid bleach in a gallon of water. [14] Non-phenol products available on the market are disinfectants and detergents but not highly corrosive.

Companies, such as Airwick, make such products. For instance, A-500 was formulated for use in hospitals, nursing homes, hotels/motels, offices, restaurants, veterinary hospitals/kennels, or any area where infection control is desired. Such products must meet four important characteristics of a detergent-disinfectant: detergency, antimicrobial capabilities, odor control, and ease of safe handling. They can be made with nonionic (no capability of carrying an electric charge) detergents for the physical removal of dirt, soil, grease, and organic matter without leaving a filter or residue buildup. The antimicrobial agent is effective against bacteria, fungi, and viruses. Some products, such as Airwick, have incorporated odor counteractants to neutralize objectionable odors without the use of perfumes or harsh chemicals. Most are also biodegradable and phosphate-free. You can purchase these products in pre-measured, water-soluble packets to reduce direct contact with the concentrated product.

When handling and cleaning deceased fingers/hands, small particles of material may fall off into the sink and go down the drain. Some have expressed concern about possible health code violations in this circumstance. If your management is concerned with this, call your local health department. However, hospitals routinely flush urine and other biological fluids down the drains. [15] A safety engineer states there is no violation of regulations or laws in our usual procedures. Sewer systems are designed to treat harmful waste and render it safe. [16] The amounts of deceased particulate that go down the drains are incidental and need not be of concern.

Take the same precautions with linens (used when handling infectious materials) as with disposable wastes. Hospitals use color-coded plastic bags. Purchase yellow or orange plastic bags labeled “Biohazard” and/or “Infectious Linen” in both English and Spanish. The same vendors who supply the infectious waste bags sell these bags. After you finish cleaning up, place all used laboratory coats and towels in one of these bags. Any industrial laundry service who does dry cleaning can launder these linens. Contact the manager of a local establishment to discuss your handling and packaging of these contaminated linens. Commercial cleaners are willing to handle your needs since they provide this service for hospitals. You simply need to inform the company of your bagging system so the manager can warn the personnel to wear gloves when unbagging the linens into their machinery. Devise a system to clean your field clothing worn at crime scenes that have hazardous contaminants. Never take such contaminated linen or clothing to your home and launder them in your own washing machine.

After you remove your gloves during or after processing and after cleanup, always wash your hands. Hand washing is one of the best protective procedures you can practice. The possibility of pin holes in gloves makes washing especially important. Germicidal hand soaps are formulated with 100% natural soaps containing moisturizers and a proven antimicrobial agent. One such soap is Epicare Antimicrobial Lotion Soap marketed by Airwick. Many of these soaps are formulated especially for hospitals, nursing homes, and other areas where frequent hand washing helps prevent cross infection. These soaps will not cause drying, irritation or dermatitis of the skin (even after frequent hand washing). If you cannot get these specially formulated soaps, regular hand soap will adequately clean your hands.

Follow all protocols regarding the use of personal protective equipment and decontamination. Seal any resulting developed fingerprints in an impervious bag and label it with a hazard warning label. Disinfect all surfaces and wash all utensils as soon as possible. Wash your hands frequently. Always assume that any deceased material is infectious and protect yourself and your co-workers from exposures.

13
Confining Contamination

Confine contamination by chemicals or biological material to specific areas or containers. This sounds very easy but actually challenges the most careful person, because he or she often cannot see the contaminant with the eyes. Since we are unable to rely on our vision for detection, the best approach is for us to isolate and control contaminated areas and items.

A good rule of thumb is to follow standard laboratory practices and universal precautions at all times. This rule helps isolate hazards and applies to all circumstances where contamination can occur. More specifically, develop protocols which encompass the following practices:

- Limit access to the laboratory to forensic identification specialists, criminalists, chemists, supervisors and other technical personnel who are properly trained in safety procedures and laboratory protocols. Janitorial staff may need access to remove waste and maintain the floor. Clerical personnel should never need access. Strictly enforce this policy. It is the only way to ensure that uninformed personnel will not spread contamination to other areas.

- Designate separate areas of the laboratory for work with biological or deceased materials and for regular chemical processing of casework. By law, you must handle and store regulated carcinogenic materials in a marked, specified area. The law requires proper ventilation systems, clean rooms for suiting up and changing contaminated clothing, and hazard-specific signs and labels. [1]

- Do not eat, drink, smoke, store food or apply cosmetics in the laboratory or any area where chemicals/biological materials are stored. Never place your lunch in the laboratory refrigerator.

- When you enter the laboratory, put on your laboratory coat or coveralls and gloves. Wear this protective equipment at all times while in the lab environment. Upon leaving the lab, remove this equipment. Laboratory coats worn in the lab should never be worn out of the lab and into non-laboratory or other common areas of the facility, including your office. You may find this protocol the easiest to violate, because it is natural behavior to wander out of the lab to your desk. Do not do it. Consider your lab coat to be contaminated. Do not spread contamination to your desk.

- After you finish processing evidence, seal the evidence in a plastic bag or cardboard container. Evidence includes fingerprint cards developed as a result of processing hands/fingers of deceased persons. Purchase hazardous warning labels commercially or develop them in your agency. Place a hazardous warning label on the outside of the bag to indicate that the container holds material which is chemically or biologically contaminated, may pose a health hazard, and gloves must be worn before handling. (See Figure 14-1.) It is your moral and legal responsibility to protect other people from exposure to contamination. Once an item leaves your facility, court bailiffs, clerks, judges, attorneys and jurists may handle it. Even with the most careful of packaging and warnings, you will often get to court to have Ninhydrin-treated documents or other evidence handed to you outside its protective wrapping. Simply, smile, retrieve a pair of gloves from your pocket and announce to the court that the item is contaminated. You will witness a drastic change in attitude by others in the courtroom who must have had intimate contact with the object.

- Consider color-coding a supply of pens and pencils which are left in the laboratory. Contaminated, gloved hands handle these implements all the time. It is easy to carry such items out of the laboratory and into other areas. If you are going to handle such contaminated items with bare hands, why wear gloves at all? Such items pose serious exposure risks to other people who do not access the laboratory and have no way of determining the presence of contaminants. Also avoid placing pens or pencils around your face or in your mouth.

- If you use a telephone in the laboratory, make it a habit to remove your gloves before handling any part of the phone. The telephone is a commonly contaminated area, handled one time with gloved hands and another time with bare hands.

- Cover all counter tops with butcher or some other type of paper when working with deceased materials or other biological items, such as blood-spattered clothing laid out to dry. After processing, decontaminate such surfaces by removing the paper and cleaning thoroughly.

- Always place disposable objects you use with biological materials into plastic bags marked "Infectious Waste." (If you lack a contract with a special waste hauler, at least seal the bags tightly.) Seal the bags and warn janitorial personnel of hazards of infectious waste. Place all linens (laboratory coats and towels) into plastic bags marked "Infectious Linen." (Figure 13-1) Have an industrial linen service clean these linens.

- After working a crime scene which involves biological materials or chemicals, confine your field clothing in a plastic bag and have an industrial dry cleaning company or linen service clean them. Never clean these items in your home laundry system. Encourage your department to supply you with at least jump suits, boots, jackets, pants and shirts for field clothing. Management may resist, but you never wear your street clothing to scenes or scene clothing back

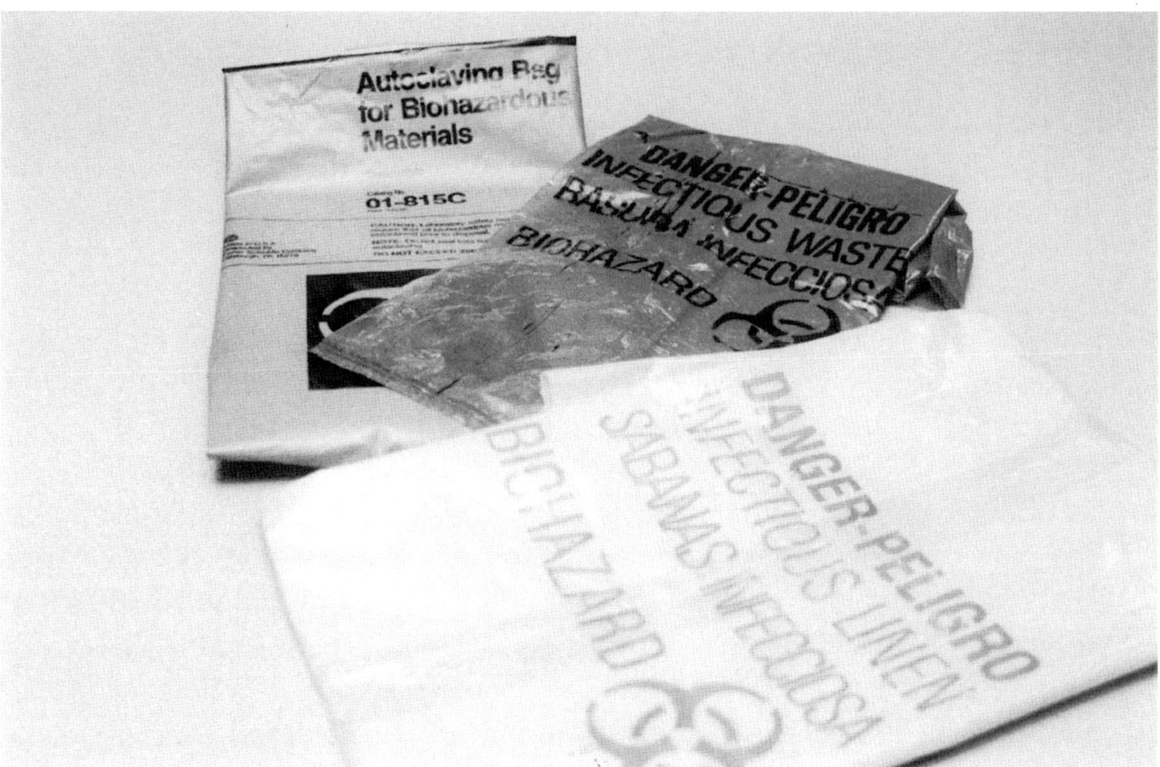

Figure 13-1: Plastic bags used for the confinement of contaminated materials (left to right): Biohazardous Materials, Infectious Waste and Infectious Linens. The first two bags are usually colored orange or red, the last is usually yellow.

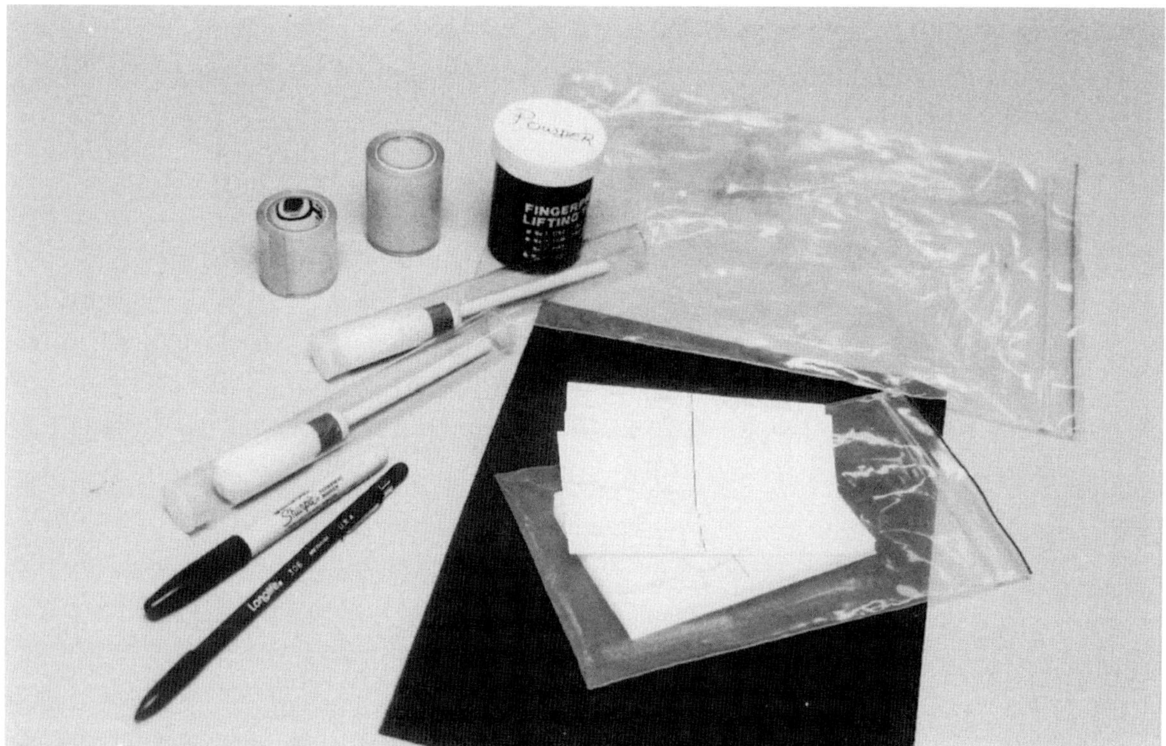

Figure 13-2: Disposable latent fingerprint kit for use at clandestine drug laboratories. After scene processing, used items are disposed of with other waste removed by licensed waste hauler. Kit contains: lift tapes, lift cards, brushes, permanent marker, ink pen, and small jar

to your office or home. The clothing may be contaminated with blood, other biological fluids or clandestine drug laboratory chemicals. You can spread contamination into your or the department's vehicle or, worse yet, your home. (Figure 13-2)

- Cover with paper or plastic any surface on which you lay chemically treated evidence. Periodically remove the coverings, decontaminate the surface and replace the covering.

- Do not take chemically treated evidence to your desk. Perform all examinations and marking in the laboratory. Do not fool yourself about this. Years ago, I would routinely take items processed with Ninhydrin to my desk for comparisons. Then came the controversy whether such treated items would contaminate other areas. The issue finally focused on Rhodamine 6G as workers debated whether the superglue had absorbed the Rhodamine dye stain and bonded with it in a way that it would not come out or rub off onto other surfaces. An examination of the non-laboratory work area (including desks) with the laser revealed beautiful fluorescing prints on these surfaces. It was a rude and unpleasant awakening for everyone. Placing such chemically treated items in common work areas will contaminate your work space and the breathing space of neighboring work partners.

- If you must take treated evidence to a common work area, protect the desk or table top from possible contamination and advise neighboring work partners of the presence of a hazardous material. You may need to use a common work area if an attorney (defense or prosecutor) or subject matter expert wishes to examine the evidence.

- Provide anyone who may handle the evidence (fellow workers or other authorized persons) with and make sure he or she wears protective gloves and a laboratory coat to avoid chemical or biological hazards from the contaminated evidence, especially any biological material that could be infectious. If clothing (or bedding, etc.) contains wet or dry biological fluid stains, provide a particulate mask and eye goggles. Once you complete examination of the evidence, package (or repackage) the evidence properly with a hazardous warning label outside.

- Reception areas are often located in the front of the laboratory for the public or law enforcement officers to access and commonly bring evidence. When you respond to a request to receive the evidence, you should determine if the evidence or its packaging requires the use of gloves and a laboratory coat. If yes, then don a clean laboratory coat and gloves to transfer the evidence to the processing area or evidence vault. Never wear lab coats/gloves which have been used in the processing area. After receiving the evidence, immediately decontaminate the reception counter. Types of evidence which need precautions are items of a biological nature (or contaminated with biological fluids) and evidence from clandestine drug laboratories.

- Even though you take great steps to deal with contamination in the laboratory, you often forget the property room. Develop a separate area in the property room for storing chemically treated items, biologically contaminated items, and chemically contaminated items. You should have properly packaged and labeled these items before leaving the laboratory, but packaging can fail. Property clerks need to be adequately informed and trained about the hazards of handling such items. You should encourage them to wear gloves when receiving or releasing such items.

- Whether your evidence is stored in a separate vault or in the property room, you must properly package the evidence to contain any biological or chemical hazards. For instance, dry out and package clothing containing blood stains before storage. If you will perform blood work or DNA work, then you must refrigerate or freeze the package. If you receive contaminated clandestine drug laboratory evidence, including chemicals for analysis, you must properly package them to contain hazards, including broken containers. If you receive liquid chemicals for analysis, seal the containers in doubled heat sealed bags.

- Lastly, always wash your hands with soap and water after handling any evidence, before leaving the laboratory or processing area, and before and after you use the restroom. I simply cannot emphasize enough this best preventative measure you can take to decrease the spread of contamination and exposures.

14
Labeling Containers

Previous sections have alluded to the importance of proper labeling of all chemical containers. But, is it really such a big deal? Consider these possible scenarios:

- You come into the laboratory to process some items of porous evidence. You will need a Ninhydrin formulation but are unable to locate a chemical container labeled as "Ninhydrin." There are some bottles in the laboratory, but some do not have any label on them. Perhaps you could mix a new formulation, but discover that the lab is out of Ninhydrin crystals. Your co-worker has left for a week's vacation. What do you do? Just pour out some solution and hope it is Ninhydrin? Should you sniff the different bottles of solutions to try and determine the contents? Can you afford to wait until your co-worker returns or until another order of Ninhydrin crystals can be received?

- You come into the laboratory to mix a formulation which calls for acetone and ethanol. After measuring out the acetone and placing it into a beaker, you reach for the bottle of ethanol. You measure out a few ml of ethanol and pour it into the acetone. A sudden explosion sends chemicals sputtering onto your body. What went wrong? You later learn that the ethanol bottle had been empty for some time and a co-worker decided to use it to store some nitric acid for use with physical developer. However, the label on the bottle was never changed. Since acetone is incompatible with concentrated nitric acid, you created a dangerous explosion. How could you have avoided that accident and your resulting pain and loss from work?

- You come into the laboratory to mix a new adhesive tape separation formula that you recently read about in a journal. You note that the reagent requires the use of chloroform. Someone tells you that there is a bottle labeled "Chloroform" in the cabinet in the chemistry lab. You mix the reagent and proceed to attempt to separate some duct tape from a rape case. As you are working, you begin to feel dizzy and you develop a terrific headache. In half an hour you must leave work and go home sick. Later, you learn that chloroform should never be inhaled, but there was nothing on the label to warn you of this hazard. How could you have avoided this situation (besides reading the MSDS on chloroform before you began working with it)?

- You are working a high profile homicide case involving a threatening letter. You process the letter with a solution of Ninhydrin but fail to develop any latent impressions. This surprises you because the case detective handed it to you with his bare fingers. While discussing the situation with some co-workers, you learn that the solution you used was actually over three years old. Someone found it in the back of the cabinet and had placed it in the fume hood for disposal. Try as you may, reprocessing with a new solution fails to develop any visible impressions because of the highly purple stained background. Were there ever any latent prints present on the evidence? Who will ever know?

Although these are invented scenarios, any of them could happen to you if procedures are not in place for proper labeling of all chemical containers. Even though the laws are very specific about labeling, a routine inspection of many laboratories will reveal violations.

What does the law dictate? The hazard communication standard intends "to address comprehensively the issue of evaluating the potential hazards of chemicals and communicating information concerning hazards and appropriate protective measures to employees." Evaluating the hazards, communicating the information as to those hazards and protective measures may include "...lists of hazardous chemicals present; labeling of containers of chemicals in the workplace, as well as of containers of chemicals being shipped to other workplaces;..." [1] The application of this standard requires "all employers to provide information to their employees about the hazardous chemicals to which they are exposed, by means of a hazard communication program, labels and other forms of warning, Material Safety Data Sheets, and information and training." [2]

The federal standard requires the chemical manufacturer, importer or distributors to determine the hazards and then develop a MSDS and a hazard warning label for all chemicals they ship. The label must identify the hazardous chemical(s), give appropriate warnings and include the name and address of the chemical manufacturer, importer, or other responsible party. [3]

Your employer also has a responsibility to insure that all incoming chemical containers are labeled and that those labels are not removed or defaced. Additionally, the labels must be legible, in English, prominently displayed on the container and available to you during your work shift. [4] You must have access to a MSDS collection and be trained in the hazards of the chemicals at your work site. A hazardous chemical is defined as any chemical which is a physical hazard or a health hazard. [5] When you receive chemicals at the laboratory, always mark them with the date of receipt before placing them in stock. This procedure assists you to evaluate any chemicals in stock for more than a year.

What is your responsibility? If you see a container which is not properly labeled, you should immediately report it to your supervisor. It is also imperative that you label all secondary containers as you place chemicals into them. In fact, all secondary containers with materials containing more than 1% of a hazardous component or combination of hazardous components which will be used for more than a single work day must be labeled with a listing of the hazardous ingredients. If the components contain as much as 0.1% of any carcinogen, it must be labeled. [6] When you mix a formula and place it into a container, you should apply a label which identifies the contents, any hazard(s) associated with that chemical, concentration, date of preparation and your initials. For instance, any chemicals which are flammable should be labeled FLAMMABLE as well as DANGER, and possibly TOXIC. This will help prevent accidental reactions and toxic exposures. Do not use grease pencils for markings, as this material may deteriorate in time. Do not use abbreviations, formulas only or code names or numbers which may lose their significance when new employees do not know these elements.

Simplify the labeling process by using preprinted labels which include the system devised by the National Fire Prevention Association (NFPA) and designated by NFPA 704. This is a visual symbol system which provides an indication of the inherent chemical hazards as well as the severity of the hazard in an emergency, of materials relating to fire prevention, exposure and control. A diamond is divided into four squares. It identifies any special hazards as well as the health, flammability, and reactivity hazards of the chemicals. A rating system of 0 to 4 indicates the severity of each,

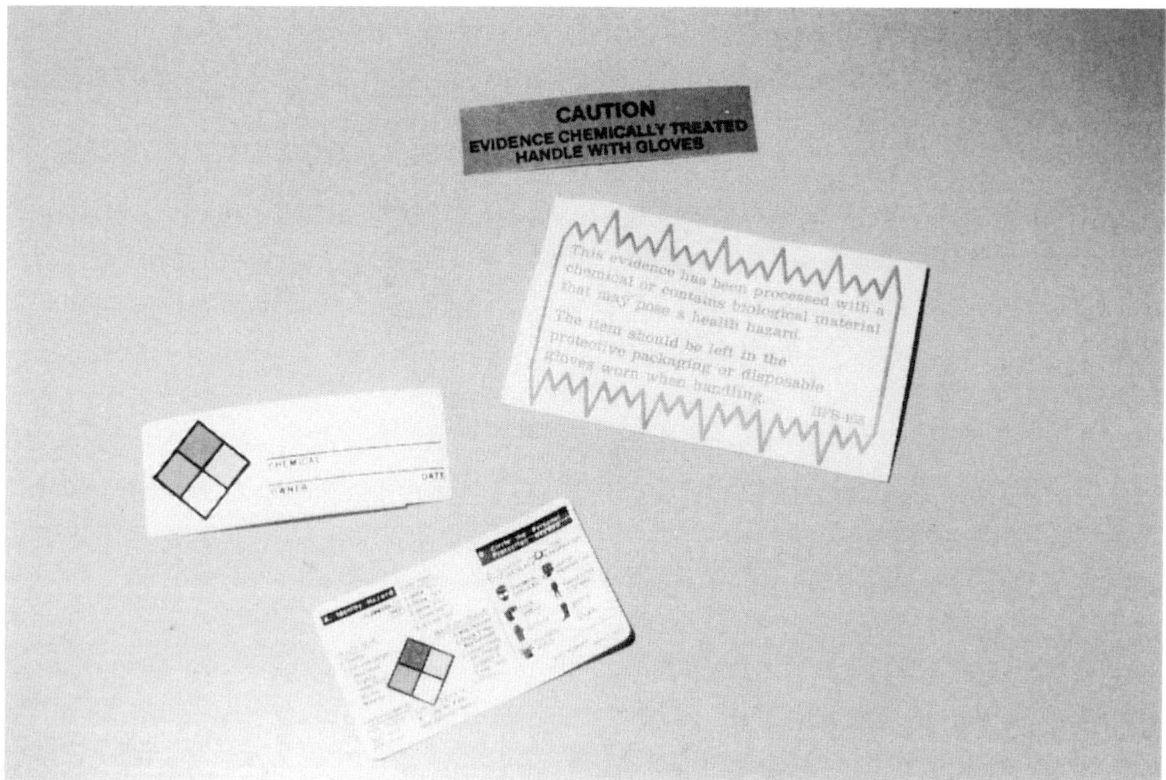

Figure 14-1: Labels (clockwise): Commercially available label to warn of contaminated contents, custom designed label, commercially available label for chemical containers which includes the NFPA hazard diamond, and an alternative label for secondary containers.

0 indicating the lowest degree of hazard and 4 the highest. This numerical rating is placed in each of the four squares of the diamond. (Figure 14-1)

In general terms, the numerical rating system has the following meaning to fire fighters:

- 0 – No special hazards; therefore, no special measures.
- 1 – Nuisance hazards present which require some care, but standard fire fighting procedures can be used.
- 2 – Can be fought with standard procedures, but hazards are present which require certain equipment or procedures to handle safely.
- 3 – Fire can be fought using methods intended for extremely hazardous situations.
- 4 – Too dangerous to approach with standard fire-fighting equipment and procedures.

The preferred way to read the diamond is to begin at the left square which designates *health* and is colored **blue**. The rating covers the degree of hazard and level of short term protection. This square is rated as follows: 0 = Ordinary combustible hazards in a fire, 1=Slightly hazardous to health, 2=Hazardous to health, but can be handled if equipped with self-contained breathing apparatus, 3=Extremely dangerous, but may be dealt with using extreme care, and 4=Deadly to fire-fighters (most protective equipment and breathing apparatus is inadequate).

The next position on the diamond is the top square which designates flammability and is colored **red**. The rating indicates the material's susceptibility to burning. The rating is as follows: 0 = Will not burn, 1 = Will ignite if preheated, 2 = Will ignite if moderately heated and can be fought with water, 3 = Will ignite in most ambient conditions (or normal temperatures) and water may be ineffective in fighting, and 4 = Burns readily at ambient temperatures, indicating material is very flammable or volatile.

The right square in the diamond designates *reactivity or instability* and is colored **yellow**. The rating identifies the level of reactivity or energy released if burned, decomposed, or mixed. The rating is as follows: 0 = Stable and not reactive with water, 1 = Normally stable but may become unstable in combination with other materials or at elevated temperatures or pressures, 2 = Violent chemical change if at elevated temperatures or pressures, but won't detonate, 3 = Shock and heat may detonate, and 4 = Readily capable of detonation at normal temperatures and pressures.

The bottom square in the diamond designates *special or other hazards* and is colored **white**. This square may have special symbols in it such as the radioactive pinwheel, OX (oxidizer) or a large "W" with a line through it indicating not to use water. [7]

The need for adequate labeling goes far beyond the considerations of the individual user in the laboratory. An individual who works in the laboratory may not be available during a fire, explosion or chemical spill. The one person who knows about a particular container and its contents may no longer be employed when a question or issue arises years later. As safety officer, I experienced this situation first hand. During an inventory of chemicals in the laboratory, I found bottles in the back of cabinets that were unrecognized by current employees. No one really knew what was in various bottles.

Again, all labels should contain the following information:

1. The name of the chemical or chemical name.
   Example: METHYL ALCOHOL OR METHANOL.

2. A warning word to indicate the severity of the hazard: such as Danger, Warning or Caution.
   Example: DANGER! MAY BE FATAL IF SWALLOWED.

3. A statement of the hazards with the most serious first: such as Flammable, Toxic, Irritant.
   Example: FLAMMABLE. TOXIC IF SWALLOWED.

4. Precautionary measures to be taken to assist in avoiding injury or damage from the indicated hazards. These would include recommendations to avoid open flame or contact with water and for use of specific personal protective equipment.
   Example: KEEP AWAY FROM HEAT, SPARKS OR FLAME. USE IN WELL VENTILATED AREA. WEAR RUBBER OR NEOPRENE GLOVES, APRON AND SAFETY GOGGLES.

5. Instructions in case of contact or exposure.
   Example: IF SWALLOWED, INDUCE VOMITING IMMEDIATELY.

As I discussed in Section 13, don't neglect the hazard warning label for containers with chemically processed evidence. Labeling of containers extends to evidence as well. This abbreviated form of label with the intent of warning others of possible contamination hazards is still a necessary label. You are morally if not legally required to provide at least minimal warning to other handlers of these materials.

Safe laboratory operations do not just happen. They result from considerable preparation, education, and compliance. Proper labeling of containers serves to protect the forensic identification specialist from being caught off guard by unexpected contents. Adequate labeling is to prevent accidental reactions and injuries. It also has the terrific advantage of preventing errors that could negatively affect the results of casework.

Nancy Masters

15
Electrical

An often overlooked area of laboratory safety is electrical safety, not given much thought and much taken for granted. In fact, electrical hazards can pose some of the most life-threatening situations.

Potential hazards include shock and/or electrocution. Electrical shorts can create fires or explosions from flammable vapors of chemicals, such as acetone and petroleum ether. Defective electrical wiring damages equipment. All personnel need general training about electrical hazards as well as specific training with equipment and instrumentation. Locate all operating manuals in a place near the equipment, so personnel can review instructions when necessary. Report immediately any problems with equipment to a supervisor and discontinue usage until the equipment is repaired.

Management should establish such engineering controls as ground fault interrupts and safety interlocks. You need some type of protective barrier where there is any risk of making contact with bare terminals or metal parts on electrical equipment. Management should provide the laboratory with insulated or rubber mats where you use electrical equipment. (Use mats also to prevent slipping in front of chemical sinks or on the floor anywhere that you use wet chemistry.)

Some laboratories lack proper wiring. All outlets should provide a grounded 3-wire arrangement for plugs. The receptacle should be adequate for any anticipated electrical load. The outlet should be tested for proper polarity when it is installed. Always know the proper voltage required for your equipment. Be aware that a 208 volt circuit will not always run a 220 volt motor. [1]

Every identification specialist should be trained in emergency shutdown procedures. Know where the electrical service panels are located in your facility. You should have access to the panel at all times. Label the inside of the panel with the names of the circuits to help locate connections rapidly.

Written policies and procedures should stipulate that only qualified personnel perform any service installation or repair on electrical equipment or the facility. Inspect wiring regularly. Install and use only equipment approved by the Underwriter's Laboratory (UL) or other recognized testing agency. Ground all equipment properly. If you can't ground the equipment, then label the electrical hazard it represents. Equipment such as fume hoods, which contain electrical motors and outlets and which may contain explosive vapors at times, must meet National Fire Protection Association (NFPA) requirements. [2]

The forensic identification specialist has specific responsibilities in this area. If using a piece of equipment with a long cord that must extend across the floor, place tape over the top of the cord to prevent someone tripping. If you note that the cord on a piece of equipment is worn or frayed, inform your supervisor. Do not use the equipment until it is repaired or replaced. Do not ever attempt to repair equipment yourself without specialized training to qualify you for the task. If you decide to modify equipment, first ask management for permission and approval.

Lastly, make an effort not to expose electrical cords to excessive heat or chemicals. Do not allow cords to become dunked in beakers of chemistry or laid over hot plates.

With these few guidelines you can avert potential disaster. Do not ever take your electrical setup for granted. Check it out before you start work as a specialist in the laboratory.

16
Chemical Storage

Chemical storage poses great potential for accidents. Two factors which can alleviate storage problems and potential accidents are to maintain and control a chemical inventory and to segregate inventoried chemicals by hazard for safe storage. Sort chemicals by their chemical characteristics into four or five categories: flammables, acids, bases, toxic substances and all other chemicals, giving special care to incompatible chemicals. Note incompatibilities shown on the MSDS and also on the label of the container when purchased. (Appendix B provides a list of the most common incompatible chemicals.) In practical terms, this means that you must store all the chemicals of a particular type together in one place and away from all other types. This is not as simple as it sounds because some chemicals possess more than one hazardous characteristic. For example, glacial acetic acid is a reducing agent and nitric acid is an oxidizing agent, so these two acids will react with each other and can never be stored together. [1] Consequently, you need to break each category into subsets for safe storage. You cannot do so without a good chemical inventory program.

Store flammables such as acetone, methanol, ethanol, and petroleum ether in a flammable storage cabinet. Store any quantities over one gallon (not each, but a total of all flammables) in a vented, flammable storage cabinet. Most state fire marshals will cite a chemical laboratory failing to provide a flammables cabinet for these chemicals. The safety cabinet designed to store flammables is constructed of fire resistant materials. The cabinet should be marked FLAMMABLES STORAGE and KEEP FIRE AWAY in large letters across the front. (Figures 16-1 and 16-2) You can store quantities of less than a gallon in the back of the fume hood or under the fume hood if the bottom cabinet is properly vented.

Permanent storage in the fume hood is not a good practice. Fume hoods were not designed to be storage receptacles. One problem is that when the hood is turned off the vapors can build up to both a toxic and dangerous level. Additionally, the

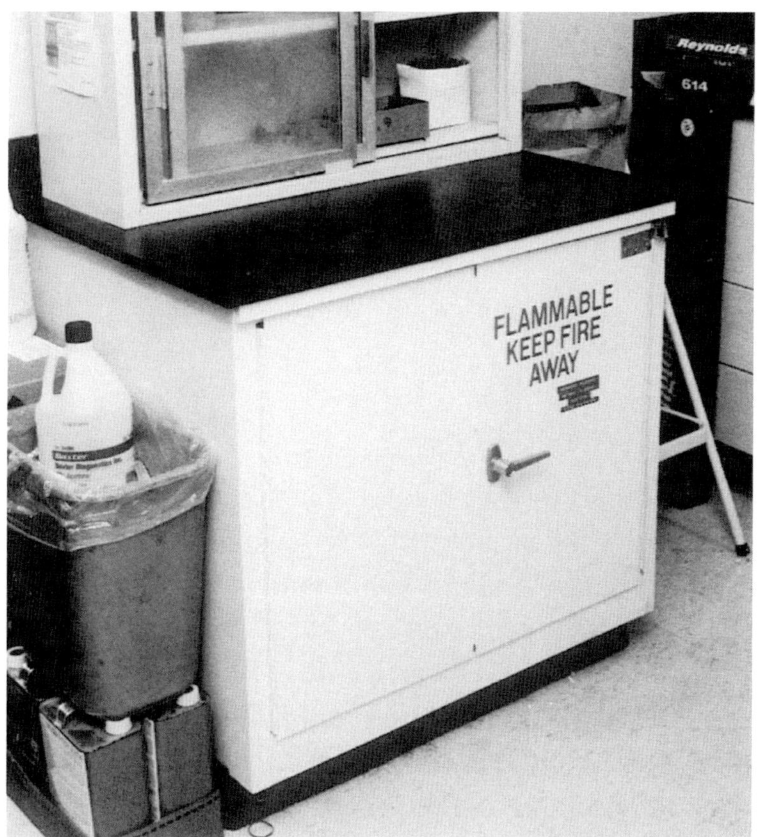

Figure 16-1: Free-standing Flammable storage cabinet.

Figure 16-2 Flammable storage cabinet installed beneath fume hood.

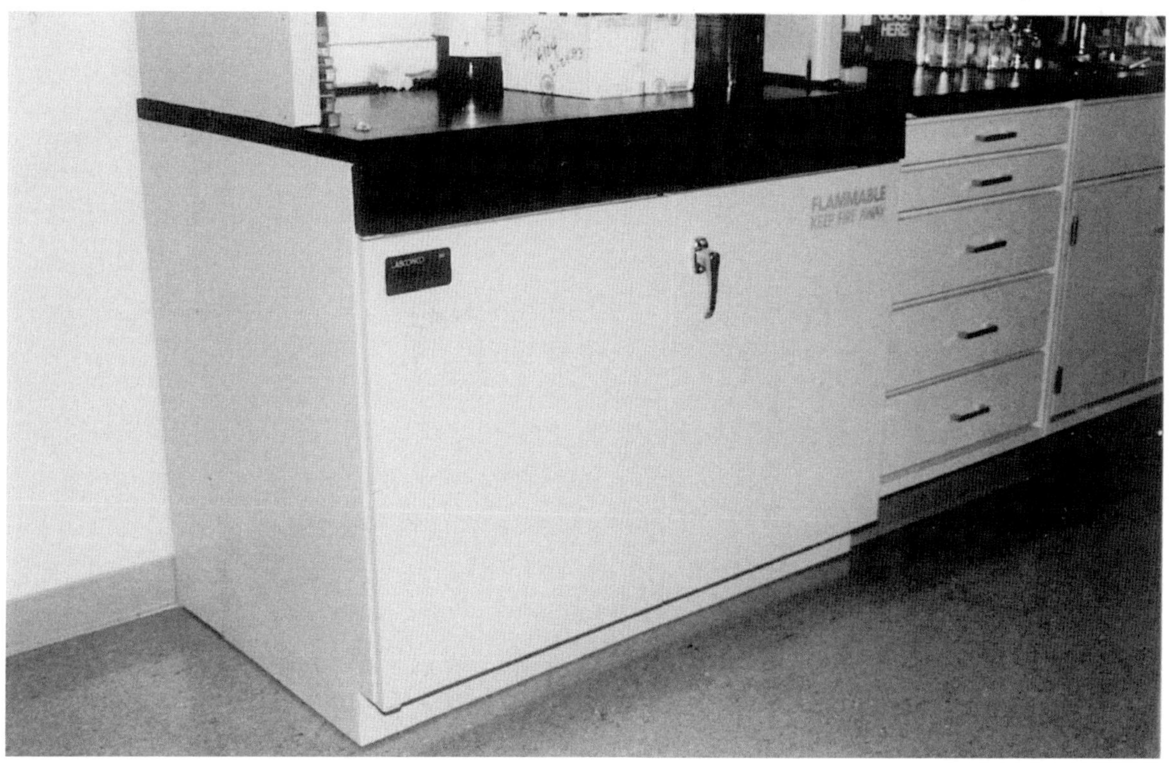

bottles and cans kept in the rear of the hood reduces the efficiency of the hood. [2] Lastly, storing chemicals in the hood can pose hazards resulting from unanticipated chemical reactions taking place during processing.

Store acids in a separate area away from all other types of chemicals. Separate acids by distance or partitions or isolate in a different cabinet. It is important for you to understand the nature of various acids. For instance, glacial acetic acid is a strong acid that is also combustible. Don't store it with other acids. While you can store it in the fume hood, you would do better to keep it in a special cabinet away from other chemicals.

Store bases away from all other types of chemicals. If an earthquake should break containers, and strong acids and bases suddenly mix, there will be explosions and spattering in the lab. The explosion resulting from sudden mixing may not be on the level with high explosives, but, any sudden chemical reaction which produces heat and energy is an explosion and causes severe burns. [3]

You can store together all other chemicals which do not have special incompatibility concerns. In the forensic identification laboratory, you should have at least three separately designated areas for chemical storage. Store all flammables such as acetone, ethanol, methanol, and petroleum ether, plus any mixed reagents with these components, in a flammables storage cabinet. Store any acids, with the exception of glacial acetic acid, in another cabinet. Store most remaining chemicals such as Ninhydrin crystals, dry chemicals for physical developer and Molybdenum, in yet another cabinet. Keep some special chemicals such as MBD and DFO crystals, Amido black and Sudan black powders in a laboratory refrigerator to increase their shelf life. Most laboratory refrigerators pose no hazards as long as you use them properly. Store any solvents in an explosion-proof refrigerator with all electrical contacts on the outside. Vapors can build up in a refrigerator and ignite. You need special electrical modifications, door latches and drain plugs to convert domestic refrigerators to laboratory use. Never store any food in a chemical refrigerator.

In order to decrease the amount of storage area required, you should order and maintain the smallest amount of chemicals needed at any given time. It is unwise to store large quantities of chemicals which cannot be used within a few months. Store the minimum of chemicals in the laboratory and maintain the larger stock in a storeroom. When you purchase and receive a chemical, assign an expiration date of no longer than one year. Inventory your chemicals at least twice a year and check the expiration dates. [4] Evaluate chemicals stored more than a year for possible disposal.

Storing chemicals on open shelves has its disadvantages. All open shelves must be bolted to the wall or floor. Each shelf should be lipped or have a restraint barrier or door so that chemical containers do not fall off when jarred. Place heavy items on lower shelves but not on the floor. It is good laboratory policy to discourage large and/or heavy items being stored at any height which requires the use of a ladder or stool for removal. The best height is eye level. Keep aisles between storage shelves clear of apparatus or equipment. Have nearby a fire extinguisher consistent for use with the type of stored chemicals. Store glassware and other laboratory equipment in an area separate from chemical storage.

Do not place any chemical without an appropriate label in storage . Always have chemicals in an adequate or appropriate container based upon the properties of the contents. Any specialist who has worked with iodine knows not to store it in a plastic container because iodine is so corrosive that it eats the container away and then goes to work on the metal shelf on which it was sitting. Be sure the container is right for the material. Purchased chemicals come in the appropriate container, but if you must transfer materials into other containers, make the container as much like the original container as possible. For example, since most components of Ninhydrin are received in glass bottles, store the mixed reagent in a glass bottle. Invest in glass bottles that are safety coated with a durable plastic covering. If the bottle is dropped, the plastic contains the contents. These coverings also resist heat and cold.

When placing liquid chemicals such as acids or solvents into storage, or removing them from storage, consider transporting them in a rubber or polyethylene bottle carrier. (Figure 16-3) This is especially important if you move them from the laboratory to another area of the facility. The carrier protects the bottle from bumping and chipping and contains the contents if the bottle breaks. The carrier also helps you hold safely to the chemical container.

I commend many forensic identification specialists for their interest in pursuing research and experimenting with special chemical formulations. However, this experimentation can create storage problems. Sometimes an individual will "hide away" bottles of special chemicals, opening the way for someone else to store highly incompatible chemicals together. If the specialist needs such chemicals, he or she should take steps to promote a safe storage scenario. Specialists also remove chemicals from storage, mix the necessary reagents and then become consumed by

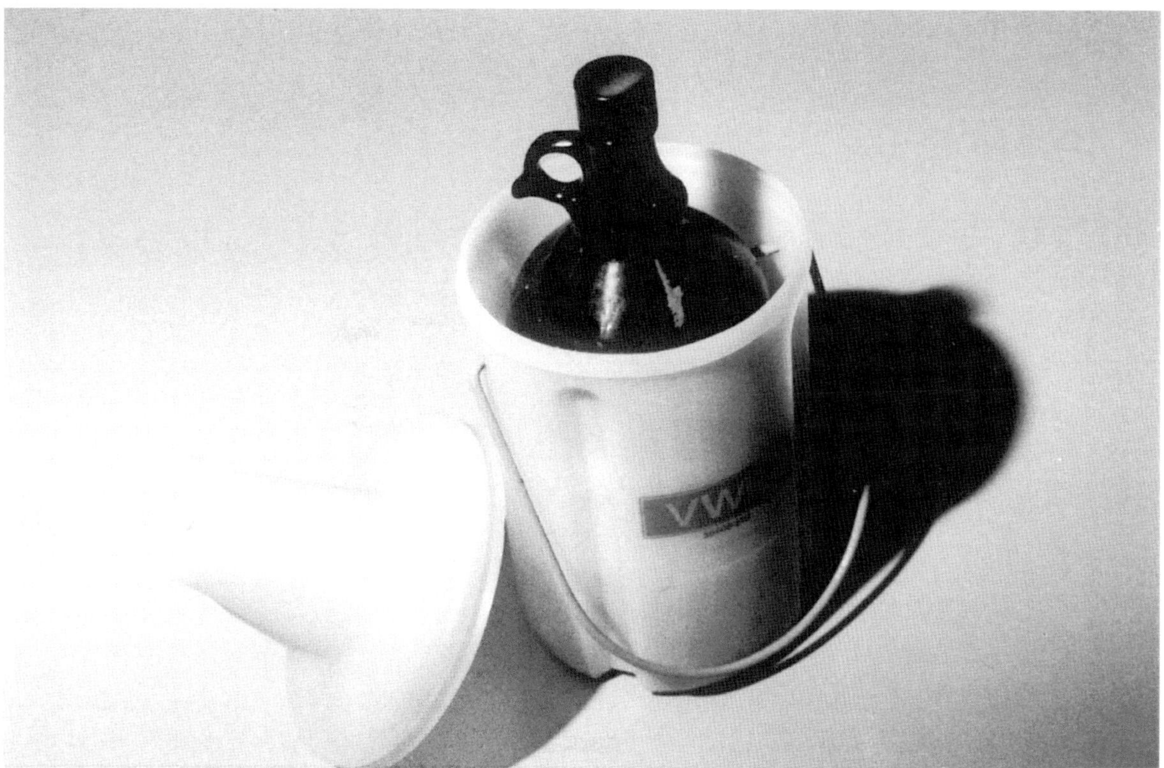

Figure 16-3: Commercially available polyethylene bottle carrier.

the processing of evidence, forgetting the chemicals out on the bench top. When you finish with chemicals, be sure to place them back into storage.

Any laboratory facility must be adequately constructed and provide necessary engineering controls. All motors, such as found in fans and ventilation equipment (including fume hoods) must be nonsparking. Each laboratory should have at least two exits. Some type of automatic sprinkler system must be in place. Electrical power, switches, lights, sockets, and appliances (such as the laboratory refrigerator) should be explosion proof. [5] These factors reduce the risk of an accident or the loss of property and life as result of an accident.

When making decisions about chemical storage, always consult the MSDS and any other source of material to educate yourself about the properties of that chemical. One comprehensive source of information is the *Handbook of Reactive Chemical Hazards,* 3rd Edition, by L. Bretherick and published by Butterworths, Stoneham, MA, 1985. Before handling chemicals, know your chemical, your container, and proper storage.

17
Spill Control and Waste Disposal

Spill Control

Chemical spills are one of the most common type of laboratory accidents and, while most spills are relatively small, all can have disastrous results. If hazardous vapors are released or toxic or corrosive materials come in contact with an individual's body, the incident is quite serious. Most spills involve small quantities of chemicals in a bottle, beaker, or flask. Each laboratory should have a spill-response person or team, as well as a spill-response plan that includes policies for the types and amounts of chemicals used, their associated hazards, and equipment used.

Although accidents can occur at any time, prevention through training, knowledge and preparation decreases the risks tremendously. Do not allow people to work in the laboratory until they have been properly trained. This training includes all procedures used to process evidence. Various engineering controls also assist to prevent spill accidents. Use plastic or plastic-coated bottles or containers, breakproof or shatterproof reagent bottles, and spill-containing or spill-proof carriers for transporting chemicals from one area to another. Use containers and/or appropriate equipment for handling hot, cold, wet or slippery containers. For example, when handling a Dewar flask of liquid nitrogen, use cryo-gloves or other low temperature gloves to protect the skin from the extreme cold. (Figure 17-1) These simple and somewhat inexpensive pieces of equipment can spare everyone the panic and problems of preventable and problematic chemical spills.

Another area not often considered is the type of footwear laboratory employees wear. Discourage slippery-soled shoes for poor traction, as well as open-toed sandals and canvas shoes for injury if chemicals are spattered or spilled onto the feet. Janitorial personnel can perform routine floor mopping during evening hours so floor surfaces have the opportunity to dry. Clean floors are essential, but

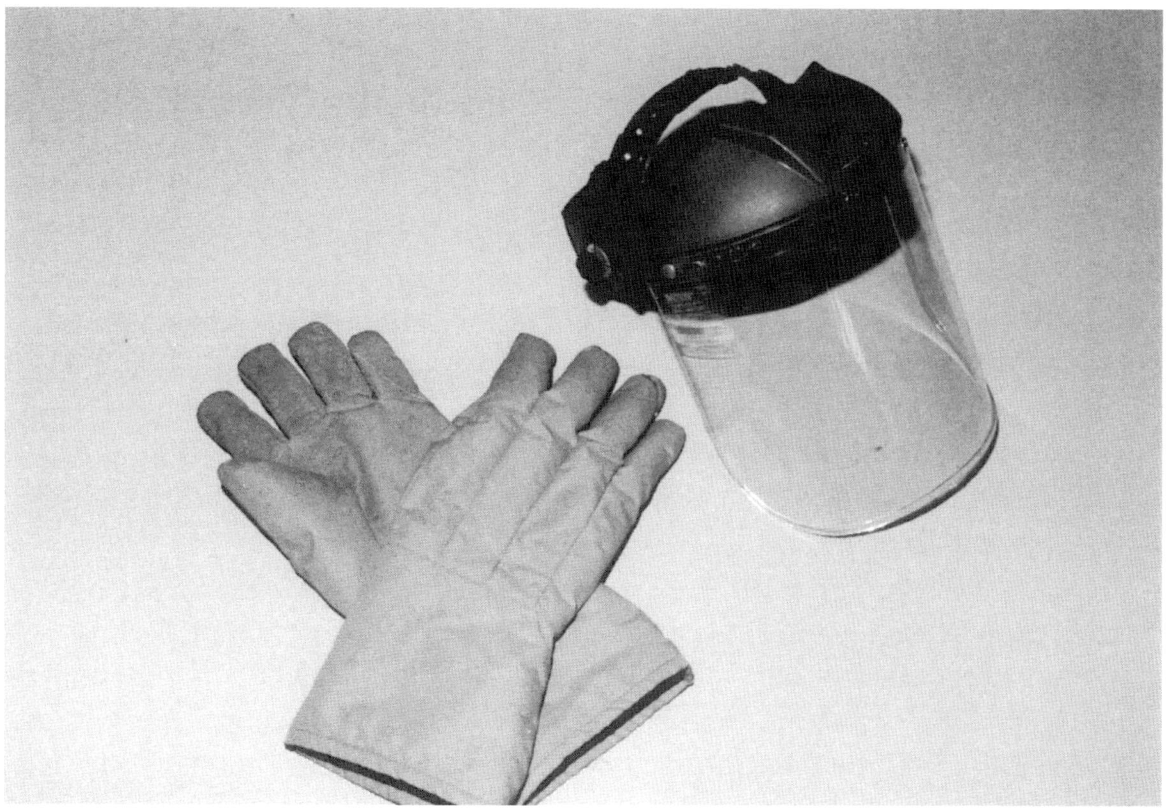

Figure 17-1: Cryo (low temperature) gloves and chemical face shield worn as protection when handling liquid nitrogen.

be careful about waxes. Only nonslip waxes will provide any assured footing, obviously important where containers of chemicals are carried from one location to another. Floor mats installed in front of sinks will alleviate wet, slippery spots in those areas.

What kinds of supplies and materials are needed for an anticipated spill? Commercial spill kits contain various tools, sorbents and personal protective equipment, but can be quite expensive. An alternative is to supply the laboratory with the necessary pieces of equipment as a part of the usual inventory. An acceptable spill kit for most situations in the forensic identification laboratory is a plastic three-to-five gallon bucket filled with plain, unscented kitty litter or sand. (They will absorb only the spill, not blanket any vapors.) Place a scoop in the bucket with the litter. Locate the spill kit at or near the entrance of your work area to allow safe access to it. Toss a scoop or two of the kitty litter over a spill to absorb and stop the spread until you can remove it. [1] For a spill of solid material, brush or sweep the material up and place it in a non-reactive container for disposal. You may want to give special consideration to an absorbent material which will not only absorb but also neutralize acids and caustics (e.g. sodium bicarbonate or sodium bisulfate). You can purchase spill kits specific to certain kinds of chemicals.

Always wear personal protective equipment during a spill cleanup. Keep on hand such equipment as chemical-resistant gloves and shoe covers, chemical-splash goggles, and respirators (organic, acid, dust, caustic) as part of the regular laboratory inventory. Additional equipment to clean up spills includes large, 6-mil polyethylene bags; a broom; a hand brush; a polyethylene bucket; 5-gallon plastic containers; lightweight and chemical-resistant coveralls; dust pan; mops; plastic-backed absorbent roll of paper; scoops; and duct tape. [2]

If chemicals are spilled on a person, strip off all contaminated clothing immediately and flush the skin with continuously running water for a minimum of 15 minutes. Run water under a safety shower (See Figure 4-3) or, if appropriate, a sink. Wash off the chemicals with soap or a mild detergent. Do not use neutralizing agents, creams, lotions or salves on the skin. [3] Seek medical attention immediately.

If chemicals are spilled, you need to have an orderly course of events. First, alert anyone in the area that a spill has occurred. Inform your supervisor immediately. Consult the Material Safety Data Sheet for information and precautions regarding the material and any procedures for cleanup. If the substance is even suspected of being a flammable, extinguish all ignition sources. Attempt to confine the spill with sorbent pads, pillows, socks, dikes, blankets, or other approved absorbent material such as kitty litter. If you are unable to determine the nature of the spilled material, do not ever take any risks. It may even be necessary to evacuate the building. [4] Confine the material if possible and get out. Otherwise, just "get out!" Some chemicals require the use of respirators or SCBA for a safe cleanup effort.

Do not leave the area of the spill without first decontaminating yourself in order to prevent the spread of contamination to other areas. Once the spilled material has been cleaned from the surface, thoroughly scrub or mop the previously contaminated area or flood with water for 15 minutes. Decontaminate all personal protective equipment that is not disposable. Determine how to dispose of waste materials, including any absorbent materials, based upon the MSDS, federal, state, and local regulations, and departmental policy.

Waste Disposal

Waste disposal is a very complex and complicated area that is heavily regulated. At one time there was no regulation. In 1976, the Environmental Protection Agency (EPA) received a mandate from Congress because of past excesses of no regulation and growing concerns over the environment. Congress enacted the Resource Conservation and Recovery Act (RCRA) to protect human life and the environment from improper waste management practices. Initially, only large quantity generators of waste were regulated. Small quantity generators, producing 100 to 1000 kg of hazardous waste in a calendar month, were exempted from most of the regulations of RCRA. (Most forensic identification laboratories fall into this category.) In 1984, amendments to the RCRA (called the Hazardous and Solid Waste Amendments) required the EPA to establish new demands on the small quantity generators. The final dictates that became law in 1986 are essentially the same as those placed upon the large quantity generators. [5]

Much like federal OSHA, the EPA regulations mandated the states to enforce all the regulations. Many states adopted the federal requirements as their standard, while other states wrote requirements that exceed federal statutes. The federal regulations should be considered the minimum requirements. Needless to say, waste disposal has become a difficult and expensive operation for all waste generators. Waste is regulated by a number of entities. Federal, state, and local regulations are intended to protect water quality, air quality, waste water quality and soil quality. [6]

What constitutes waste? The EPA classifies waste as any material that usually is discarded or has no economic value. [7] Hazardous material does not become hazardous waste as long as it has value and the generator has not declared it waste. [8] Previously used (whether in part or total) or unused surplus chemicals become hazardous waste. This is why it is so important to keep a chemical inventory and not be burdened with unopened, expired chemicals which require expensive disposal. The EPA would interpret all waste products and surplus chemicals from forensic laboratories to be hazardous. There are basically three classifications of waste:

1. **Characteristic waste** (40 CFR 261.10) is any material that is

- Ignitable or capable of fire hazard under normal conditions or operations (40 CFR 261.21).
- Corrosive or capable of eating through normal containers (40 CFR 261.22).
- Reactive or has a tendency to explode under normal use conditions, to react violently with water, or to generate toxic gases under specified conditions (40 CFR 261.23).
- Extraction procedure toxic as such that it contains certain toxic materials that can be released in acidic water (40 CFR 261.24).

2. **Listed waste** applies to anything which occurs on the EPA's "F" list (40 CFR 261.31), "P" list (40 CFR 261.33 (e)), and "U" list (40 CFR 261.33 (f)), respectively hazardous wastes, toxic wastes and acutely hazardous wastes.

3. **Statutory waste** is any material which may pose a threat or cause harm to human health and the environment. There are substances in this category which are not listed in the above two. [9]

The bottom line is that almost any material can be classified as hazardous waste. A licensed waste transporter must collect and haul the waste to a licensed waste processing facility. You must identify every waste product, including its various chemical components, to the transporter because it is unlawful for the transporter or facility to receive any unknown chemicals for disposal. Consequently, as you place waste materials into waste bottles (or other containers), you must identify the chemical name, components, the volume and concentration of the material. Usually store these waste containers in the back of a fume hood until removal for transporting to a waste disposal facility.

Another serious ramification to generating waste is that the RCRA stipulated a "cradle-to-grave" responsibility for all hazardous waste generators. In other words, once a material is declared hazardous waste, even though hauled away, possibly stored and finally disposed of, liability remains with the initiator as long as the origin is able to be determined. This liability coupled with the costs of waste hauling and disposal, is the reason why the laboratory should attempt to create as little waste as possible. Do not order more chemicals than you can use in a few months. Capture and reuse any reagents that are reusable, such as Sudan black, Rhodamine 6G and other fluorescing dye stains, Gentian Violet, Small

Particle Reagent, etc. If you have more chemicals than can be used, pass them on to other units or laboratories. The time is long past when you could pour chemicals down the sink. Allowing solvent to evaporate out a fume hood is not an acceptable means of disposal for excess solvents.

Use a medical hazardous waste program to dispose of biological materials. Only a licensed medical hazardous waste hauler can remove wastes containing or contaminated with biological materials such as urine and blood. Give consideration to what items you place in bags marked as biological waste. You can dispose of some material, such as paper towels, latex gloves, and lift tape used in the processing of deceased fingers/hands through the laboratory's garbage system.

The laboratory must inventory the amounts of hazardous waste it produces throughout the year. Inventory determines the lab's status of small or large quantity waste generator. Every laboratory must obtain an EPA Identification Number. This number assists the EPA and the state to determine hazardous waste activity. There are also limits on the amount of waste that you can store in-house and on the period of time you can store it before removal.

Needless to say, waste management and disposal are expensive propositions that are heavily regulated with no end in sight. Minimize your expenses and problems with detailed planning and application of process design (including on-line processes), conservative purchasing procedures and policies, inventory control, safe and legal material storage, recycling and reuse of spent materials, and competent, safe and legal disposal. [10]

18
Light Sources

Since 1976, with the advent of the argon-ion laser for detection of inherent luminescence of organic compounds in fingerprint residues, [1] light sources have come into their own as a technique in forensic identification. While the use of light was not a new concept, the tremendous amount of research and experimentation in the use of lasers, filters and fluorescing chemistry for the development of latent prints opened up this "new" frontier. Whether performing latent print examinations, document examinations or photography, numerous specialists use one light source or another.

Forensic latent print specialists use these light sources to detect and/or enhance latent prints through the fluorescence of natural constituents of sweat and contaminants, dye stains, amino acid reactive reagents, and background substrates. They also use light sources to enhance contrast of backgrounds against materials which absorb the light (consequently appearing darker), such as blood or Ninhydrin; or to fluoresce backgrounds to make reflective prints more visible. [2] Incidental to latent print detection, these light sources are often effective in the visualization of fibers, cosmetics, blood, semen and other body fluids.

In forensic document examination, luminescence and reflectance have been used as detection techniques for about forty years. Various wavelengths of light are employed to differentiate varieties of inks from one another and to separate inks from backgrounds. The technique is important in detecting and restoring or enhancing alterations, obliterations and other ink problems. This could include entries on medical charts and accounting ledgers or possible forgeries. Ultraviolet is effective in the differentiation of paper and in determining the mucilage (adhesive) patterns on envelopes. Theoretically, discrete wavelengths of light can assist in the sequencing of strokes on a surface and in eliminating color in backgrounds with indented writing. [3]

Photographers, who may also be forensic identification specialists, employ light sources to visualize all the above-mentioned fluorescing targets as a means of documentation. They may also use ultraviolet light to document bruises or impressions on human skin.

The manual published by the Police Scientific Development Branch of the United Kingdom gives an excellent explanation of fluorescence, as follows:

> Fluorescence is the property that some chemicals possess of being able to absorb light of a specific color and then convert some of this absorbed energy into light of a different color of longer wavelength. The time delay between absorption and emission is only a fraction of a second (less than 10^{-8} seconds) so that when the illuminating light is removed the emission apparently stops.
>
> Typically, light in the ultraviolet, blue or green parts of the spectrum is used to excite fluorescence which may result in the emission of light in the yellow, orange, red or infrared parts of the spectrum.
>
> Most of the illuminating light is usually not absorbed but is scattered or reflected from the surface being examined. Filters which transmit the fluorescence but not the illuminating light are therefore placed in front of the eye and camera to enable the fluorescence to be seen and recorded.
>
> Different chemicals require illumination with light from different regions of the spectrum to excite fluorescence and the wavelength (color) of the emitted light varies from one chemical to another. [4]

The light sources which are used to excite fluorescence are typically lasers, alternate light sources or high intensity lamp systems and ultraviolet lights. While each of these sources differs in the power of emitted light and wavelengths of light, they all pose health hazards to the user. In addition to the hazards of the light, there are also associated electrical hazards and dangers in using the various developing or fluorescing chemicals.

Lasers

To understand the workings of a laser, it is important to first understand the nature of light, the nature of atoms and the interaction of atoms with light and other forms of energy. Simply stated, light is a form of energy which acts as both a wave and a particle and is released from individual atoms or molecules in substances. In providing a brief but concise explanation of atomic behavior and light emissions, Insun Chang stated:

> Every atom is a storehouse of energy. The amount of energy in an atom depends in part on the motion of the electrons that orbit the atom's nucleus. When an atom absorbs energy, the energy levels of the electrons increase, and the atom is said to be excited. The atoms of a substance become excited when they absorb heat, light, or other forms of energy that pass through the substance. An excited atom can return to its normal energy level by releasing its excess energy in the form of light. This release of light is called *spontaneous emission*.
>
> In spontaneous emission, excited atoms release light irregularly. As a result, the light has different frequencies, different phases, and travels in different directions. Light released in this way is called *incoherent light*. Such light is produced by the sun and by ordinary electric bulbs.
>
> Excited atoms also may release light systematically. This kind of release, called *stimulated emission*, is the main process that takes place in a laser. Stimulated emission occurs when the energy released from one atom interacts with another atom that is still excited. The interaction stimulates the excited atom into releasing its own energy as light. Most of the light produced by stimulated emission has the same frequency and same phase as the stimulating light. It also travels in the same direction, and so it combines with and amplifies the triggering light Such light is called *coherent radiation*. [5]

Lasers produce coherent radiation where other light sources produce incoherent light. While all light poses health hazards, the light concentrating and focusing effect of coherent radiation is what makes it the most dangerous.

As more lasers and laser applications were developed, it became necessary to make distinctions between the various systems and the safety protocols needed for safe practices. A hazard classification system was devised to assist the user in applying the proper set of safety rules and was based upon the hazards the laser poses. The American National Standards Institute (ANSI) developed the first classification system. The Bureau of Radiological Health (BRH) modified the ANSI standards to what we use today. While there are basically four classifications of lasers, most used in forensic identification work are either Class III-B or Class IV. Class III-B, or medium powered systems, consists of lasers which can accidentally injure an individual when directly viewed. A direct or reflected beam can cause injury. Warning labels are necessary. The Laserprint 1000 is such a laser and notes the various hazards on the warning label. The manufacturer also notes that it meets U.S. Food and Drug Administration (FDA) requirements under 21 CFR 1040. Class IV lasers are also referred to as "high powered systems." These lasers require controls to prevent eye and skin exposure to both direct and reflected beams. Most stationary, high-powered lasers used in forensic identification work are of this type.

In the late 1970s and 1980s, many agencies invested in lasers. Some purchased the large Argon-ion lasers while others obtained Copper vapor or Neodymium: YAG lasers. A few facilities, usually research in nature, obtained dye lasers. The large Argon-ion laser has a power output between 4 and 25 watts. While these lasers can be tuned in a single line that would allow for up to 9 discrete wavelengths, many are used with all-lines lasing at one time. They are also capable of producing ultraviolet light if an alternate set of mirrors is used. These lasers are stationary and are water-cooled. An alternate to the large Argon-ion laser is the small, low-powered (output between 50 and 200 milliwatts) portable laser such as the Laserprint 1000 made by Omnichrome. This laser provides an all-lines lasing mode and is air-cooled. [6]

There are not many Copper vapor lasers still in use in the United States. These lasers have an output as high as 10 to 40 watts and are either water-cooled or air-cooled. While two lines are available, the 510.6 nm is the only one used for latent print work. [7] The 578.2 nm line can be used in forensic document work.

The Neodymium: YAG (Yttrium Aluminum Garnet) lasers are either small air-cooled systems or can be more powerful water-cooled systems. This laser was one of the first portable systems that could be taken by cart to a crime scene. The visible light output is "achieved at 532 nm by frequency doubling. These lasers have a pulsed emission with time-averaged continuous power up to about 1 watt." [8] The pulsed emission (a flickering effect of the light) is difficult for some people to tolerate and may increase their eye fatigue. Other people seem unaffected. [9]

Dye lasers are usually used with another laser, such as the Argon-ion, which pumps it. Various dyes, such as Rhodamine 6G, can be used. The dye provides the ability to tune the laser continuously over a range of discrete laser lines. [10]

All of the above-mentioned lasers pose hazards. Since the eye is often more vulnerable than the skin to injury from visible and near-infrared radiation, it is considered the organ most important to protect from all wavelengths of laser radiation. Because the eye focuses radiation in the visible and near visible region of the spectrum, the irradiance at the retina may be several orders of magnitude greater than at the cornea. [11] A beam of laser light directly to the eye can be devastating. Such an accident was experienced by the manager of an electro-optics laboratory belonging to GTE, the American telecommunications company. The accident occurred when he was unexpectedly called into the laboratory. Approximately 10 seconds after coming through the door, he recalls, he was partially blinded in his left eye by a pulse of invisible light, at a wavelength in the near-infrared range of the spectrum, from a neodymium: YAG laser. Read his description of the event:

> When the beam struck my eye, I heard a distinct popping sound caused by a laser-induced explosion at the back of my eyeball. My vision was obscured almost immediately by streams of blood floating in the vitreous humour and by what appeared to be particulate matter suspended in the vitreous humour. It was like viewing the world through a round fishbowl full of glycerol into which a quart of blood and a handful of black pepper have been partially mixed. There was a local pain within a few minutes of the accident, but it did not become excruciating. The most immediate response after such an accident is horror. As a Vietnam War veteran, I have seen several terrible scenes of human carnage, but none affected me more than viewing the world through my blood-filled eyeball. In the aftermath of the accident, I went into shock as is typical in personal injury accidents.

As it turns out, my injury was severe but not nearly as bad as it might have been. I was not looking directly at the prism from which the beam had reflected, so the retinal damage is not in the fovea. The beam struck my retina between the fovea and the optic nerve, missing the optic nerve by about three millimeters. Had the focused beam struck the fovea, I would have sustained a blind spot in the center of my field of vision. Had it struck the optic nerve, I probably would have lost the sight of that eye.

The beam did strike so close to the optic nerve, however, that it severed nerve-fiber bundles radiating from the optic nerve. This has resulted in a crescent-shaped blind spot many times the size of the lesion.... The effect of the large blind area is much like having a finger placed over one's field of vision. [12]

The parallel or collimated rays of visible light from a laser, regardless of distance, can be imaged on the retina in a very small area. This focusing effect of the cornea and lens of the eye will concentrate these light rays by an enormous

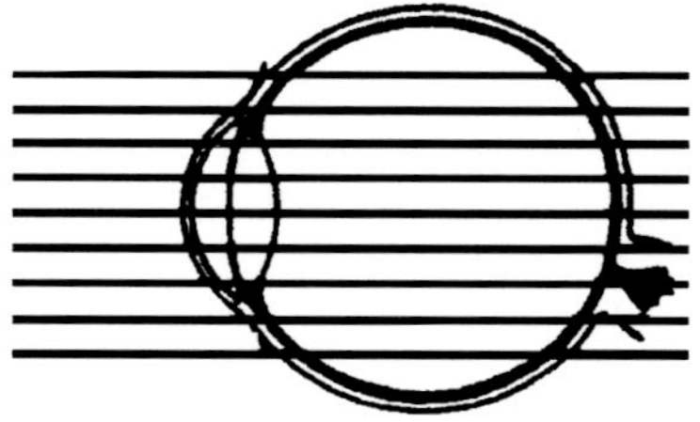

a. Microwaves and Gamma Rays

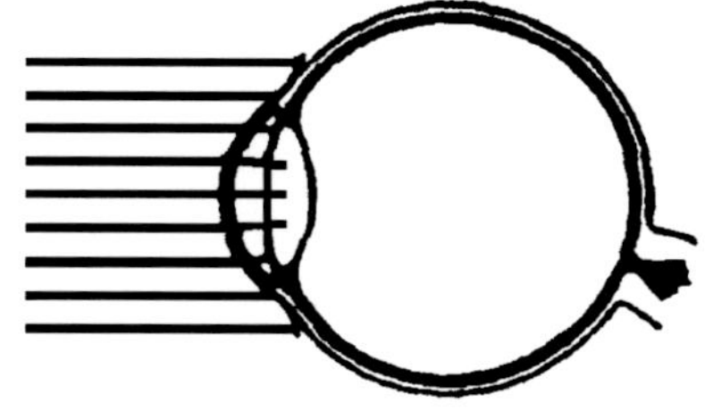

c. Near Ultraviolet

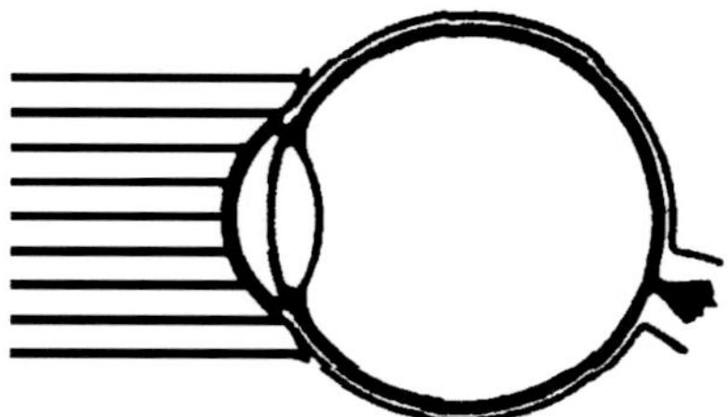

b. Far Ultraviolet and Far Infrared

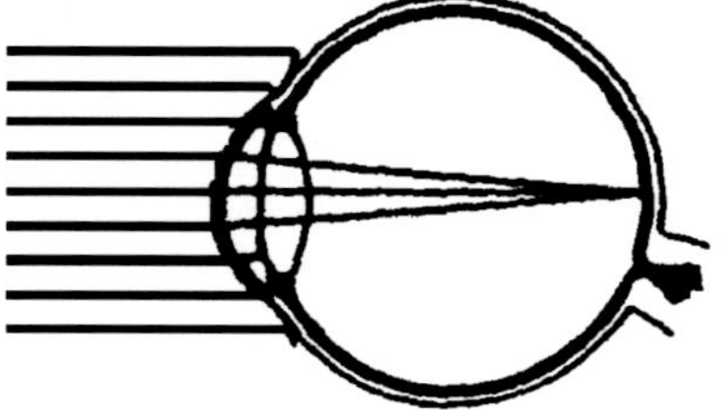

d. Visible and Near Infrared

Figure 18-1: A 1-W visible laser beam represents a far greater hazard to the retina than a 100-W light bulb. The brightness of the collimated beam is more than one billion times greater than the light bulb. (Reprinted with permission from Plenum Press.)

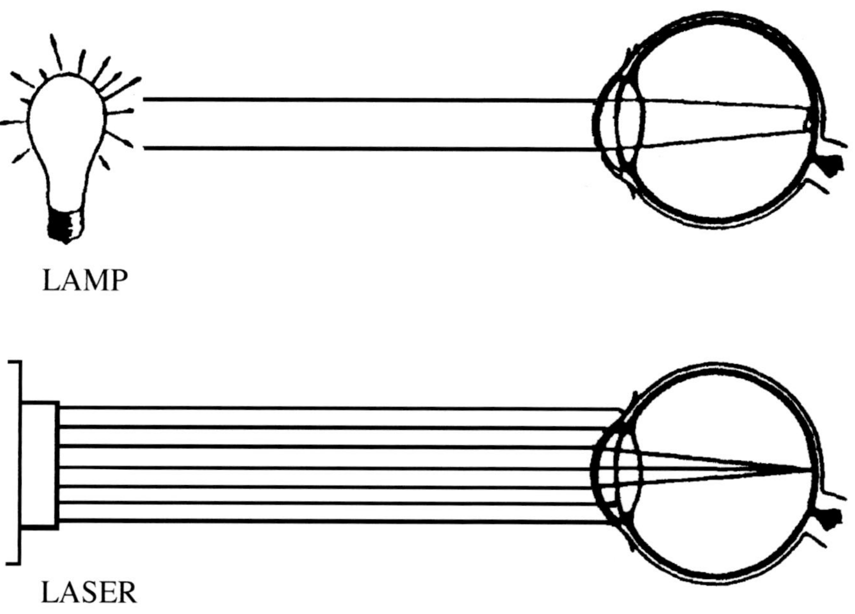

Figure 18-2: Schematic diagram of the absorption of electromagnetic radiation in the eye. (Reprinted with permission from Plenum Press.)

factor of 100,000 times. This means that the light leaving the laser and entering the eye is pinpointed down onto the retina at 100,000 times the brightness (intensity) which left the laser. (Figure 18-1) The brightness of a laser source is greater than all known natural and man-made light sources, including the sun or xenon-arc lamp. The concentration of light falling upon the retina is dependent upon the brightness of the object being viewed. (Figure 18-2) [13]

As noted in the work by Hardwick, Kent and Sears, "the intensity of the light emitted from the powerful sources required for fluorescence examination can present potentially dangerous levels of light to unprotected eyes, even though a diverging beam of light is used." And, "when the eyes are exposed to very bright sources the natural response is to close them; typically this takes a quarter of a second. The light sources required for fluorescence examination, however, may cause retinal damage during exposure times of less than 0.25 second. Under no circumstances must the light be viewed directly at short distances, even for a fraction of a second, without eye protection." [14]

Other than a direct hit from the beam, the hazard in forensic latent print identification and photography comes from the incidental light. This damage occurs when the specialist views surfaces closely while making an examination. The close viewing may continue for a prolonged period of time when many exhibits are being scanned or photographed.

The best methods for preventing eye damage are to use the appropriate viewing filters to reduce the intensity of light (to the eyes) and always to observe from an established safe distance. Most laser manufacturers will provide viewing goggles. Require all personnel to wear protective goggles when using the laser. (Figure 18-3) The manager at the GTE laboratory would never have been injured had he entered the laboratory with goggles over his eyes.

A special room should be allocated for laser (or other high intensity light source) examinations. Cover any windows for safety and examination purposes. Post a warning sign on the door when the laser is operating. Lock any door to the laser examination room while the laser is operating. Restrict entry to the laser area

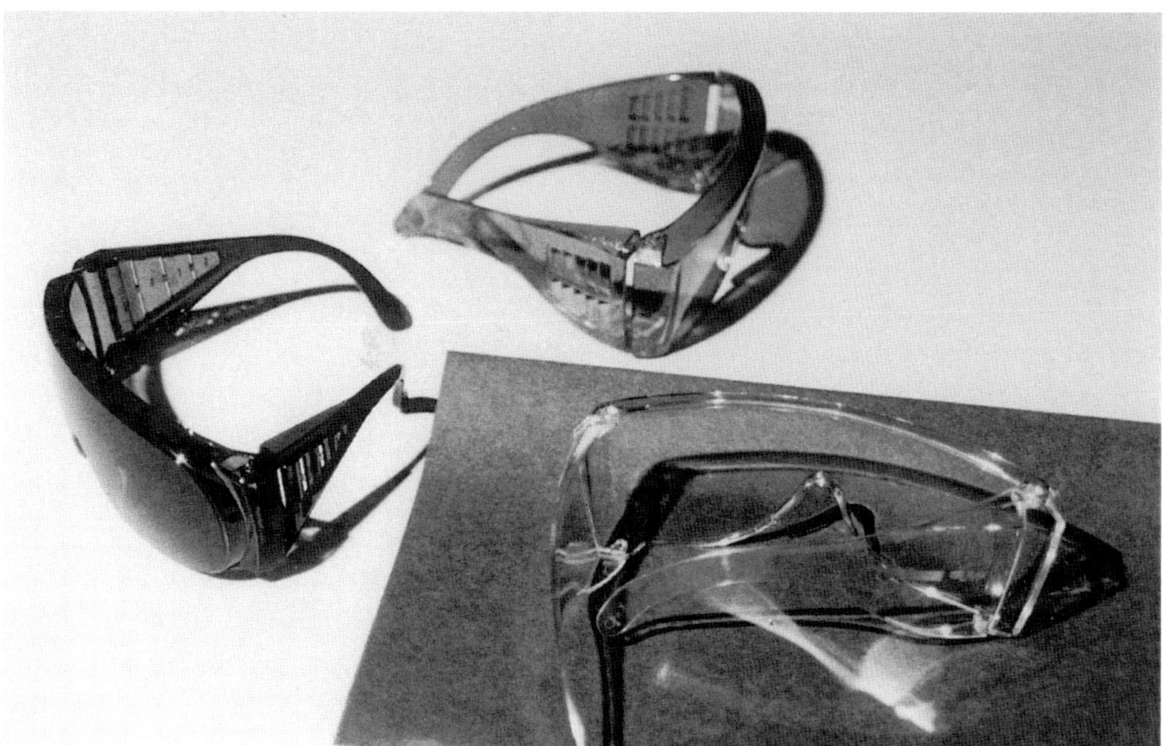

Figure 18-3: Commercially available goggles: Top – orange filtered; right – UV filtered; left – red filtered.

to authorized people who have been trained in the safe operation of lasers. Cover surfaces with a disposable material that you can frequently replace to control contamination in the laser area. Purchase rolls of black paper for low background fluorescence.

If the laser must be taken into the field for crime scene work, prominently post the laser area to alert others to the hazards. There is a minimum safe distance beyond which goggles are not needed. According to manufacturers of the Omnichrome Laserprint 1000, this distance is 15 feet from the location of the hand piece. [15] (For the high powered Argon-ion laser in the laboratory, the minimum safe distance is approximately 60 feet.) [16]

Injury to the skin by laser radiation is considered secondary to injury to the eye. The thresholds of injury to the eye and skin are much alike except in the area of hazards to the retina (400 - 1400 nm). There is a far greater probability of exposure to skin areas than to the eye because of the skin's greater surface area. Hazardous levels of illumination can occur during the examination of evidence if the light guide is held close to any skin. Injury to the skin may range from minor changes in the "horny layer" of skin cells from short exposures to more severe injuries from longer exposures. Most injuries will heal with no long-term damage, but injury to larger areas of skin can be far more serious and may lead to serious loss of body fluids, bacterial poisoning of the body and infections of vital body systems. [17] (It is unlikely this type of injury would occur in the forensic latent print laboratory, but you should be aware of the potentials of this light.) In other words, the skin gets burned. This occurs by the same mechanism as excess heat in the tissues (thermal burning) or a sunburn (photochemical effect).

To avoid burns to the skin, always wear either nitrile or latex gloves and a long-sleeved laboratory coat. If you are examining fibers or other trace evidence where there is no biological hazard, you can wear cotton gloves. Hardwick, Kent and Sears make the point that "since the light should always be directed towards the surface under examination and not the face, the face should not normally be exposed to hazardous levels. A possible exception to this is the examination of highly reflective surfaces such as mirrors or polished metal. In such circumstances the total distance between the light guide and the face via the surface must exceed 250 mm (or 350 mm)." [18] This distance would be between 9 to 10 inches or 13 to 14 inches depending upon the actual emitted power of the laser. Even if you do not know the power of your laser, use this guideline.

Always cover any areas of the skin or eyes that the light beam could touch.

So use any necessary personal protective equipment to cover eyes, arms and hands. Always wear an appropriately filtered viewing goggle. Never aim a laser beam at a person's eyes or face. Never intentionally irradiate unprotected skin. Always think of others in the area. Devise a system for alerting co-workers in the laboratory that the laser is in use, so they do not enter the laser room without proper protection. At the crime scene, establish the safe minimum distance from the lasing area and do not allow improperly protected individuals to approach. Ensure that spectators are not exposed to a hazardous condition.

High Intensity Lamp Systems

In the 1980s, a new type of light source appeared on the market as an alternative to a laser. This system became known in the United States as alternate light sources or ALS. Most are air-cooled and use a xenon, xenon/mercury arc lamp or metal halide lamp. [19] They use a series of filters, or a filter wheel, of different wavelengths and bandwidths. Moving the filters in front of the illuminated lamp produces a variety of wavelengths. Many agencies prefer these devices rather than the laser for decreased maintenance, cost and hazards.

Initially, many users thought that these light sources posed no health hazard. This misconception resulted from years of using common lamp systems. When electric lamps were first developed, they were mass produced in a time when product standards and safety standards were essentially unknown. It was not until lasers were developed (single-wavelength systems) that the public became alarmed about potential hazards. Evaluating and controlling lamp hazards is more complicated. Making the required radiometric (light energy) measurements of these various lamp systems is very intricate and detailed because they do not involve the simple optics of a point source, but rather they deal with an extended source which may or may not be altered by a projection system. Supplementary optical elements, diffusers, lenses, etc., [20] may alter the wavelength distribution.

Hardwick, Kent and Sears have documented their in-depth research in evaluating light sources in the publication, *Fingerprint Detection By Fluorescence Examination*. This tremendous accomplishment should be included in all forensic identification libraries. The authors address the difficulties of assessing the various lamp systems. They took the following factors into account: "spectral emission of the light source, amount of emitted light, beam divergence of the light delivery system, output aperture dimension, proximity of the light to the eyes or skin, period of exposure, and whether the output is continuous or pulsed." [21] They also make the very important point that

> the intensity and spectral output of the radiation must be measured since manufacturer's information is frequently inadequate for safety assessment: for example, a new laser may emit twice the specified output power or a lamp may emit some light outside the spectral region quoted in the literature. The maximum emission, usually when the system is new and the optical components are clean and optimally aligned, must be used to allow for the worst possible hazard. [22]

Therefore, the manufacturer may not have included adequate information to assess all of the potential hazards of lamp usage. This is not to imply that the manufacturer is "hiding" anything. Very possibly, the lamp was not tested for all of the above-mentioned factors. In evaluating the users manual for one light source, I was unable to ascertain whether the manufacturer had conducted such tests. The only warning pertained to directing the light from the light guide into the eye. Hardwick, Kent and Sears recommend that you assess thoroughly for optical radiation hazards all high intensity lamps used for fingerprint detection. Consider the optical configuration in which you are to use the lamps and filters. [23]

To ensure the safest possible viewing of fluorescing materials, the Police Scientific Development Branch of the Home Office developed the Quaser systems. These high-intensity lamp systems use semi- or fully-enclosed viewing housings. Light is fed into the housing, usually by use of a light guide, to illuminate the target which is viewed through windows containing viewing filter glass. This system eliminates the need for goggles. This is one of the safest alternate light sources devised. You can use viewing housings with lasers or high intensity light sources. They are compatible with fiber optic or liquid light guide light delivery systems. [24]

Many forensic document examiners use the Visual Spectral Comparator (VSC 1 and VSC 4) This instrument combines a video camera with a light source and series of filters. The filters provide wavelengths mainly in the blue-green and infrared ranges. All light is housed in an enclosed unit that provides a barrier between the target and the viewer.

Since high intensity light sources do pose health hazards to the eyes and the skin, they require the same safety considerations as lasers. The nature and extent of all potential hazards is not known because in-depth assessments have not been made of most of the high intensity lights used in forensic identification work. Exposures to ultraviolet and infrared light can be damaging. If the light source is not contained in a viewing housing system, then use any necessary personal protective equipment to cover your eyes, arms and hands. Always wear an appropriately filtered viewing goggle. Never aim a light beam at a person's eyes or face. Never irradiate unprotected skin. Always think of others in the area. Devise a system for alerting others in the laboratory that the light source is in use so they do not enter the examination room without proper protection. At the crime scene, establish the safe minimum distance from the examination area, and do not allow improperly protected individuals to approach. Ensure that any spectators are not exposed.

Ultraviolet Lamps

Ultraviolet light has been used for many years for a wide variety of purposes from sterilization to black lights. In forensic identification work, it is very effective in the laboratory or at the crime scene. Human physiological fluids, such as semen, urine, saliva, and vaginal fluids will fluoresce. Many of the fluorescent dye stains (Ardrox, Thionyl Europium Chelate, Rhodamine 6G) and fluorescent powders used in latent print development will give good fluorescing results with UV light. Bruising, bite marks and other impression marks, hairs, fibers, and ligature marks also become visible with UV light. Rape victims as well as deceased victims are examined under UV light for trace evidence. Ultraviolet has been used in forensic document examinations for years. Even with all these positive attributes, the ultraviolet lamp has been much underrated in its usefulness. With the advent of lasers and other high intensity light sources, UV lamps became almost forgotten. There is now a resurgence in the use of these lamps. More research is being conducted in the use of high-power ultraviolet such as that which can be produced by an argon laser. An ultraviolet lamp appeals as a light source to agencies with small equipment budgets, because the lamps are basically inexpensive and yet highly efficient. However, they also pose serious eye and skin hazards that went unnoticed for years.

Ultraviolet radiation is part of our natural outdoor environment as sunlight.

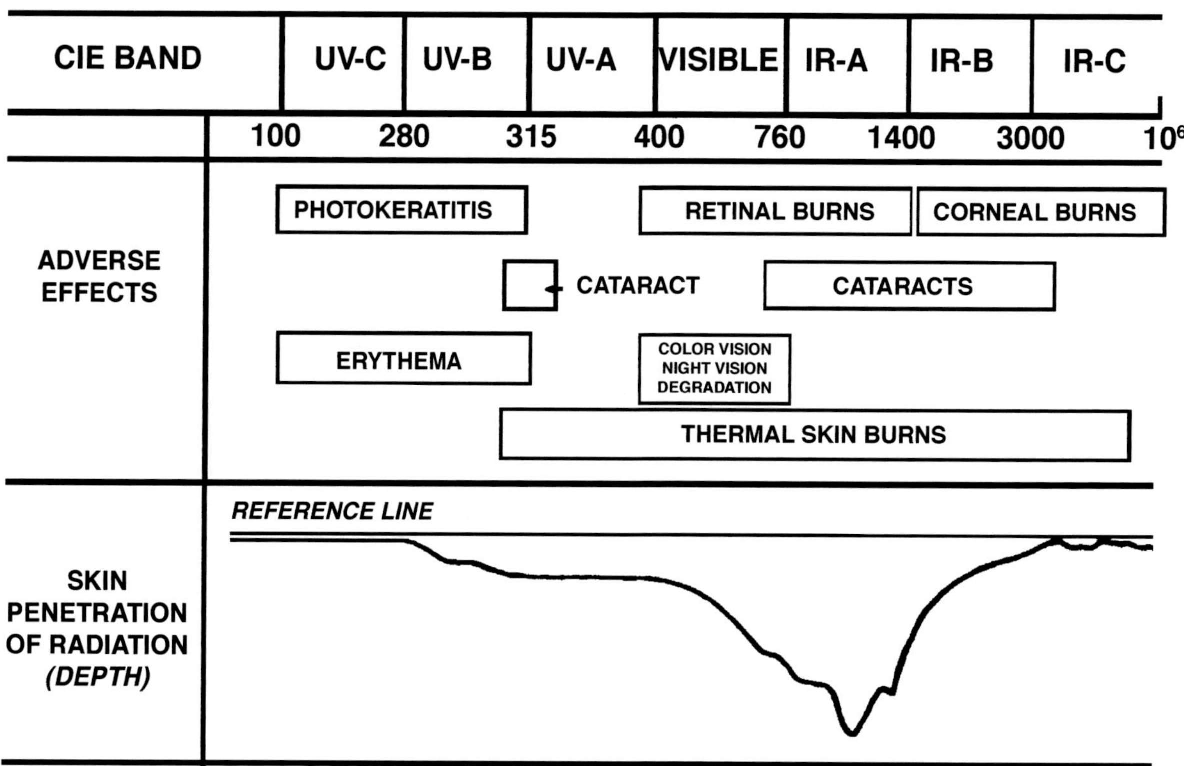

Figure 18-4: The International Commission on Illumination (CIE) divides the optical spectrum into seven spectral bands. Most biologic effects are limited to two to three spectral bands. (Reprinted with permission from Plenum Press.)

Although the ozone layer protects us from most shortwave ultraviolet radiation (UV-B and UV-C), a harmful amount of UV-B does reach the earth. Most of us are familiar with the effects of UV-B: a sunburn. UV-B radiation in the solar spectrum causes such burns of the skin and can seriously affect the eye as well, as seen in snow blindness (an inflammation of the conjunctiva and cornea from reflection of the sunlight on the snow into the eye). Chronic exposures to the ultraviolet rays of the sun can result in cancer and accelerated aging of the skin, and corneal degeneration and lens cataract in the eye. Additionally, most people know the effects on the retina of staring directly into the sun. Every solar eclipse results in reported cases of eclipse blindness. Short wavelengths within the visible spectrum (400 to 500 nm) may be responsible for certain types of retinal degeneration and for accelerating other retinal disease states. [25]

The International Commission on Illumination (CIE) divides the optical spectrum into seven spectral bands. (Figure 18-4) The three areas of ultraviolet radiation are UV-C at 100 to 280 nm, UV-B at 280 to 315 nm, and UV-A at 315 to 400 nm. UV-C is the shortest wave ultraviolet and UV-A is the longest wave ultraviolet. The retina of the eye is not very vulnerable in the ultraviolet or far-infrared portions of the spectrum. It is the cornea and lens that absorb ultraviolet light. High exposure levels can permanently damage these structures of the eye. Intermediate levels in the UV (200 - 320 nm) cause greater injury to the cornea, which is severe but temporary. The injury, photokeratitis, may last for only one or two days but is extremely painful. (Snow blindness and welder's flash are examples of this type of injury.) This type of injury results from excessive exposure to these wavelengths of light. [26]

Near-ultraviolet (long wavelength) and near-infrared radiation (UV-A, IR-A, and possibly IR-B) are absorbed heavily in the lens of the eye. Damage to this structure is of greater concern. The lens has a very long memory. An exposure from one day may have effects that are not evident for many years. While new tissue is continually added around the outside of the lens, the interior tissues remain in the lens for the lifetime of the individual, chronic exposures produce delayed effects. [27]

Human skin shares the same susceptibility to injury as the cornea. This susceptibility occurs in the range of radiant energy present in the ultraviolet spectral region of 200 to 320 nm. This type of radiation causes sunburn and many types of skin cancer. Certain photosensitizing chemicals greatly increase the sensitivity of the skin. Previous exposure to specific wavelength bands that are generally in the long wavelength ultraviolet and visible portion of the spectrum also sensitize skin. The light-sensitizing substances can occur in the skin as a result of diseases such as lupus erythematosus and herpes simplex. Other photosensitizing chemicals reach the skin either directly from contact or indirectly through oral administration: certain fungicides, plants and plant extracts, and the pitch and bacteriostatic agents, such as hexachlorophene, used in soaps. Some orally administered drugs such as tetracyclines also cause this photosensitization. [28]

The factors predisposing you to harm vary with the sensitivity of each individual, the length of exposure and intensity of the ultraviolet light source.

Take the following precautions with the thought in mind that ultraviolet light, at most wavelengths, poses hazards to eyes and skin. Always wear filtered viewing goggles when working with ultraviolet light. Purchase safety goggles that filter UV wavelengths. Always cover unprotected skin with gloves and a laboratory coat. If incidental radiation can be reflected onto the face, wear a face shield made for filtering UV wavelengths. If you are taking a medication that causes photosensitivity, make an extra effort to follow all the mentioned precautions. You may even wish to wear a protective skin cream, such as sun screen, if an ultraviolet shield is not available. Ultraviolet light was once thought to be innocuous, but we now know that it presents some serious hazards.

Electrical Hazards

All light sources that require electricity pose an electrical hazard. High-voltage power supplies make the laser the highest risk. Almost all laser power supplies can cause severe electrical shock and death from electrocution. At least four individuals in the United States have been electrocuted as result of carelessness while working around their lasers, usually when the untrained individual attempt to open and repair the laser. Hardwick, Kent and Sears point out that "all the various types of light source have associated high voltage power supplies. Many of these lamps are ignited by voltages of up to 40,000 volts. Lethally high residual voltages may be present even when the power supply is disconnected from the main supply. On no account should unqualified staff attempt any servicing or repair." [29]

Follow safety standards for electrical safety when using any electrical equipment. Pay special attention to any warnings the manufacturer provides. Before using any electrical equipment, look for warning statements or labels. For instance, the Laserprint 1000 portable laser has a warning label which reads "High voltages - Can be Lethal." Avoid carelessness. Remember that all energy, not just light energy, can pose a hazard to your health and safety.

Chemical Hazards

Although forensic identification specialists use lasers and other high intensity light sources on untreated surfaces to illuminate or stimulate inherent luminescence, they frequently use them in conjunction with other processes, such as cyanoacrylate esters and fluorescent dye stains or powders. Most fluorescent powders are nontoxic, manufactured from lycopodium, a club moss spore. However, the fluorescing agent used as the pigment may not be safe. Rhodamine B, 6G and other dye materials are in questionable status regarding carcinogenicity. Many dye stains, while not carcinogenic, are toxic. Always read the material safety data sheet on any fluorescent powder before usage. If the MSDS indicates any toxicity, use the recommended personal protective equipment, at least a dust/mist respirator and protective clothing. You should automatically wear gloves. Cotton, nitrile or latex gloves are adequate when working with powders.

Before applying a fluorescent dye stain, evidence is fumed with cyanoacrylate esters (superglue) in either a vacuum or an atmospheric chamber. Unless the chamber is built with an extraction system which allows the fumes to vent into a water or charcoal filter or into a fume hood, the fumes present a serious breathing (inhalation) hazard. (If an extraction system is present, extract at least 60 chamber volumes after treatment before opening the chamber.) [30] Upon evaporation, cyanoacrylate esters, either ethyl or methyl, produce fumes that will irritate your mucous membranes, creating an intense burning sensation. Since moisture is a key element to the polymerization of superglue [31], there is every reason to believe that the vapors of cyanoacrylate will also bond with moisture in the eyes and bronchial tubes. Consequently, if your chamber lacks an extraction system, plan your approach to the chamber after the fuming process. Wear an air purifying respirator with an organic vapor cartridge and non-vented goggles. As an alternative, you can use a full face air purifying respirator with the organic vapor canister to offer protection to both your eyes and respiratory system. Place the chamber in front of a fume hood or other ventilation device to trap the vapors and not merely release them out into the laboratory area when you open the chamber.

There have not been any good studies to test the toxicity of cyanoacrylate. It is reported as either not a serious toxicity hazard or carcinogenic. Cyanoacrylate's property of bonding skin to skin and skin to other objects does cause a problem. Always use care when working with cyanoacrylates, and wear cotton, nitrile or latex gloves. Wear safety glasses to help protect your eyes from any potential splashing of liquid glues. Wear a laboratory coat whenever you work in the laboratory.

The remaining problem of working with cyanoacrylate is that of excessive heat. Since heat is often applied to speed up the vaporization of this material, it is important to be aware of the hazard coming from glue which has polymerized [32], such as on a piece of aluminum foil from a past processing. In other words, if you heat hardened glue above 205° C, or 401° F, it will decompose to cyanide gas. Cyanide gas is deadly. Do not reuse any containers which have any hardened residue of glue in them. Handle carefully any hot plates or other heating devices to avoid a serious burn. Make sure all such devices are in good working order and do not create any electrical hazards.

The solvents used to mix fluorescing dye stains pose even more serious and immediate hazards. Commonly used solvents, petroleum ether, ethanol, and methanol, are highly flammable and very poisonous. Wear neoprene or other chemically impervious gloves any time you work with dye stains containing any of these materials. When processing with the dye stain, process in a fume hood or wear an air-purifying respirator with an organic vapor cartridge. Wear chemical splash goggles. You can wear a chemical splash shield for additional face protection. Wear a laboratory coat to protect your clothing and any bare skin.

An amino acid reactive reagent such as 1,8-diazafluoren-9-one (DFO) can be used on porous items such as paper and cardboard. The advantage of this type of fluorescing formulation is in the increased sensitivity of the reagent as well as overcoming difficult background problems. However, handle these types of materials with the same precautions as other amino acid reactive chemicals such as ninhydrin and its analogs. Additionally, the solvents used in the formulations pose serious immediate health hazards. Some solvents may be 2-propanol, petroleum ether, methanol, xylene, ethyl acetate, acetone and acetic acid, toxic and flammable chemicals. When mixing or applying fluorescent chemistry such as DFO, wear neoprene or other chemically impervious gloves. Process in a fume hood, or wear an air purifying respirator with an organic vapor cartridge. Wear chemical splash goggles. You can wear a chemical splash shield for additional face protection. Wear a laboratory coat to protect your clothing and any bare skin.

When examining items already processed with dye stains or other fluorescent chemicals, wear a laboratory coat and at least nitrile or latex gloves. Remember to cover surfaces in the examination area with a material which can be changed and removed routinely. When you finish working the evidence, place it into a protective container and put hazard warning labels on the outside.

Training

Train every forensic identification specialist who is going to work with lasers or other light sources. The training can include an evaluation of the frequency of use and types of the various light sources in the work place. Training programs should encompass a basic explanation of the physics of light, the different classes of lasers, types of light sources, and the use and selection of filters. Explaining engineering controls is an important aspect of safety and accident prevention, helping specialists understand their environment. Reading and discussing the safety manual, viewing a slide presentation and reading and discussing various technical articles or texts may comprise training. Certainly, consider the amount of training an individual may have already received.

Train any individual who may work in and around the laser/light source laboratory, including support personnel who may wish to deliver a telephone message to a specialist and the supervisor who does not routinely perform case work. Develop a training program for all the potential hazards, as well as for all laboratory and office personnel.

Lasers and alternate light sources are one of the most marvelous technologies available to the forensic identification specialist. They have helped solve many cases that would have gone unsolved a mere ten years ago. They should be used at every appropriate opportunity. However, the technology comes with a price and presents very serious safety concerns. With training and knowledge, safety protocols and engineering controls, these light sources can prove to be one of the best tools to date. While not the technology to end all technologies, while not appropriate in all instances nor successful in all cases, they can pull a piece of evidence out of the black hole of "no results" and provide the clues that clench the case. Use them wisely and carefully.

19
Training

Previous sections mention the necessity for training all forensic identification specialists. Training is the key to reducing accidents and illnesses as well as to increasing quality of work. Police departments should not arm officers without first training them in the safe handling and use of weapons. By the same token, laboratories should not put forensic identification specialists to work without training in health and safety. The tide is beginning to turn. The process is slow and tedious because most supervisors are as uninformed on safety issues as their employees. Effective training is ongoing and includes both supervisors and employees. The manager of the facility has the primary responsibility for training. What are the requirements for training? What does the law mandate that employees be taught?

Management must inform employees firstly of any operations in the work area involving hazardous chemicals and secondly, of the location and availability of the written hazard communication program, including the required lists of hazardous chemicals and Material Safety Data Sheets. As 29 CFR 1910.1200, this act has become known as "Right to Know."

The law lists the following areas which must be covered in any training program:

1. Methods and observations that may be used to detect the presence or release of a hazardous (toxic) chemical in the work area. This should include methods directly available to the employee, such as odor or visual appearance of hazardous chemicals being released or the presence of a respiratory irritant or other various symptoms, such as dizziness, weariness or exhaustion. It should also include types of monitoring which can be done whether by the employee, other laboratory personnel or outside public and private agencies.

2. The physical and health effects of the hazardous chemicals which the employees may use or to which they may be exposed.

3. Measures or means of reducing or eliminating the exposure of employees to the risks associated with the hazardous chemicals in the workplace. This includes specific procedures or work practices (such as using solvents in a fume hood instead of in an open room) which will reduce exposures. It also includes the use of personal protective equipment.

4. Details of the Hazard Communication Program developed by the employer, including an explanation of the labeling system and the MSDS, and how employees can obtain and use appropriate hazard information. In practical terms, this relates to the actions the department has taken to minimize the exposure of employees to the chemical hazards. This can include implemented engineering controls, such as fume hoods, ventilation, and other safety-related features of the facility. It can also include policies which encourage compliance (through incentives) to follow/practice safe work practices and penalties for those who violate safe practices.

5. Emergency procedures to follow in the event of an accidental exposure to a hazardous substance.

6. Procedures to warn the non-forensic identification personnel (such as clerical and janitorial), working in the area, of potential exposures.

7. Measures to provide information as to the hazards and the protective measures which can be taken by both the employees and employer to reduce or eliminate hazards associated with non-routine tasks involving chemicals. [1]

Training programs must, at a minimum, provide training and instruction to all employees when the safety program is first established. All new employees, as well as all employees given new job assignments for which training has not been previously provided, must receive training. Whenever new substances, processes, procedures or equipment are introduced to the workplace and present a hazard, management must provide training. Whenever new personal protective equipment or different work practices are used on existing hazards, management must provide training. Whenever an employee or employer (supervisor) learns of a new or previously unrecognized hazard, management must provide training. All supervisors should receive training to assure they are familiar with the safety and health hazards to which employees under their immediate direction and control may be exposed. [2] Safety training should be repeated periodically (many recommend annually) and "provided at no cost to the employee and at a reasonable time and place. It should be tailored to the education and language level of the employee, and offered during the normal work shift." [3]

Training programs should serve as a mechanism to let supervisors know:

- They are key figures responsible for establishment and success of the injury and illness prevention program.

- The importance of establishing and maintaining safe and healthful working conditions.

- They are responsible for being familiar with safety and health hazards to which their employees are exposed, for recognizing them and the potential effects these hazards have on the employees, and for imposing rules, procedures and work practices for controlling exposure to those hazards.

- How to convey this information to employees by setting good examples, instructing them, making sure they fully understand and follow safe procedures.

- How to investigate accidents and take corrective and preventative action. [4]

Training programs should serve as a mechanism to let employees know:

- The success of the department's injury- and illness-prevention program depends on their actions as well as on the actions of the employers.

- The safe work procedures required for their jobs and how these procedures protect them against exposures.

- When personal protective equipment is required or needed, how to use it and maintain it in good condition.

- What to do if emergencies occur in the workplace. [5]

Additionally, each employee needs to understand that:

- No employee is expected to undertake a job until he or she has received instructions on how to do it properly and safely and is authorized to perform the job.

- No employee should undertake a job that appears to be unsafe.

- No employee should use chemicals without fully understanding their toxic properties and without the knowledge required to work with them safely.

- Mechanical safeguards must always be in place and kept in place.

- Employees are to report to a supervisor or designated individual all unsafe conditions encountered during work.

- Any work-related injury or illness suffered, however slight, must be reported to management at once.

- Personal protective equipment must be used when and where required and properly maintained. [6]

In order to accomplish fully the mandates, a number of safety policies must be written and implemented. Once implemented, all employees must receive training on those policies. Such policies should include an injury and illness prevention program, a hazard communication program, an emergency evacuation plan for the facility, and a fire prevention plan. Additional training for the forensic identification specialist should include bloodborne pathogens, chemical hygiene plan, firearms safety, and respiratory protection. These programs will educate individuals in fire safety, personal protective equipment, safe work practices, electrical safety, fume hoods, pressurized systems, and storage of chemicals. At the discretion of the supervisor, some individuals should be trained in CPR and first aid. Any specialists who drive vehicles provided by their agency should receive defensive driving training. Those specialists who process clandestine drug laboratories should also receive training in hazard waste operations and emergency response. [7]

Safety training can be acquired in a number of ways. Firstly, centralize all information on safety policies and organization, emergency procedures, accident reporting, protective clothing and equipment, safety rules for the laboratory, and appropriate specific information on chemical and equipment hazards in a safety manual. Issue every forensic identification specialist a copy of the manual. [8]

Organize training sessions around a variety of methods. Use video tapes to communicate basic safety information. Commercial tapes are available on right-to-know and bloodborne pathogens information. There are many video tapes about safety; however, many are produced for industry and are not really appropriate for the forensic identification laboratory. Some commercial providers will allow their tapes to be reviewed at a small charge. Lectures and presentations by guest speakers can be very effective. Slide presentations allow for audience participation. Hands-on demonstrations effectively introduce individuals to new equipment, materials and processes. Develop drills to familiarize people with emergency situations. Quizzes and questionnaires assist employees to recognize areas of knowledge or deficiency. All these methods are proven effective. Some require more planning than others. In my opinion, you are not trained by simply reading a document and then signing a paper indicating you have read it. You should always have an opportunity to ask questions.

Once s/he completes training for a given area, the employee should document that training was provided [9] by signing a dated statement which identifies the training received. Retain these documents for the duration of the person's employment. If the specialist was exposed to materials known to pose problems with chronic health effects, maintain the records for as long as five years longer. [10]

You must have a training program to have a complete safety program. Training provides the pathway to knowledge and accident prevention.

20
Applications

This section briefly recommends safety equipment used during many forensic identification processes. Some departments will require their specialists to wear more equipment. The information should serve as a guideline for mixing or using the reagents or performing the procedures. This information is based on laboratory applications. Processing in the field often changes the equipment requirements.

Amido Black (Naphthalene Black)	Wear a laboratory coat, neoprene or other chemically impervious gloves and chemical safety goggles. This technique is used on items containing blood, so employ universal precautions. Do all processing in a fume hood because of methanol and acetic acid. Methanol is flammable and toxic. Acetic acid is corrosive and combustible. If a fume hood is not available, wear an air purifying respirator equipped with an organic vapor cartridge in an area with good local ventilation. Always wash hands before leaving the laboratory.
Blood Reactive Reagents (Diaminobenzidine) (Tetramethylbenzidine) (Leucomalachite Green) (O-Tolidine)	Wear a laboratory coat, neoprene or other chemically impervious gloves and chemical safety goggles. This technique is used on items containing blood, so employ universal precautions. Do all processing in a fume hood because of alcohols and/ or acids. Alcohols are flammable and toxic. Acids are corrosive and possibly combustible. Some of these reagents are suspected carcinogens. Do not spray these reagents, because they react with constituents of blood. Instead of spraying, pipette the reagent over the

	surface. If a fume hood is not available, wear an air purifying respirator equipped with an organic vapor cartridge in an area with good local ventilation. Always wash hands before leaving the laboratory.
Crystal (Gentian) Violet	Wear a laboratory coat, neoprene or other chemically impervious gloves and safety goggles. Do all processing in a fume hood, if you use ethanol formulation. Ethanol is flammable and toxic. Phenol is very toxic. Always wash hands before leaving the laboratory.
Cyanoacrylate Ester (Superglue)	Wear a laboratory coat and latex or nitrile gloves. Wear safety glasses while working in the laboratory, or non-vented safety goggles, if there is any hazard of exposure to the fumes. Design a system for exhaust ventilation of fumes with the atmospheric chamber. Before building a vacuum cyanoacrylate chamber, thoroughly research construction materials. Organic acids in CAE will cause PVC pipe to lose its integrity, posing a serious implosion hazard. Never place closed containers such as aerosol cans, bottles with caps, light bulbs or batteries in the vacuum system, because they may explode. Cyanoacrylate ester fumes are an irritant to the respiratory system in concentrations above 2 ppm, about the minimum level that can be detected by smell. Cyanoacrylate products will bond skin to skin and skin to other objects. Excessive heat can be a problem with polymerized or hardened glue. Cured glue that is heated above 205° C, 401° F, will decompose to deadly cyanide gas. Use caution when handling any hot plates or other heating devices to avoid a serious burn. Make sure all such devices are in good working order and do not create any electrical hazards. Always wash hands before leaving the laboratory.

Deceased Casework	Wear a laboratory coat and nitrile gloves. Wear chemical splash goggles and a particulate mask. A nuisance odor mask may help alleviate unpleasant odors. Do not place Vicks in the nostrils. Vicks or peppermint oil can be placed in the particulate mask. For extreme conditions, use an air purifying respirator equipped with an organic vapor cartridge. Work in a well ventilated area. Always apply universal precautions when working with human flesh and body fluids. Avoid use of formalin or formaldehyde solutions. Some ridge building materials may be toxic. Always wash hands before leaving the laboratory.
DFO (1,8-Diazafluoren-9-one)	Wear a laboratory coat, neoprene or other chemically impervious gloves and safety goggles. Do all processing in a fume hood. If a fume hood is not available, wear an air purifying respirator equipped with an organic vapor cartridge in an area with good local ventilation. Do not spray this material, because it reacts with amino acids. Health studies are incomplete on DFO crystals, so treat them the same as Ninhydrin. Most solvents, with the exception of 1,1,2 Trichlorotrifluoroethane, are flammable. All solvents are toxic. Always wash hands before leaving the laboratory.
ESDA (Electrostatic Detection Apparatus)	Wear a laboratory coat and latex nitrile or cotton gloves. Use in a well-ventilated room with good local exhaust ventilation, because the process generates ozone, a severe respiratory hazard. Toning beads used in process are of questionable toxicity. Always wash hands before leaving the laboratory.
Fluorescent Dye Stains	Wear a laboratory coat, neoprene or other chemically impervious gloves and safety goggles. Do all processing in a fume hood. If a fume hood is not available, wear an air purifying respirator equipped with an organic vapor cartridge in an area with good local ventilation. Most of these dye stains are mixed with solvents such as ethanol and methanol. Ethanol and

methanol are flammable and toxic. Some of these stains are suspected carcinogens. Always wash hands before leaving the laboratory.

Hot Flame Method	Wear a laboratory coat, latex or nitrile gloves, and safety goggles if any risk of getting smoke into eyes. Otherwise, wear safety glasses while using procedure. Do all processing in a fume hood with the ventilation turned off or in an area with good local exhaust ventilation, because you produce smoke. Wear a particulate mask, if not using a fume hood. Don't inhale smoke from materials used in this process (camphor or magnesium). Take extra care to work in an area away from any possible flammables. Always wash hands before leaving the laboratory.
Ink Analysis	Wear a laboratory coat, neoprene or other chemically impervious gloves and safety goggles. Do all processing in a fume hood. Some chemicals used are toxic and/or corrosive. Always wash hands before leaving the laboratory.
Iodine	Wear a laboratory coat, neoprene, nitrile or other chemically impervious gloves and safety goggles when preparing/using fixing solutions. Otherwise, latex gloves are sufficient. Do all processing in a fume hood. Iodine is very corrosive and toxic. Iodine fixing solutions are considered toxic. Always wash hands before leaving the laboratory.
Light Examination (ALS, Laser, UV)	Wear a laboratory coat and latex or nitrile gloves. Wear laser or UV approved safety goggles. Avoid shining light into eyes or on skin; especially avoid shining UV light onto skin anywhere on the body. If conducting extended examination, wear a UV approved safety shield. Always wash hands before leaving the laboratory.

Ninhydrin	Wear a laboratory coat, neoprene or other chemically impervious gloves and chemical safety goggles. Do all processing in a fume hood. If a fume hood is not available, wear an air purifying respirator equipped with an organic vapor cartridge in an area with good local ventilation. Do not spray this material, because it reacts with amino acids. Instead of spraying, pipette the reagent over the surface. Ninhydrin is toxic and an irritant. Most solvents, with the exception of 1,1,2 Trichlorotrifluoro-ethane, are flammable. All solvents are toxic. Always wash hands before leaving the laboratory.
Photography	Wear a laboratory coat and latex or nitrile gloves. While mixing photographic chemicals, wear safety goggles and a particulate mask. When photographing fluorescing prints, wear laser or UV approved safety goggles. Fume-sensitive specialists have reacted with tears, coughs, or labored breathing to reheated, dried Ninhydrin deposits. If you experience such reactions when you photograph chemically developed evidence prints under high intensity lights, use an air purifying respirator equipped with high efficiency particulate air filter (HEPA) cartridges to trap the airborne contaminate. [1] Always wash hands before leaving the laboratory.
Physical Developer	Wear a laboratory coat, nitrile gloves and chemical safety goggles or safety glasses. Mix the reagent and process evidence in an area with good general ventilation. Various components of the formulation are corrosive, irritants or toxic. Silver nitrate is especially toxic. Acids used for pre-wash are corrosive. Always wash hands before leaving the laboratory.
Powders	Wear a laboratory coat and latex or nitrile gloves. Safety goggles are optional but help protect your eyes from airborne powder particulate. Process evidence in a fume hood or at a slot hood. If no local ventilation

system is available, wear a particulate mask, always when working with metal powders (aluminum, etc.). Some powders are quite toxic if they contain polynuclear aromatic hydrocarbons or cadmium. These chemicals have been identified as carcinogens. Most fluorescent powders are non-toxic. Always consult the MSDS on any powder before use to determine possible toxicity. Always wash hands before leaving the laboratory.

Silver Nitrate	Wear a laboratory coat, neoprene or other chemically impervious gloves and chemical safety goggles. Do all processing in a fume hood, if using formulations which contain ethanol or methanol. If a fume hood is not available, wear an air purifying respirator equipped with an organic vapor cartridge in an area with good local ventilation. Ethanol and methanol are flammable and toxic. Silver nitrate is toxic. If developing prints with an ultra violet lamp, use caution not to expose bare skin to light. Use UV approved safety glasses. Always wash hands before leaving the laboratory.
Small Particle Reagent (Molybdenum Disulfide)	Wear a laboratory coat, latex or nitrile gloves and chemical safety goggles. Use in area with good general ventilation. Molybdenum can be toxic. Always wash hands before leaving the laboratory.
Sticky-Side Powder	Wear laboratory coat, latex or nitrile gloves and chemical safety goggles when mixing formulation. Wear safety glasses while applying. Safety studies are not complete on the toner material. It may be an irritant or toxic. Always wash hands before leaving the laboratory.
Sudan Black	Wear a laboratory coat, neoprene or other chemically impervious gloves and chemical safety goggles. Do all processing in a fume hood because of ethanol. If

a fume hood is not available, wear an air purifying respirator equipped with an organic vapor cartridge in an area with good local ventilation. Sudan Black B is toxic. Ethanol is flammable and toxic. Always wash hands before leaving the laboratory.

Vacuum Metal Deposition

Wear a laboratory coat, nitrile gloves and safety glasses. Wear low temperature gloves, face shield and apron when handling liquid nitrogen. Wear particulate mask when cleaning chamber in a manner which may generate dust. Never put closed containers such as aerosol cans, bottles with caps, light bulbs or batteries in the vacuum system, because they may explode. Zinc is toxic. Liquid nitrogen causes severe burns. Use liquid nitrogen in areas with good general ventilation and never inhale the vapors. If using other sequences with vacuum metal deposition, such as cyanoacrylate fuming and fluorescent dye staining, follow the safety guidelines for those procedures. Always wash hands before leaving the laboratory.

Zinc Chloride

Wear a laboratory coat, neoprene or other chemically impervious gloves and chemical safety goggles. Do all processing in a fume hood, because of solvents such as methanol or petroleum ether. If a fume hood is not available, wear an air purifying respirator equipped with an organic vapor cartridge in an area with good local ventilation. Methanol and petroleum ether are flammable and toxic. If using liquid nitrogen to stimulate fluorescence, follow all guidelines listed above in vacuum metal deposition. Use laser safety goggles when making fluorescence examinations or performing fluorescence photography. Always wash hands before leaving the laboratory.

21 Aspergillus

During the 19th century, there was a boom of archaeological interest in Egypt and the old tombs and crypts buried within the desert. In 1891, Englishman Howard Carter arrived in Egypt in search of the undiscovered tomb of the somewhat unknown boy-King, Pharaoh Tutankhamen. Relying upon the financial backing of wealthy Lord Carnarvon, Carter spent over five years digging for the missing Pharaoh. In 1922, Carter's workmen finally unearthed an ancient doorway bearing the name Tutankhamen. Within hours, a curse was pronounced by some of the more superstitious workmen upon any persons disturbing the tomb. Carter wired Lord Carnarvon to come to Egypt for the opening of the tomb and discovery of the inevitable treasures. Carnarvon arrived and stood behind Carter as he opened the door for the first time in centuries. The tomb was intact and contained all the treasures and riches the royal one would need in the next life. This includes grains and other organic items for the after life.

A few months later Lord Carnarvon, 57, was tragically taken ill and rushed to Cairo. He died within days. While the exact cause of death was unknown, it seemed related to an infection from a mosquito bite opened while shaving. Carnarvon, with his resistance lowered, succumbed to pneumonia. For many years, some people insisted that Lord Carnarvon had fallen victim of the mummy's curse.

In 1999, German microbiologist, Gotthard Kramer of the University of Leipzig, suggested a scientific explanation for the death. Analysis of 40 mummies resulted in the identification of several potentially dangerous mold spores on each. Mold spores are tenacious and can survive thousands of years in a dark, dry environment. Kramer opined that when the tombs were first opened and fresh air gusted inside, these mold spores could have been blown up into the air. "When spores enter the body through the nose, mouth or eye mucous membranes," he adds, "they can lead to organ failure or even death, particularly in individuals with weakened immune systems." [1]

Specifically for this reason, archaeologists today wear protective gear such as masks and gloves when unwrapping mummies. Some believe the curse of the mummy was possibly a mold spore named *Aspergillus flavus*.

While there are some 100,000 types of molds in existence, only a few dozen produce toxins. *Aspergillus* is just such a group of molds that can pose pathogenic problems. These "opportunistic fungi" exist worldwide, especially in the Northern Hemisphere. They are a natural part of the ecosystem and assist in the decomposition of decaying matter. *Aspergillus* infestations have been documented throughout the United States and Canada in houses, schools and colleges, office buildings, police facilities and hospitals. It has been found thriving in wallboard and plywood, stucco, insulation, carpets and the underside of roof sheathing. Air conditioners can become infested with mold and then spread the spores into ventilated rooms.

While *Aspergillus* grows in decaying vegetation, this mold concerns the law enforcement community because of its documented growth in marijuana. Marijuana is an abundant and richly organic material perfect for introducing *Aspergillus* into the police facility. Decay occurs as result of harvested green plant material not being adequately dried. The problem is most prevalent when marijuana is placed in plastic bags. However, there is potential for fungus development in quantities of moist marijuana placed in paper. Residual moisture in the marijuana encourages bacterial growth, which in turn facilitates the growth of molds. Current knowledge indicates that "this fungi can thrive at elevated temperatures. It tends to be abundant in damp, decaying vegetation heated by bacterial fermentation. As the temperature rises, other micro-organisms cease to grow, but Aspergilli will flourish under these conditions and can almost become a pure culture."[2] Only a few of these molds can cause disease in humans.

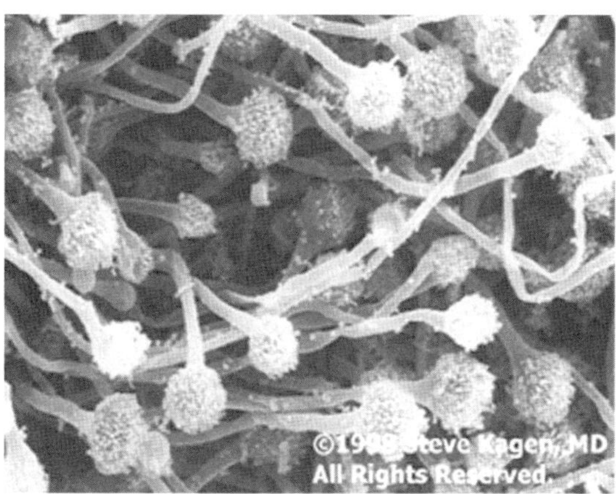

Figure 21-1: Aspergillus mold.

<u>*Aspergillus Fumigatus*</u> is diagnosed in 90% of all *Aspergillus* infections. Initially a threadlike flat white growth, it becomes a powdery, blue-green mold as consequence of production of spores. Handling the decaying material can re-

sult in an inhalation exposure to the spores. Anyone working with such decaying plant material may be subject to potential health hazards arising from *Aspergillus*. Physicians have found these spores in the ears, nose and lungs of humans. In fact, Dr. Steve Kagen, a well published physician and professor of Allergy/Immunology at the Medical College of Wisconsin, informed the author, "We identified *Aspergillus* in every sample of marijuana that we cultured in our research studies in 1980-81. *Aspergillus* is a potent cause of asthma, and as many as 10% of all patients with asthma have it living in their airways - and they are allergic to it. The disease is called ABPA, or Allergic Bronchopulmonary Aspergillosis." [3] While some may consider marijuana an innocuous material, it poses real health hazards to individuals working around it at crime scenes and in evidence vaults or property rooms.

While *Aspergillus* is considered opportunistic fungi, most people are naturally immune to the mycotoxins and do not develop *Aspergillus* related disease, Aspergillosis. The severity of Aspergillosis is related to various factors including the state of an individual's immune system or the presence of a predisposed condition. Thus, persons with compromised immune systems are at greater risk of infection. Most initial infections are as result of inhalation of spores and involve the respiratory system. When the disease does occur, it takes several forms.

Aspergillosis can range from sinusitis conditions to pulmonary infections as severe as pneumonia. Allergic aspergillosis typically becomes chronic. Continued colonization of the spores in the body may result in the continuation of a chronic condition or can become invasive. [4]

Aspergillus disease can occur in the sinuses leading to *Aspergillus* Sinusitis. In individuals with <u>normal</u> immune systems, stuffiness of the nose, chronic headache or discomfort of the face is common. Drainage of the sinus, by surgery, usually cures the problem, unless the *Aspergillus* has entered the sinuses deep inside the skull. Then antifungal drugs and surgery are usually successful. When individuals have <u>damaged</u> immune systems such as is caused by leukemia or a bone marrow transplant, *Aspergillus* Sinusitis is more threatening. This type of sinusitis is a form of invasive aspergillosis. Symptoms include fever, facial pain, nasal discharge and headaches. Diagnosis is made by finding the fungus in fluid or tissue from the sinuses and with scans. Powerful antifungal drugs are essential in the treatment. Surgery is done in most cases as a step in determining exactly the nature of the problem and is often helpful in eradicating the fungus. [5]

Allergic bronchopulmonary aspergillosis (ABPA) results where an allergy

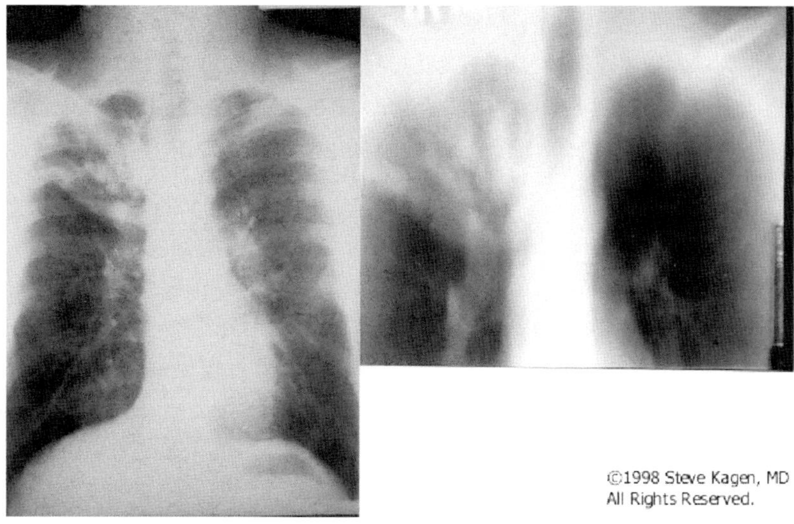

Figure 21-2: Left X-ray shows healthy lung while right X-ray shows Aspergillus infected lung.

to the mold spores develops. This condition is quite common in asthmatics; up to 20% of asthmatics might get this at some time during their lives. The symptoms are similar to those of asthma; intermittent episodes of feeling unwell, coughing and wheezing. Some patients cough up brown colored plugs of mucus. Diagnosis can be made by X-ray or by sputum, skin and blood tests. If untreated, long term ABPA can lead to permanent lung damage. [6]

Many people with damaged or impaired immune systems die from invasive aspergillosis. The earlier the diagnosis is made the higher their chance of survival. Unfortunately, there is no good diagnostic test. Often, treatment has to be initiated when the condition is only suspected. This condition is usually clinically diagnosed in persons with low defenses resulting from medical conditions such as bone marrow transplant, low white cells after chemotherapy, AIDS or major burns are at moderate risk of infection. A rare inherited condition that gives people low immunity (chronic granulomatous disease) also puts these people at moderate risk. Individuals with invasive aspergillosis usually have a fever and symptoms from the lungs (cough, chest pain or discomfort or breathlessness) which do not respond to standard antibiotics. [7]

In extreme cases, the fungus can transfer from the lung through the blood stream to the brain and other organs, including the eye, the heart, the kidneys and the skin. Usually this is a sign that the individual has a severe infection with a higher risk of death. However, sometimes infection of the skin enables an earlier diagnosis and treatment. [8]

This is a rather extensive explanation of *Aspergillus* and the resulting Aspergillosis conditions. It is not intended to create fear and panic but rather to begin necessary dialogue and awareness. Most individuals will never be confronted with the more serious aspergillosis conditions. However, many people are potentially at risk for *Aspergillus* exposure in the laboratory, at crime scenes and in the property and evidence room. Such exposures could result in developing a sensitivity to this fungus. In fact, I have spoken with a number of individuals across the United States who have suffered serious health problems as result of exposure to an *Aspergillus* rich enviroment while at work. So, the core issue is what can be done to avoid *Aspergillus* exposures and other ancillary problems.

The real issue is not the existence of *Aspergillus* but the reality of dealing with these fungal spores in the work environment. *Aspergillus* problems in the police facility, the laboratory or at crime scenes can be attributed to the following problems:

- An *Aspergillus* rich culture in the environment.
- Inadequate ventilation in the environment
- Improperly packaged marijuana being stored.
- Large quantities of marijuana being stored.
- Inadequate housekeeping in the evidence/property area.
- Inadequate use of personal protective equipment.
- Rodent infestation and the Hantavirus

It has already been established that *Aspergillus* will thrive in an environment that is warm and provides area for the spores to continue developing. When marijuana has become extensively contaminated with *Aspergillus*, it becomes a living receptacle and potential amplifier for microorganisms. Once spores have escaped the initial environment (i.e., packaging or container), they will layer out on any available surface. The matrix of the police facility whether the laboratory or evidence area often provides these surfaces. Walls and floors consisting of concrete that exhibit small openings in the matrix provide an excellent area for fungal spores to lodge. Porous surfaces such as cardboard boxes, leather, paper and burlap bags, and building insulation support and serve as a reservoir for microorganisms when dirt and debris become trapped in the pores. [9] Activity in and around these reservoirs of spores and dust disturbs the particulate layers and they become airborne. This provides an excellent opportunity for personnel to receive inhalation exposures. These exposures are not necessarily confined to the forensic identification specialist or property room officers. Once *Aspergillus* is thriving, it can make its way into other areas of the building. Since crime scenes are uncontrolled sites and any condition can prevail, the best prevention strategy is to use appropriate personal protective equipment to protect the eyes and any mucous membrane.

Ventilation plays a key role in maintaining an *Aspergillus* free environment. Forensic identification laboratories, as well as property and evidence facilities should have a separate, negative pressure ventilation system that vents outside the building. Inadequate ventilation promotes the multiplication of microorganisms which in turn allows them to become highly concentrated. Where HVAC systems are in place, the filters must be replaced on strictly scheduled intervals. Dirty, contaminated filters reduce the effective filtration and causes microorganisms to reproduce and recirculate into the work area. [10] Suitable clean, filtered outside makeup air must be provided. While local codes may vary, a minimum should be at least 10 liters per second per occupant. Inadequate ventilation systems should be upgraded as soon as possible.

Marijuana is often submitted as evidence in burlap or paper bags. Unfortunately, these packaging materials provide an excellent matrix for the escape of *Aspergillus* spores. The real problem with marijuana, as a decomposing plant material, is the moisture content left in the plant. Living marijuana plants contain about 80% water. Fungi cannot grow below 15% moisture content. Perfectly dried marijuana contains about 10% -15% water. [11] Most growers of illicit marijuana market their product above 15% since it is sold as soon as possible and by weight and not volume. This is the product that is submitted to the evidence facility. In addition to the problem of yet moist, packaged marijuana is the often-whole plant that has been pulled up from a cultivation site. Both scenarios present the impossible question: how much moisture content is still present in any given amount of marijuana being submitted into evidence? The answer is unknowable. The only adequately dried marijuana is that which is brittle. Since the moisture content is an uncontrollable factor, packaging becomes the only solution to the problem.

Proper packaging presents its own dilemma. Burlap and paper provide an inadequate barrier to contain *Aspergillus* spores. The only material left is an impermeable bag. Such bags are usually manufactured of plastic. Plastics create the problem that moisture-laden marijuana enclosed in such material will eventually decompose into a material equivalent to mush and soup. Once in this state, its evidentiary value may come into question. Management must make the decision regarding packaging versus the potential for introduction of *Aspergillus* spores into the law enforcement facility.

In fact, most agencies store quantities of marijuana that may not need to be maintained in their facility. Firstly, marijuana should not continue to be stored if the case has been adjudicated. Such marijuana should be sent for destruction as soon as reasonably possible. Secondly, agencies should make a commitment to maintain only the amount of marijuana required by law to adjudicate the case. Why not document and photograph the excessive amounts of marijuana, take necessary samples for laboratory analysis, and then destroy it. Considering the potential health hazards presented by quantities of marijuana, why take the risk of becoming infested with *Aspergillus* spores. All efforts should be made to reduce the amount of marijuana being held in the evidence facility. Evidence should be inspected as it is delivered and cleaned and sealed appropriately before being stored.

Air monitoring of a facility will detect suspected molds. (If mold spores are found to be present at a level of 100,000 spores per cubic meter, then mold is probably growing in the environment.) However, unless mold is suspected in a facility, air monitoring will be unlikely to transpire. Such monitoring is usually performed by an Industrial Hygienist and has all the associated costs. Prevention is the key. Housekeeping procedures present one of the best solutions and preventative measures available for contamination problems in the police facility.

If a building or area of the building is suspected of being contaminated, corrective measures can be taken. Discard all porous building materials and property that are visually contaminated with fungi. Remove baseboards, walls and insulation. Wash the entire area down with a dilute bleach solution (1 cup per gallon of water). All smooth surfaces potentially contaminated with fungus should be included in the decontamination. Replace H-VAC filters and disinfect or replace the entire system. Workers performing decontamination must be provided with adequate personal protective equipment including protective clothing, gloves, goggles, shoe covers and particulate masks.

Discarded items should be placed in plastic bags and carefully disposed of as a biohazard. If the contaminated area is 10 to 30 feet square, hang a plastic sheet around the area being cleaned to capture disrupted spores. If the contaminated area is larger than 10 to 30 square feet, trained technicians should professionally clean it.

Once decontamination is complete, seal all porous surfaces such as concrete walls to eliminate dust and debris settling points. These settling areas provide reservoirs for microbial growth. Vacuum and wet wipe (with an anti-fungal agent) all building and content surfaces in the evidence facility. [12]

It is imperative that a regular schedule for housekeeping be developed that includes vacuuming and surface cleaning with appropriate disinfectants. This may require an attitude upgrade on the part of the evidence facility personnel. Housekeeping should never be viewed as an extra responsibility. It is an integral part of her/his job and is a standard part of operations.

Personal protective equipment is the mainstay of protection for personnel in providing necessary protective barriers between them and a potentially damaging material. When handling or storing marijuana, long sleeves, gloves and a dust/particulate respirator should be worn. Disposable sleeves can be purchased through many safety equipment suppliers. A jump suit or protective coat/smock will provide such protection. Latex gloves are adequate but a no powder vinyl or nitrile glove may be preferable where latex sensitivity is a concern. While a standard dust/particulate mask is adequate, some individuals may prefer to use a High Efficiency Particulate (HEPA) mask. Personnel who exhibit microbial sensitivities are often more confident of protection with this type of mask. As added protection, eye goggles (chemical splash) can be worn to assure that no *Aspergillus* spores can lodge in the moist areas of the eyes while handling marijuana.

Since crime scenes containing marijuana are uncontrolled sites and any condition can prevail, the best protection available to identification personnel is to use protective clothing, gloves, goggles, shoe covers and particulate masks. Again, if an *Aspergillus* rich environment is suspected, a HEPA mask would provide better protection to the respiratory system.

As previously noted, personal protective equipment should always be worn during decontamination of the storage facility. Management must encourage all employees to review labels on disinfecting agents prior to use. Adequate ventilation must be provided when performing decontamination.

If you suspect you have Aspergillosis, an allergist or immunologist must see you. Most family practice physicians will diagnose your symptoms as flu. An allergist will do a panel on you for *Aspergillus* to determine its presence in your system. How do you know if you have it? If you are always sick at work or seem to react to "something" in areas where marijuana is or has been stored, you need to see a physician. If you ever dig a black ball of material from your ears or nose (with the exception of fingerprint powder), by all means, see a physician immediately! Once you have an *Aspergillus* infection, you may have to take medication long term and get allergy shots. You may be permanently asthmatic. If your immune system is seriously compromised, an infection could be life threatening. This is a serious matter and should never be taken lightly.

An ancillary problem related to marijuana storage is the problem of rodents. Unfortunately, mice like to eat and nest in marijuana. The most obvious sign of mouse infestation is the appearance of droppings. The health hazard comes with the infestation by the common deer mouse. This mouse is prevalent throughout the United States. It is also a carrier of the Hantavirus, which attacks the respiratory system. The resulting disease, Hantavirus Pulmonary Syndrome (HPS), caused the death of a number of people in the Four Corners area of the United States in 1993 and cases continue to be reported to this day. In fact, as of April 2001, 283 Hantavirus cases were confirmed in 31 states. [13]

The hazard is associated with an accumulation of mouse droppings and urine and saliva. The virus gets into the air as mist from urine and saliva or dust from feces. Breathing in air borne particulate from the droppings when swept up or moved around is the most common way of becoming infected. Additionally, you can receive a contact exposure by touching your mouth or nose after handling contaminated items. And lastly, a rodent bite can also cause infection with the virus.

Symptoms of Hantavirus include fever (101°-104° F) and aching muscles as well as abdominal, joint and lower back pain. Many people experience chills, cough, headache and intestinal problems such as nausea, vomiting or diarrhea. The incubation period can be as short as three days or as long as six weeks. Once there is an onset of symptoms, the disease worsens rapidly. As fluid enters the lungs, patients develop breathing difficulties. Treatment requires intensive care, supplemental oxygen and ventilator support. [14]

If the laboratory or property and evidence areas display obvious signs of mouse droppings or infestation, measures should be taken immediately to eliminate these rodents. The mice are best removed by trapping. Once trapped, they should be sprayed with a disinfectant solution of 1 cup bleach to 10 cups of water. Always wear rubber gloves where handling any dead rodents or traps. Any traps, dead rodents or other contaminated materials must be placed in plastic bags, sealed and disposed of in the garbage.

Personal protective equipment should be worn during any cleaning procedures. This would include rubber gloves, protective clothing, goggles, shoe covers and particulate masks with a rating of N95. According to Dawn Viebrock and Mary Ann O'Garro of the Grant County Health District in Washington, buildings should be aired out for at least one hour prior to entering to clean. "Any dead rodents, droppings, and nesting materials in the building should be wet down with a bleach solution and the debris scooped up with a shovel. Dusting, sweeping, vacuuming or any other activity that would stir up dust should be avoided if at all possible." [15]

Again, prevention is the best strategy for avoiding infestations. Sealing all openings and cracks in walls, floors, foundations and pipe openings will remove possible rodent access points. The exterior of the building should also be maintained in a manner that discourages rodents from nesting. Debris should be removed and weeds, brush and grass should be kept cut.

It truly is imperative that forensic identification specialists and evidence facility personnel and their management recognize the hazards of handling and storing marijuana. Once the awareness is there, preventative steps can be taken to ensure a healthier work environment.

22
Crime Scene Safety

I strongly recommend that individuals working crime scenes take the time to read all the other sections of this book. Most safety issues that arise at crime scenes also occur in the laboratory and are addressed in detail in other sections. Such detail will not be repeated in this section.

Crime scene safety is an enormous topic. Every scene is different and can pose a variety of different hazards. Concerns regarding the potential for biological hazards remain the same regardless of the scene. However, other scenes, such as arsons, often pose entirely different hazards due to weakened structures. As result, the forensic identification specialist must also be aware of possible falling materials and trip hazards. Clandestine drug laboratories bring in another array of concerns from booby traps and explosive devices to acid fumes and thermal stress. Consequently, this section will address general safety issues such as biological hazards, chemical hazards, contamination, personal protective equipment, safety protocols and hazardous waste. Additionally, hazards specific to arsons and bombings, autopsies, clandestine laboratories, disasters, exhumations, homicides and suicides, and underwater scenes will also be discussed.

The crime scene is an extension of the work place. Safety requirements placed on employers also apply at crime scenes. All law enforcement agencies that provide forensic identification personnel for processing scenes should have written guidelines and procedures as a part of their Hazard Communication Program. Employees must be educated and trained on the hazards of any type of crime scene they may be expected to attend as a part of their job duties. The Occupational Health and Safety Administration (OSHA) is very clear on these requirements as spelled out by 29 CFR(Code of Federal Regulations) 1910. This standard requires written policies and training for any potential chemical hazards (including latent fingerprint powders) or bloodborne pathogens. This is the first step in crime scene safety!

Bloodborne Hazards

Universal Precautions

While the issues surrounding bloodborne pathogens is detailed in Section 5, some safety protocols bear repeating. When in an environment where potentially infectious materials (PIMs) may exist, ALWAYS apply **universal precautions** (a safety strategy used for infection control). This means that all blood; human tissue and other body fluids, which contain visible blood, must be treated as though they are infected. In other words, treat these materials as if they are known to be infectious for HBV, HCV, HIV and other bloodborne pathogens.

Engineering and Work Practice Controls

Engineering and work practice controls are the best defense to infection and contamination problems. Adequate hand washing includes the use of antibacterial soap and running water for at least two or three minutes. If antibacterial soap is not available, traditional bar soaps are as adequate. The most important aspect is that plenty of soap is applied and all surfaces of the hands and fingers are cleansed.

Use mechanical means to pick up broken glass or other sharp objects. NEVER use the hands only. This can be accomplished with forceps, a "grabber" tool or a dust pan and broom. Always use a leakproof/puncture resistant container capable of being closed tightly for collecting and transporting Sharps. Never reach into dark or concealed areas searching for evidence. Use flashlights, mirrors and paint stirrers (or other available implements) to search confined spaces.

Make it a practice to post hazard warning signs with the Universal Biohazard symbol on access doors where biological fluids are present at scenes. Remember that "safety begins with YOU" and each of us also has a moral obligation to look out for other people as well. If you are aware of a potential hazard, spread the word to anyone else who could be at risk. The beauty of hazard signs is that they remain at the scene after you leave. So individuals who must access the scene for other functions, whether investigative or sanitation, are also informed of the hazards.

Never eat, drink, smoke or apply contact lenses or cosmetics at the scene where PIMs may exist. Do not place your personal clothing (jackets, gloves, etc.) or items (purses, lunch, etc.) at scene areas. Leave these items in your vehicle until needed. Avoid touching clean surfaces with contaminated gloves. Never place items such as pens or pencils in your mouth. (This seems a pretty basic and straightforward thought but some people do habitually and subconsciously put things in their mouths.) Make sure that you follow proper procedures in removing personal protective equipment at the end of scene processing. Not following proper procedure may result in the contamination of unprotected skin or clothing.

Personal Protective Equipment (PPE)

The purpose of personal protective equipment is to prevent PIMs from passing through or reaching personal clothing, skin and mucous membranes such as the eyes, nose and mouth. A detailed description of PPE can be found in Section 8. However, the following points are especially important to remember.

- Protective Clothing is a must at scenes. Personal clothing and footwear should never be worn exclusively without additional protection. Disposable fluid-resistant gowns, coveralls or jump suits should be worn over personal clothing. Disposable shoe covers prevent the transfer of contaminates to vehicles, the laboratory, headquarters and your home. In situations where ceilings are blood spattered, wear a disposable hair cover. When selecting protective clothing, take into consideration the working environment and any temperature extremes. Some materials do not breathe and can add to heat stress.

- Gloves are one of the most important pieces of PPE. Latex or vinyl gloves are worn for anticipated hand contact with PIMs, contaminated items or surfaces. Any glove used should be 8 to 10 mils thick at a minimum. Latex gloves have a documented history of problems. High temperature, Ultra-Violet light (including sunlight) or prolonged storage will cause the gloves to deteriorate. Try blowing into the gloves before donning them. This will assist you in assessing the integrity of the glove for obvious flaws. One thing to keep in mind is the nature of the latex material. Unfortunately, if a pinhole has developed, the latex tends to self-seal, making the flaw very difficult to detect. This has led some people to double gloving. They mistakenly feel that they are better protected wearing two pair of gloves rather than one pair. There are reasons and occasions in which double gloving is recommended. However, protection from PIMs is not such an occasion. Wearing two pair of gloves gives a false sense of security. Following the same logic, if two pair is safer than one, why not don five or six pair? Rather than go down this path of "how many are enough?"; choose a better glove. An alternate glove to latex is nitrile. The nitrile glove gives the same protection against PIMs but has the added quality of ripping when donned if a flaw is present in the material.

- Latex sensitivity is an additional consideration when selecting latex gloves. People who are exposed to latex gloves (and other products containing natural rubber latex) can develop allergic reactions including skin rashes, hives, nasal, sinus or eye symptoms, asthma and even shock. If you choose latex gloves, use powder-free gloves with reduced protein content. (The allergy-causing proteins or antigens are the problem.) Learn to recognize symptoms of latex allergy: skin rashes; flushing; itching; nasal, eye, or sinus symptoms. Some people know they have this sensitivity and use other gloves. But for others, the sensitivity comes on suddenly and unexpectedly. One forensic identification specialist had to be rushed to the hospital within minutes of donning her latex gloves. She had never had any past problems but on this particular day, she ended up in anaphylactic shock, gasping for air, face swollen and eyes nearly swollen shut. She did recover but be aware that once a latex sensitivity rears its ugly head, you can never come in contact with latex again. If you develop symptoms of latex allergy, avoid direct contact with latex gloves and products until you can see a physician experienced in treating latex allergy. If you have latex allergy, consult your physician regarding taking precautions. These may include: avoiding contact with latex gloves and products; avoiding areas where you might inhale the powder from the latex gloves worn by others; telling your employer, physicians, nurses, and dentists that you have latex allergy; and wearing a medical alert bracelet. Take advantage of all latex allergy education and any training provided by your employer. [1]

- Face and Eye Protection are necessary to protect the mucous membranes of the eyes, nose and mouth from potential contact with HBV, HCV, HIV and other bloodborne pathogens. Wear a face mask (particulate) combined with safety glasses having solid side shields, or goggles, where splashes, sprays or droplets of PIMs may be generated (as in autopsies). Face shields offer added protection when worn in addition to eye protection and a particulate facemask. Wear eye and face protection when ever there is a potential to encounter an exposure to dry blood particles.

Biological Hazards

Crime scenes may pose biological hazards other than those from bloodborne pathogens. These can include diseases from vectors such as ticks, funguses, infected animals and resinous plants. Scenes are often located in outside locations or in filthy environments. All forensic identification specialists should be aware of the hazards that could be present in such environments and take a preventative approach to the scene. While unable to discuss every possible hazard, following are some notable hazards worth mention.

Ticks and Lyme Disease

Ticks can present the potential for contracting Lyme Disease. This disease is transmitted by a spirochete organism called *Borrelia burgdorferi*. It is carried by a very small tick *Ixodes dammini* and similar ticks (the Deer Tick, *Ixodes pacificus* in the western states). [2] The first sign of Lyme Disease after a tick bite appears within a few weeks. A red rash starts with a small red spot that expands over a period of days or months to become a circular, triangular or oval rash. It may resemble a bull's eye. Arthritis occurs in slightly more than half of those not receiving treatment. This will cause recurring attacks of painful and swollen joints that last a few days to a few months. Neurological symptoms include a stiff neck and severe headache; temporary paralysis of facial muscles (Bell's palsy); numbness, pain or weakness in the limbs and poor motor co-ordination; and memory loss, difficulty with concentration, and a change in mood or sleeping habits. The heart can become stressed and exhibit irregular heartbeat. Dizziness or shortness of breath may result. Other symptoms may include eye inflammation, hepatitis and/or severe fatigue. Lyme Disease can be treated with nonsteroidal anti-inflammatory agents and antibiotics. However, the effects of the disease will probably continue for the remainder of one's lifetime.

Prevention is the best approach. When working a crime scene in an environment that may promote tick infestation, consider taking a few protective measures. If walking through the woods or brush, stay in the middle of the trail. Wear long pants and sleeves and tuck pant legs into your socks. Wear light colored clothing for ease of detection of ticks on your clothing. Spray clothing with an insecticide and use insect repellants on your skin on any uncovered areas. There is a vaccine available and if you are going to be at risk for tick bites, consider getting it through your insurance carrier.

Valley Fever

Two funguses are of particular concern to crime scene personnel. One is *Aspergillus* and is discussed at length in Section 21. Please take time to read this section and educate yourself on this hazard. The other fungus is called *Coccidioides immitis* [3] and causes Coccidioidomycosis, also known as Valley Fever. This fungus grows as a mold in soil and is primarily found in desert soils where there is low rainfall, high summer temperatures and moderate winter temperatures. Its highest documented concentrations are in the San Joaquin Valley of California, southern portions of Nevada and Utah, Arizona, New Mexico and west Texas. It may also be found in parts of Mexico, Central and South America. The fungus affects humans by way of the respiratory system. Infection occurs when a spore is inhaled. Once in the lung, "the spore changes into a larger, multicellular structure called a spherule. The spherule grows and bursts, releasing endospores which develop into spherules." [4] Dust control is critical in reducing risk. While called a "fever", it is not spread from one person to another. The incident rate of Valley Fever varies seasonally. It is highest in the late summer and early fall when the driest soil conditions prevail. Dust storms can lead to outbreaks and historically have caused an increase of cases of the fever in California. Earthquakes creating landslides (of soils) have also caused increased outbreaks. California statistics have been documented as high as 35,000 new cases in a year.

Occupational exposures to dust can come as result of working a scene in a windy environment or driving to and from a scene through dusty areas. If Valley Fever is contracted and develops in the primary form, the illness will only effect the respiratory system. One can experience a range from flu-like symptoms to pneumonia, but this form of the disease is self-limiting. In less than 5% of cases, people develop the disseminated form of the disease which includes bone and joint infection, skin disease, soft tissue abscesses, meningitis and often death. [5] As with Aspergillus, individuals with suppressed immune systems are at greater risk of developing the progressive disease. While no treatment is required for the primary form of Valley Fever, the progressive form is quite serious. Various anti-fungal drugs have proven moderately effective. Drugs such as Amphotericin B (used only to treat the progressive form) must be given intravenously and are highly toxic. If the disease becomes systemic, cerebrospinal fluids must be monitored. Unfortunately, Valley Fever is frequently misdiagnosed. It can be confused, symptomatically, with cancer, tuberculosis, chronic obstructive pulmonary disease, chronic fatigue syndrome and others. It can be confirmed with a specific blood test (cocci serology) to measure antibodies against the fungus, along with chest x-rays, and appropriate skin tests. When these medical results are coupled with a history of travel in areas prevalent with Valley Fever fungus, a diagnosis is made.

Prevention can be difficult in the crime scene setting. Fungal spores become airborne when winds, construction, farming and other activities disturb the soil. Dust control is the best method to minimize potential exposures but this is quite impossible if driving through dusty areas. There is little guidance available regarding respiratory protection. A physician from the University of California, Department of Pathology and Medicine asserts that "any mask that is OSHA approved for respiratory pathogens will work fine". [6] There are ongoing efforts to develop experimental vaccines for Valley Fever but at this writing, there is no vaccine.

Poison Ivy, Poison Oak and Poison Sumac

Poison Ivy, Poison Oak and Poison Sumac all present a potential biological hazard to individuals coming into contact with them. Poison Ivy is a climbing vine found in numerous areas of America. Poison Oak is a shrubby form of Poison Ivy, which is found in western America from British Columbia to Baja. It grows in a wide variety of settings from sea level to 5000 feet elevation. It may be located in grasslands, woodlands, chaparral and forests. Poison Sumac is a swamp shrub with a slightly different leaf arrangement than ivy and oak. They all belong to the genus *Toxicodendron*. These plants cause over 2 million cases of dermatitis a year in the United States. Due to the number of lost work hours, they are often considered the most hazardous plants in the country.

The plants produce oil in the sap called Urushiol. This is an extremely irritating oily resin that may also be a potent sensitizer since in many cases subsequent contacts produce increasingly severe reactions. The oil (Urushiol) is clear to light yellow, odorless, and turns dark upon exposure to air. It is rapidly absorbed through the skin. An itchy rash will develop within a few hours to several days and form water blisters in one to six days. The blisters usually rupture and are followed by oozing of serum and subsequent encrusting. The dermatitis usually disappears within 10 days. Transmission of the allergen can occur from exposure to smoke, clothing, tools and pets. [7] Anyone who has ever suffered the resulting dermatitis from contact with one of these plants knows about the accompanying misery. I have contracted it while tramping through the woods and from touching my dogs, cats and goats that so lovingly brought it home to me on their coats!

Because the Urushiol can carry in smoke in the form of small droplets, NEVER burn these plants. Severe respiratory irritation can occur. In fact, my grandfather was hospitalized a number of times with poison oak in his lungs because Oregonians would burn brush containing the dreaded plant!

While the U.S. Army has researched the problem for years in an attempt to develop an antidote, prevention is still the best approach to the problem. Wear long sleeves and pant legs when traveling through areas that may contain these plants. If you come into contact with the oily resin, WASH AFFECTED AREA AS SOON AS POSSIBLE (within 5 minutes of exposure). Use a mild solvent such as Isopropyl alcohol followed with copious amounts of cold water. Do NOT use warm or hot water. A small amount of water, or handi-wipes, are more likely to spread the allergen than remove it. If you develop the rash, available treatments range from the use of lotions such as Calomine to alleviate itching to a regimen of corticosteroids such as Prednisone. Regardless of the treatment, the dermatitis must run its course. To date, there is no medication which will stop the progression of events after a contact exposure.

Animals

Animals at crime scenes pose a host of potential problems. Animal contact can result in bites, scratches and kicks. If you participate in the processing of clandestine drug laboratories, you know how very often the suspects have dogs, cats and horses. Some scenes may also have exotic birds such as parrots, cockatoos or macaws. I attended a scene where the suspect kept emus! (You do not want to be bitten or clawed by an emu.) Animals at crime scenes, through bites or scratches, can transmit organisms that cause disease (rabies, cat scratch fever, and parrot fever). The best preventative measure is to avoid contact with animals unfamiliar to you. If you must handle them, wear protective clothing and gloves to cover as much exposed skin area as possible.

Hanta Virus

The common deer mouse also presents potential health hazards. This mouse is prevalent throughout the United States and is a carrier of the hantavirus, which attacks the respiratory system. This virus caused the death of a number of people in the Four Corners area of the country a few years ago and cases continue to be reported to this day. The hazard is associated with an accumulation of mouse droppings and subsequent exposure to those droppings when swept up or moved around. Crime scenes located in a structure that is filthy or where marijuana is dried and stored encourage the habitation of deer mice. The most obvious sign of mouse infestation is the appearance of droppings. If in such an environment, try not to disturb any obvious mouse droppings. Always wear a particulate mask to decrease the possibility of inhaling any particulate from the mouse feces. Hantavirus is discussed in more detail in Section 21.

Chemical Hazards

Most chemicals used in the field are also used in the forensic laboratory. The same safety protocols and safe work practices used in the laboratory apply to working at crime scenes. **Whenever possible, remove evidence requiring chemical processing from the scene and return it to the laboratory for processing**. Processing evidence with chemicals in the field increases risks and problems including exposures and contamination.

If the decision is made to do chemical processing at the scene, then a series of actions should be taken first. Determine the perimeter of the Safety Zone. Evacuate immediate neighbors if necessary. Demand that the police agency in control of the scene enforce outside scene security. Review ALL safety measures with the police and fire department personnel prior to entry.

Material Safety Data Sheets

The crime scene vehicle should contain a collection of Material Safety Data Sheets (MSDSs) for ALL chemicals used in the field. MSDSs should also be available in the collection for ALL anticipated chemicals at clandestine drug laboratories. Prior to using any chemicals in the field, it is recommended that the forensic identification specialist review the appropriate MSDS for potential hazards. The most common and careless mistake made with chemicals is developing an overly confident attitude. Some individuals may feel that a hazard is not a true hazard because they never experienced a problem when ignoring past warnings. Interestingly, the Chernobyl plant explosion in the Ukraine in 1986, is "often described as the world's worst nuclear accident. A report on the disaster speaks of a catalogue of reckless operating procedures and the repeated flouting of safety precautions." [8] We often become oblivious to the hazards when we have worked with chemicals accident-free over a period of time. The fact that an accident or exposure has never happened in the past is no guarantee that some event will not occur in the future. A review of MSDSs gives you a good edge on safety.

Flammable Chemicals

Chemical formulations for field use (ninhydrin, amido black, dye stains, etc.) should be prepared in the laboratory prior to accessing the crime scene unless procedure indicates otherwise. Most chemical mixtures used in the field contain flammable solvents such as acetone, ethanol, methanol, petroleum ether or hexane. Consequently, mixtures or components for mixtures should be transported in rugged, pressure-resistant and non-venting containers. Use non-breakable or plastic coated containers. Always transport chemical mixtures in vehicles equipped for such transport. This requires that such vehicles are well ventilated, cool, and the chemicals can be located in a separate compartment from the driver. Eliminate all potential ignition sources. At the scene, when working with flammable chemicals, DISCONNECT, REMOVE OR SHUT DOWN ALL SOURCES OF POSSIBLE SPARKS OR IGNITION. In fact, there are documented cases of forensic identification specialists involved in massive explosions while spraying ninhydrin because this precaution was not taken at the scene. Do not allow smoking around a scene where flammable or combustible chemicals are being used or stored.

Do NOT store or use the ninhydrin/freon formulation in the same contained environment that houses any metal object too hot to touch. Phosgene gas will result. This is an extremely toxic gas in very small quantities.

Personal Protective Equipment

Use all necessary personal protective equipment where chemicals are present. At a minimum, protective clothing, gloves and eye protection should be worn. Respirators may be necessary.

The employer should provide protective clothing for use in the field. This clothing should only be worn at crime scenes and never for personal, non-work related use. Such clothing could include shirts, pants, belts, jackets, hats, jumpsuits and footwear such as steel-toed boots. Disposable protective clothing should also be provided for crime scene processing where necessary.

Disposable clothing should be fluid resistant and include gowns, coveralls, jumpsuits, head/shoe covers. Always wear disposable clothing at scenes where chemicals are used or present or where PIMs are present. When selecting clothing, temperature extremes need to be considered. Some materials do NOT breathe and may cause an increase in body temperature and subsequent dehydration.

Gloves are a must for the forensic identification specialist. Even if no apparent safety hazard is present, wearing gloves is the only way to reduce the risk of contaminating potential evidence with fingerprints not relevant to the case. From a safety perspective, glove materials should be matched to the potential hazard and/or types of contamination. Chemical resistant gloves made of butyl rubber, neoprene or nitrile are worn when processing scenes with chemicals. Latex or vinyl gloves should be worn when working with potentially infectious materials. These gloves (latex, vinyl) however, will NOT provide protection from solvents such as acetone, methanol, ethanol, hexane, heptane or petroleum ether. Latex gloves should not be worn if any rash or other allergic reaction occurs. Nitrile or vinyl can be used in the event of a latex sensitivity. Always remove any jewelry that may puncture the gloves. Remember to cover any cuts, scratches or other skin breaks with a bandage or tape before gloving; especially if working around PIMs. Latex, vinyl or cotton gloves should be worn when working with alternate light sources and Ultra Violet wavelengths. If a break or tear occurs in a glove, remove it and don a new glove immediately.

Eye protection may be necessary at some scenes. Chemical splash goggles should be worn when applying chemicals at a scene. Goggles equipped with appropriate barrier filters are put on if working with or around a laser, alternate light source or ultraviolet lamp. Chemical splash shields offer further protection when worn in addition to goggles or safety glasses. Face shields are never donned as a replacement for goggles or safety glasses. Ultraviolet filtering shields are good for working with UV.

Respirators protect the nose, throat and lungs from exposures to hazardous materials. They are used when it is impractical to remove dust, mist, fumes, vapors or gases at their source. They are also necessary for emergency or brief events. (Departments assigning respirators to crime scene personnel must have a Written Respiratory Program (RRP). Personnel expected to wear a respirator must be certified as medically fit by a physician.) Failure to use a respirator can result in damage to the respiratory system due to irritation, inflammation or increase in mucous secretions. Results of some illnesses can threaten an individual's health or life.

Respirators are used when working in: oxygen deficient environment (less than 20%); materials in the environment have no warning properties; or chemicals in the environment are present in unknown concentrations. Respirator selection is based on a number of factors. One factor is the type of work being performed whether dusting with powders or processing with chemicals. Another factor is the type and concentration of the hazard. An additional consideration is the distance from the work site to a safe area. Selection is also based on the amount of time the respirator must be worn. Only use respirators that are approved by Mine Safety and Health Administration (MSHA) and/or the National Institute for Occupational Safety and Health (NIOSH).

Only persons who have a functional sense of smell should wear respirators. Again, a physician must medically approve these individuals as having a respiratory status commensurate with respirator usage. They must also be trained in the use, maintenance and inspection of respirators.

The types of respirators are varied and selection must be appropriate to the scene. (See Section 8 for greater detail.) Facemasks (particulate masks) are worn in confined spaces or areas of poor ventilation when using latent print powders. These masks are disposable equipment and should never be reused or passed back and forth between specialists. Half or full-face, air-purifying respirators (APR) are worn where known chemicals exist that exhibit warning properties. Cartridges or canisters that filter out specific chemicals are attached to the face piece. The selection of cartridge/canister is based on the hazardous chemicals in the environment. If the chemical is known but no filter exists for that chemical, then an air-purifying respirator cannot be used. Wearing this type of respirator requires an immediate change of cartridge/canister when the wearer detects a "break through". (Break through is when a chemical odor can be detected by smell when wearing the respirator.) Self-Contained Breathing Apparatus (SCBA) is a positive pressure apparatus worn when performing chemical processing in confined spaces. It is always used if chemicals present exhibit NO warning properties or in an oxygen deficient environment. SCBAs have the air supplied from a tank carried by the user. It is a positive pressure system that prevents contaminated air from leaking into the system. The air supply is limited and not indefinite. Most tanks are adequate for 20 to 30 minutes. This type of equipment protects against all respiratory hazards. If using an SCBA, safety protocol requires the use of the "Buddy System". This means that a second individual monitors the actions of the person in the SCBA in case any problems or trouble develops. A stand-by person with suitable rescue equipment, including an SCBA, must be prepared to enter and rescue if necessary.

Supplied-air devices may be used rather than SCBAs. This is a positive pressure apparatus that is appropriate for use where chemical processing is performed in confined spaces. It is also employed where chemicals have no warning properties or in an oxygen deficient environment. The air supply is connected by hoses and comes from a source outside the area of contamination. The positive pressure prevents contaminated air from leaking into the system. The negative aspect of these devices is the restrictive movement created by the hoses (300 feet long). Hoses can kink or be damaged. When exiting an area, you must retrace your steps. The air supplied to the respirator must be of high purity. Air compressors for this purpose must be equipped with high temperature and carbon monoxide alarms. These devices protect against all respiratory hazards. As with the SCBA, the "Buddy System" must be employed.

Chemical Processing/Blood Reactive Reagents

Blood reactive reagents include **Diaminobenzidine, Tetramethyl-benzidine, Leucomalachite Green, O-Tolidine, Leuco Crystal Violet, Amido Black, Fluorescin, Ninhydrin** (including **Ninhydrin Analogs), and Merbromin**. Take any blood samples for DNA tests prior to processing with any of these reagents. Some of these reagents are suspected carcinogens so consult the MSDS prior to use. It is always preferable NOT to spray the reagent. If possible, apply by pipette, dip or brush over the surface.

Since these techniques are used on items containing blood, always employ universal precautions. Remember that the alcohol in the mixtures is flammable and toxic. Acids used in the mixtures are corrosive and possibly combustible. Wear protective clothing, neoprene or other chemically impervious gloves and chemical safety goggles. An air-purifying respirator equipped with an organic vapor cartridge or an SCBA must be worn during processing.

Chemical Processing/Cyanoacrylate Ester (CAE)

Fumes from cyanoacrylate are an irritant to the respiratory system in concentrations above 2 ppm. Unfortunately, this is also the level at which the material is detected by the nose. So, once you can smell it, you have received an exposure. Take precautions prior to use! Cyanoacrylate products will bond skin to skin and skin to other objects. Cured (polymerized or hardened) glue heated above 205 degrees Centigrade or 401 degrees Fahrenheit will decompose to deadly cyanide gas. Never heat polymerized glue deposits. Use new aluminum trays for each application. For processing with this material, wear protective clothing and latex or nitrile gloves. Don non-vented chemical safety goggles to keep fumes out of the eyes. Wear an air-purifying respirator with an organic vapor cartridge or an SCBA. Because water is the catalyst for polymerization, moisture in the eyes and lungs present a perfect CAE environment for things to happen. Protect your eyes, nose and lungs!

Chemical Processing/Fluorescent Dye Stains

Fluorescent dye stains used in the field would include **Rhodamine 6G, RAM** (Rhodamine 6G, Ardrox and MBD), and the ultraviolet dye **Ardrox**. Most fluorescent dye stains are mixed with solvents such as ethanol and methanol. These solvents are flammable and toxic. Some stains are suspected carcinogens. Wear protective clothing and neoprene or other chemically impervious gloves. Wear chemical safety goggles and an air-purifying respirator with an organic vapor cartridge or an SCBA.

Chemical Processing/Ninhydrin and Analogs

These materials react with amino acids. Ninhydrin is toxic and a known irritant. Most solvents used in the formulations, with the exceptions of 1,1,2 Trichlorotrifluoroethane or one of the new freon replacement materials, are flammable. All are toxic. Spraying is the LEAST desirable means of application to a surface. If possible, apply by pipette, dip or brush over the surface. Wear protective clothing, preferably a saranex-type suit (suit impregnated with plastic coating). Wear neoprene or other chemically impervious gloves. Don non-vented chemical safety goggles and an air-purifying respirator with an organic vapor cartridge or preferably, an SCBA.

Chemical Processing/Fingerprint Powders

Powders are the most commonly used chemicals in the field. We use powders so frequently that we tend not to even consider them chemicals. However, they are classed as chemical compounds and can pose serious health risks. Some latent fingerprint powders ARE toxic; those containing polynuclear aromatic hydrocarbons or cadmium present carcinogenity hazards. Powders containing metals present toxicity hazards. For instance, silver powder contains aluminum, which has a potential link to Alzheimer's. Other metals that may be in powders include mercury, zinc, iron, lead and manganese. Most fluorescent powders are non-toxic. Always consult the MSDS before use to determine possible toxicity. It is a good practice to don a particulate mask when using powders, especially if working in confined spaces. ALWAYS use a particulate mask when working with metal powders.

PPE includes dust/mist respirators (also called a particulate mask) to protect your lungs from inhaled powder particles. Additionally, wear protective clothing, latex or nitrile gloves and non-vented chemical safety goggles. Fingerprint brushes and powder containers often become contaminated with chemicals or body fluids at scenes. Do not keep any contaminated equipment. Dispose of such equipment either before leaving the scene (clan labs) or after returning to the laboratory (bloodborne pathogens).

Chemical Processing/Small Particle Reagent

Small Particle Reagent is a solution containing Molybdenum Disulfide. It is used on articles that are or have been wet. It is best suited to surfaces that have either a non-porous (vehicles) or semi-porous (concrete) matrix. Molybdenum disulfide, as well as the detergent solution, is an irritant and toxic. Some sources indicate that Molybdenum disulfide is a suspected mutagen. [9] Always wear protective clothing, latex or nitrile gloves, and chemical safety goggles. Use in a well-ventilated area. If ethanol is added to the formulation to prevent the solution from freezing in extremely cold environments, wear neoprene or other chemically impervious gloves. And keep in mind that ethanol is flammable. Take all necessary precautions.

Chemical Processing/Sudan Black

Sudan Black is a dye that stains fatty components of sebaceous sweat. It is very effective on surfaces contaminated with materials such as grease, foodstuffs, and soft drink deposits. It is also used to enhance cyanoacrylate prints. Sudan Black (Sudan Black B) is toxic. The reagent is mixed with ethanol, which is also toxic and flammable. Wear protective clothing, neoprene or other chemically impervious gloves and chemical safety goggles. Also wear an air-purifying respirator with an organic vapor cartridge or an SCBA.

Chemical Contamination/Decontamination

Prior to processing the scene with chemicals (such as ninhydrin, cyanoacrylate, amido black, etc.); inform the investigating officer that the processing will result in contamination of property and evidence and MAY result in unknown health hazards. During the discussions with the investigating officer, explain the effects of the chemical and any clean-up or follow-up procedures. As stated in Section 13, the best approach to dealing with contamination is to isolate and control contaminated areas and items. Confine contamination whenever possible. This is accomplished by placing contaminated items into containers or bags and placing a warning label on the outside.

Chemically contaminated items (from chemical processing) being returned to your department must be properly sealed in protective containers or bags. Affix a hazard warning label on the outside. Potentially biologically contaminated items being returned to your department must also be sealed in protective wrapping, container or bag. Affix a biohazard warning label on the outside. Latent lift cards or paper containing latent lifts being returned to the department that have contamination from chemicals or biological materials must be properly sealed in a protective container or bag. A warning label is affixed to the outside depending upon the type of hazard. Separate contaminated sharp objects (broken glass, needles, knives or razors) from other items. Place sharps in a closable, leakproof, puncture-resistant container. Affix a biohazard and sharps warning label on the outside.

Place contaminated PPE in approved protective containers and affix a warning label on the outside. Dispose of these containers/bags or clean (decontaminate) the contents per departmental policy. If your department has no policy, this does not mean that nothing need be done. Demand that your department develop and enforce a policy. The consequential health risks of improper handling of contamination can affect not only the forensic identification specialist, but also every person who may come in contact with the material at a later point in time. This could include other forensic scientists, officers, property room personnel, attorneys, courtroom personnel, jury members and the victim(s) or general public.

Homicides and clandestine drug laboratories present greater contamination hazards than scenes that require no chemical processing or have no potentially infectious materials. At scenes where these contaminates are present, decontamination must be initiated prior to leaving the site. Personal clothing should NEVER be worn to scenes of homicides or clandestine drug laboratories. Unless outer disposable protective clothing (Tyvek®, Saranex® fluid-resistant gowns, etc.) is worn, clothing should be considered contaminated. Crime scene personnel should decontaminate themselves and any used equipment before returning to the department or personal residence. Where chemical contamination is present, place disposable protective clothing in a plastic bag for disposal by a properly licensed waste hauler at the scene or according to departmental policy. Used fingerprint materials and sampling equipment is discarded with other hazardous waste.

Remove contaminated clothing while wearing gloves. (If you have donned two pair of gloves such as latex under neoprene, remove the outer pair but retain the inner pair for stripping out of protective clothing.) Remove gloves last. If personal clothing is contaminated, place it in a protective bag and affix a warning label to the outside. Have any contaminated personal clothing laundered by a contracted linen service. NEVER take these items home and launder them in your own washing machine. If you do, you will likely spread the contamination to your personal household equipment and then to items subsequently washed in it. As result, you have introduced the crime scene contamination into your home!

Safety Protocols

Follow all safety protocols in the field. Remember that "safety begins with you".

- Demand that officers at the scene establish safe scene perimeters and limit access to the site.
- Inform the lead investigating officer of any hazards or resulting contamination from chemical processing.
- Consult your Chemist or Criminalist regarding any scene hazards and necessary approaches if appropriate.
- Alert the Fire Department if flammable chemicals are used in processing the scene.
- Ensure that a qualified person at the scene has a working knowledge of First Aid and CPR.

Hazardous Waste

All hazardous waste from scenes can be divided into two categories:

biological and chemical. Determinations on the handling of such wastes are based on the type of waste. While these materials share some common elements and concerns, they are handled differently.

Biological wastes include sharps. All sharps are placed in sharps containers and disposed of as biohazardous, solid waste. Other contaminated, disposable items are double bagged in puncture-resistant plastic bags and labeled. These bags are disposed of the same as sharps. In the event of a spill of blood or body fluids, clean all surfaces with soap and water or household detergent. Wipe the cleaned area with a fresh solution of sodium hypochlorite (bleach).

Chemical wastes include the formulations of latent print processing chemicals. NEVER pour these chemicals down a sink or floor drain. Return chemicals to the laboratory. In the laboratory, place chemicals in containers marked "Waste" and hold for removal by a properly licensed waste hauler. Always safeguard against fire and sources of ignition. All chemicals from clandestine drug laboratories (with the exception of evidential samples taken for analysis) are removed from the scene by a licensed hazardous waste hauler.

Physical and Mechanical Hazards

Lasers, Alternate Light Sources and Ultraviolet Lamps

Lasers, Alternate Light Sources (ALS) and Ultraviolet (UV) Lamps are used at scenes and autopsies. Specifically, they are used to detect trace evidence, blood and body fluids, bruises, inherently luminescent latent prints, contaminants, ligature marks, bitemarks and chemically developed fluorescing latent prints.

Lasers produce coherent or collimated light. Alternate light sources are high intensity lamps but do not produce coherent light. Ultraviolet lamps also do not produce coherent light. Most of these light sources require electricity unless battery powered. All light sources that require electricity can pose significant electrical hazards. Power supplies for these light sources have the potential of causing severe electrical shock. Always check the light source for bad connections and loose, damaged or frayed wires. Report any needed repairs to a supervisor. Never open or attempt to service or repair any light source unless trained and authorized to do so. (There are documented cases of persons being electrocuted trying to repair their laser.) Never place light sources against a conductive surface. Do NOT use light sources at an outdoor scene if existing conditions are wet.

Establish a safe viewing perimeter at a minimum safe distance with barrier tape. Do NOT allow persons NOT wearing eye protection to enter inside the established perimeter. Light generated by an intense light source can cause permanent eye damage as result of direct illumination to the eye or reflected or refractive light hitting the eye. Goggles (or barrier filters) are selected to match the wavelengths of light being used in the examination. Eye protection is always necessary when using light sources. Whether you elect to use goggles or viewing shields will probably depend upon the setting and situation. Always wear UV filtered goggles when working with UV light. UV has negative health effects on eyes. UV-C (100-280 nm) and UV-B (280-315 nm) can cause inflammation of the cornea causing a condition called Photokeratitis. This type of injury is severe but temporary. Intermediate range UV light causes Conjunctivitis of the eye. Prolonged exposure can result in cataracts. Never look directly into the light or beam and never point the light at another person.

Always wear protective clothing and gloves to cover all exposed areas of skin. Glove selection is based on the nature of the scene. When using Ultraviolet light, wear a face shield made for filtering UV. Susceptibility to skin injury occurs in the range of radiant energy in the UV spectral region of 200-320 nm. Exposures are cumulative and can lead to skin cancer. Photosensitizing chemicals greatly increase the sensitivity of the skin. The skin reacts abnormally to light, especially ultraviolet rays or sunlight; due to the presence of drugs, hormones, or heavy metals in the system. [10] This photosensitization can come as result of diseases such as Lupus and Herpes or from drugs, plant extracts, pitch, fungicides, or bacteriostatic agents such as hexachlorophene.

Horseplay should never be tolerated when working with light sources. Indiscriminate pointing or waving of the light wand presents hazards to others at the scene. Safe work practices should be strictly enforced.

Fire Safety and Suppression

Following protocols for other aspects of crime scene safety will serve as the best prevention for potential fires. Smoking should never be allowed at a scene in proximity to flammable or combustible chemicals being stored or used for processing. When working with flammable chemicals, disconnect, remove or shut down all sources of possible sparks or ignition. This may require contacting the local utility companies to disconnect electrical, gas, water and telephone services. Remember that photographic equipment can ignite gases; so ensure that any equipment being used does not pose this hazard.

Insuring that all electrical equipment is in good working condition will help prevent electrical fires. Never use a piece of equipment that does not function properly. Check any electrical outlets before use and determine whether it is grounded or on a ground fault interrupter. Locate any fuse boxes or circuit breaker boxes so you can shut down the power if necessary.

All crime scene personnel should be trained in the use and handling of fire extinguishers and fire suppression. ALL crime scene vehicles should have a fire extinguisher which is inspected at least annually. Any fans used for ventilation at a scene where chemicals are present must be spark proof. These fans can often be obtained from the local fire department.

Lighting Considerations

Adequate lighting is necessary for scene processing, documentation, evidence collection and hazard awareness. Portable lights (task lights or banks of lights) may be used if additional lighting is necessary. Fluorescent lights are cooler and give better visibility. Poor lighting will result in evidence not being detected that would be seen in better lit conditions. Chemicals should never be handled at a scene without adequate lighting. Labels on containers and MSDSs must be clearly visible. Poor lighting can also lead to trip and fall hazards or the inability to see hazards such as broken glass or spilled materials. If adequate lighting can not be accomplished, the scene should be secured until a later time. Lighting issues are often resolved by simply waiting until daylight.

Ventilation

Adequate ventilation can be accomplished by natural or mechanical means.

Some scenes only need for doors and windows to be opened to make a workable environment. Other scenes such as clandestine drug laboratories and scenes where the forensic identification specialist is using chemical processing may require the use of ventilation fans. If ventilation fans are used, they must be spark proof. All fire departments have spark proof fans and are willing to provide them as needed. Never work in an inadequately ventilated area. A lack of ventilation will increase the risk of heat stress and breathing problems from air that is either inadequate in quality or quantity. The ambient environment must have at least 20% oxygen to sustain life. If the oxygen should fall below the required 20% level, wearing a self-contained breathing apparatus will be necessary.

Clandestine drug laboratories usually present the worst scenarios for poor ventilation due to the quantity of chemicals and/or the drug manufacturing process at the scene. If a clandestine drug laboratory is located inside a structure and is an operating lab; the interior must be evaluated and air monitored prior to entry by the identification specialist. The scene should be well ventilated before any processing for latent prints. It is always preferable to remove the evidence from the interior of the scene and process it outside the structure. Sometimes this is not possible due to large reaction vessels being full of chemicals. Moving such vessels can pose greater hazards than working the items inside. If items must be worked inside, there should be an ongoing air monitoring and ventilation process until the waste haulers remove all materials from the site.

Firearms

Firearms at crime scenes and in property rooms or evidence vaults pose tremendous hazards. An unbelievable number of property room technicians (also forensic identification specialists) are shot in the property room by accidentally discharged firearms being stored for evidential purposes. Any firearm located at a scene must be rendered "safe" before it is collected, transported or processed. Rendering a firearm safe means that all ammunition is removed, the chamber cleared and opened. Any ammunition in the chamber, cylinder or magazine can be documented with sketches and photographs before being removed. There are a wide variety of firearms, both handguns and long guns, with differing firing mechanisms, safeties and magazines. Most forensic identification specialists handle firearms as a part of the job but are not firearm experts. If a firearm is encountered and has not been rendered safe, get the assistance of a sworn officer or a Criminalist. Refuse to handle any firearm with an uncertain status.

When handling firearms (including ones rendered safe), always know what is down range of the barrel. Remember the standard rule of handling firearms: Never point it at anyone or anything you do not intend to shoot. Carelessness is your worst enemy and is responsible for most accidents. It is easy to wave a firearm around in one direction or another while examining it. Additionally, a gun not rendered safe and dropped can discharge. ALL firearms pose a risk, including zip guns, BB guns and pellet guns.

Thermal: Heat and Cold Stress

Crime scenes can occur in an outdoor environment or inside some type of structure or container. The ambient temperature is not always ideal for working. Furthermore, personal protective equipment worn at certain types of scenes may add the factor of additional heat. Heat stress or cold stress can seriously inhibit body function and make working impossible. These stresses can also be threatening to the health and/or life of the forensic identification specialist at a crime scene. The following is a general discussion of heat and cold stress. For your own safety and well being, become familiar with the signs and symptoms of thermal stresses. Keep an eye on colleagues at scenes where extreme temperature is a factor. People can begin to suffer from thermal stress and not realize they are in trouble. Be aware of changes in behavior that seem inappropriate for that individual; such as sleepiness or irrational responses. An individual experiencing thermal stress needs **immediate** assistance to reverse the problem. If not remedied, thermal stress can cause permanent damage or death.

When wearing personal protective equipment such as Tyvek® or Saranex® suits, **Heat Stress** should be considered a physical hazard throughout the duration of work when the ambient temperature is 70° F or higher. (Protective clothing can induce heat stress, as the body is unable to breathe. At clandestine drug laboratory scenes, the body is covered with overalls, the cuffs and ankles sealed with duct tape and a full-face respirator in place.) If working in an enclosed area, take a temperature reading. The ambient temperature outdoors could be 68° F, while the ambient temperature inside a boxcar or shipping container may be 80° F. The best approach for dealing with heat stress is <u>prevention</u> of the problem. Wearing personal protective equipment is a necessity. However, there are methods that can decrease the associated safety risks.

Some prescription drugs can impair your physiological response to heat. These include heart drugs, oral hypoglycemics, antidepressants and antiphychotics, anticholinergics and belladonna alkaloids, antihistamines and antiparkinsonians.

If you are on prescribed medication, consult your doctor or pharmacist regarding any drug related problems you may anticipate if you are in a heat stress situation.

All employees should be trained to recognize the signs of heat stress and steps to take in prevention. A system must be in place to have frequent monitoring of individuals during work periods while wearing PPE. Replacement of lost body fluids from sweating is essential to maintaining the physical integrity of water and electrolyte balance in the body. The employer should provide the necessary liquids. Such replacement fluids include potable water or commercial preparations such as Gatorade™ . A combination of such liquids can be used but must be taken in excess of what seems required to satisfy thirst. Drinking to satisfaction of thirst is an unreliable indicator of whether or not adequate fluid and salt have been replaced. Drink at least a gallon of liquid a day when the outside temperature is above 90° F. Never drink alcoholic beverages (beer, wine or liquor) for fluid replacement. The alcohol causes further dehydration. Drinks containing caffeine such as coffee and sodas are also not recommended. The best fluid replacement is water and drinks manufactured to replace lost electrolytes. A depletion of electrolytes will effect brain function and can lead to hallucinations, convulsions, heart attack or stroke. (This was experienced by one of my brothers, and he barely survived the experience.)

Avoid unnecessary over exertion during work. There must be an allowance for adequate rest periods for cooling down. Some environments may be so hot that work periods will consist of fifteen-minute intervals with forty five-minute breaks. During this time, PPE can be opened or removed to allow the body an opportunity to ventilate and cool down. Take cooling down breaks in a shaded or protected area out of the direct sun. If possible, use electric fans to promote cooling. If fans are not an option, cool down with the use of wet towels, ice bags or dampen inner layers of clothing. Staff can be rotated to accomplish the work at a scene where there is potential heat stress. Plan the processing of such a scene to use shade and avoid midday temperatures whenever possible.

Guidelines are available to assist in the monitoring of heat stress. The following table gives a guide for a work and rest schedule. In heat stress conditions, an individual's heart rate can be monitored to determine the ability to work and work intervals.

Ambient Temperature	Work Time	Rest Time
77° F or above	After each 15 min	Rest for 45 min

74.5° F - 77° F	After each 30 min	Rest for 30 min
69.5° F - 74.5° F	After each 45 min	Rest for 15 min

An individual's pulse rate should be measured at the beginning of the rest period. If the heart rate exceeds 110 beats per minute, the next work cycle should be shortened by one third (1/3). Keep the same rest period. Should the heart rate exceed 110 beats per minute at the beginning of the next rest period, then shorten the work cycle by one third (1/3). Continue monitoring and shortening the work cycle until the heart rate is reduced to less than 110 beats per minute. These guidelines were established from the NIOSH Heat Stress criterion (1985) and are used by California's Bureau of Narcotic Enforcement when working drug labs.

The signs and symptoms of heat stress are recognizable to the trained eye. They are divided into four categories ranging from the mildest symptoms to the most deleterious. Heat stress, if not met with intervention, will progress to the worst stages. This is why it is so important to recognize it in the early stages. While this information is available from many sources, the following detail is quoted from the California Department of Justice, Bureau of Narcotic Enforcement's Clandestine Laboratory Safety Certification training manual.

- Heat Rash can be caused by continuous exposure to hot and/or humid air. This condition is characterized by a localized red skin rash and reduced sweating.

- Heat Cramps can be caused by profuse perspiration with inadequate fluid and salt replacement. Muscle spasms and pain in the extremities and stomach characterize this condition.

- Heat Exhaustion is a mild form of shock, caused by substantial physical activity in heat and profuse perspiration without adequate fluid and salt replacement. The signs and symptoms include pale, cool, moist skin, heavy sweating, dizziness, nausea and fainting.

- Heat Stroke is the most serious form of heat stress. Temperature regulation fails and the body temperature rises to critical levels. Immediate action must be taken to cool the body before serious injury and death occurs. Medical help must be obtained immediately. Signs and symptoms include red, hot, unusually dry skin, lack of or reduced perspiration, nausea, dizziness and confusion, strong, rapid pulse and coma.

Working in outside environments in cold-weather conditions can present problems of **Cold Stress**. Employers are tasked with responsibility for ensuring the employee can stay safe and healthy in extreme temperatures. While there are few fatalities each year (according to the Bureau of Labor Statistics) from working in extreme cold temperatures, there are many lost workdays due to cold-related illnesses. Additionally, accidents result when people suffer from hypothermia and become disoriented. Again, prevention is the best remedy. Employees must be trained to understand and recognize the elements of cold stress. Departmental policy must support the establishing of work and rest schedules at scenes that present cold stress hazards. People must be allowed to stop and rest and warm up when working in extreme environments. Yes, it does take longer to process a crime scene, but the savings in human misery far outweigh any extra hours on site.

The thermal condition of cold can be divided into two separate categories. These are dry cold and wet cold. **Dry cold** results from two factors: ambient temperature and wind velocity. A combination of these two elements creates the wind chill factor. The term "wind chill" describes the chilling effect of a combination of moving air with low temperature. As the wind chill increases, it also increases the chilling effect to the air. As an example, an ambient temperature of 10° F combined with a wind of 15 miles per hour creates an equivalent in chilling effect to still air at -18° F. This factor is significant when considering that nearly 60 percent of an individual's energy is metabolized to keep the body warm. Exposure to cold causes body temperature to decrease. Decrease in body temperature results in blood vessel constriction, which in turn slows blood flow to the skin. Under such circumstances, exposed skin can lead to frostbite and hypothermia.

The best prevention to dry cold stress is the selection of clothing. Wool or thermal synthetics are the most effective insulating materials and should be layered to enhance maintenance of dead air space. An outer layer of woven nylon or Gore-Tex™ will protect against wind and allow ventilation. These materials breathe but also protect against water penetration. Wool or synthetic fiber garments are beneficial as an insulating middle layer. While down is a good insulator, it is ineffective if it gets wet. Thermal underwear is commonly worn as an inner layer. The key to keeping the skin as dry as possible is to allow good ventilation around the torso. The head, hands and feet must also be covered with warm, layered garments. Footwear should always be waterproof and insulated for protection against dampness and cold. Often overlooked is the factor of heat loss through the surface of the head. Due to the large quantities of blood that circulate to the brain, as much as 40 percent of body heat can be lost when the head is exposed. Cold weather head covering such as knit caps or ski masks can be combined with hooded jackets. In cold and wet weather, insulated waterproof gloves provide the best protection. Glove liners can be worn in addition to gloves. During rest periods, mittens can be worn to increase warmth to the fingers.

Proper hydration is as important in cold environments as it is in hot. Fluids are a must but may be preferred if heated before consumption. Never drink alcoholic beverages to warm up. The feeling of warmth is misleading. Again, alcohol leads to dehydration.

Wet cold results from a direct contact with water, immersion in water, or contact with dampness in the air from freezing rain or sleet. Wet cold robs the body of heat even faster than dry cold. Information from OSHA indicates that a body in wet clothing can lose heat up to 24 times faster than one in dry clothing. Cold, wet environments present a challenge to keep clothing dry. Again, dressing in layers is the best prevention for problems.

Recognition of the signs and symptoms of cold stress are an important element in the prevention of serious injury. As with heat stress, cold stress unchecked can progress into the worst and most life threatening stages. Following are the recognized stages of cold stress to the body.

- Frost nip or incipient frostbite is characterized by suddenly blanching or whitening of the skin. Warming at this stage results in no permanent damage.

- Superficial frostbite causes the skin to have a waxy or white appearance and is firm to the touch. The tissue beneath remains resilient.

- Deep frostbite causes the tissues to be cold, pale and solid. This is result of the freezing or effect of freezing a part of the body. Exposed areas such as ears, cheeks, nose, fingers and toes are usually effected. Deep frostbite is an extremely serious injury and can result in gangrene and amputation.

- Hypothermia occurs when an individual is exposed to prolonged cold and the body temperature falls below what is normal; or the safe "core" body temperature. Hypothermia causes drowsiness and disorientation. A person can experience hallucinations and become delusional. Hypothermia unchecked results in death.

Educate yourself about thermal stress and do not become a victim. Take all possible stress prevention measures at crime scenes.

Vehicles

Every law enforcement agency has the responsibility of providing safe vehicles for use at crime scenes. However, vehicle maintenance can often fall through the proverbial "crack" and not happen on a scheduled basis. This shifts a measure of responsibility to the forensic identification specialist to check a vehicle before driving it.

Always walk around the vehicle and check the tires for pressure and wear. Never drive a departmental vehicle equipped with bald tires or separated tread. Refuse to drive any vehicle with obvious fluid leaks such as gasoline, oil, antifreeze or transmission or steering fluid. If you leave headquarters and note the vehicle to have any type of mechanical problems such as difficult steering, bad brakes, wobbly wheels or strong gasoline fumes return to headquarters for another vehicle. Insist the returned vehicle be removed from service until necessary repairs are completed. All vehicles should be properly equipped with road flares, spare tire and jack, chains (if in snow country), a blanket and first aid kit at a minimum. Additional items can be added based on vehicle use and environment.

Always wear a seat belt when driving or riding in a moving vehicle. Drive defensively and take your time traveling to the scene. There is never a reason to speed or drive in a careless or reckless manner. If you must drive long distances or are especially fatigued (call out in the middle of the night with little sleep), take rest stops to stretch your legs and get some fresh air. If you are seriously fatigued, pull over and take a 10 to 20 minute nap to refresh yourself. Drinking caffeinated beverages, turning up the radio or opening a window for fresh air can not be relied upon to keep you awake. You must always put your safety first in any situation and not take any risks when driving.

Be aware of the effects of weather conditions on the vehicle. In hot weather, regularly monitor the vehicle's gauges for any problems. Road surfaces generally reflect the effects of weather. Mud, pot holes, slick pavement due to rain, ice, and snow are surface hazards to anticipate. Be familiar with the response of the vehicle and adverse road conditions in your area. Make a request for training for driving in such adverse conditions if not already educated on safe handling of the vehicle. It is important that you know how to operate a vehicle in the safest manner in any of these conditions. When traveling in fog, use extreme caution. Slow down and use only the amount of lighting needed since light reflects off fog and can create a greater visibility hazard.

Never take a vehicle where it is not designed to travel. If a scene is in an area requiring offroad capabilities, or 4-wheel drive, an appropriate vehicle must be used. However, anyone using a 4-wheel drive should be trained in 4-wheel drive operations. Remember that 4 wheel drive vehicles are top heavy and should never be driven on more than a 25-degree lateral grade as it could create a rollover situation.

For ease of access to equipment, park as close to the scene as is safely possible. Set the parking brake any time the vehicle is in park whether or not the engine is running. And naturally, make sure to release the parking brake before moving the vehicle.

While many of these suggestions seem simplistic, they are worthy of review. If you have an accident or are injured in any manner related to the departmental vehicle, there will be issues because there are liabilities. Accidents are incredibly expensive in terms of lost life or health, loss of time from work, loss of equipment and the financial burden of resolving liabilities. Accident prevention is certainly the more prudent approach.

Arson and Bomb Scenes

Never enter a bombing scene unless it has been cleared by bomb experts. There may be more than one explosive device, especially in this day of terrorism. A series of bombs may be set with delayed timing devices with the intent of killing or maiming responding crime scene personnel. And sometimes, devices fail to explode by plan or design but may detonate upon being disturbed or handled.

Scenes involving bombings or arsons present potential hazards from falling debris. Scenes at construction sites or disasters also present these hazards. Wear a hard hat at such scenes. Always inspect your hard hat before donning it. The plastics can deteriorate over time. Inspect the shell of the hard hat for "cracks, nicks, gouges, dents or damage caused by impact, penetration or abrasions. If the hat is made of polyethylene or polycarbonate, it should also be checked for stiffness, brittleness, fading, dull color or a chalky appearance." [11] Hats displaying any of these conditions should be replaced immediately. The hat suspension should be "free of cracks or tears and the suspension straps free of any cuts or fraying. The suspension should be pliable and show no signs of wear. All points in the suspension should fit tightly in their respective slots." If the suspension is lacking in any way, it must be replaced with one appropriate for that shell. [12] Other safety considerations with hard hats include not carrying items in the hard hat and not drilling ventilation holes in it. Hard hats can not be worn backwards unless the manufacturer states explicitly that the hat has been tested and passed in that manner and the suspension is positioned as required by that test. Additionally, be aware that a hard hat dropped more than 8 to 10 feet or that has been struck forcibly should be replaced immediately.

Autopsies

Autopsies present the greatest potential for exposure to biological materials. These could be potentially infectious materials from human tissue, blood and other body fluids containing traces of blood, and bone dust. Bone dust provides a potential exposure to HBV, HCV and tuberculosis. (When the pathologist starts the Striker saw to cut and remove the cranial cap, make it a point not to be positioned in the area of flying bone dust.)

At a minimum, the forensic identification specialist, pathologist and any assistants should wear the same PPE. Unfortunately, past experiences revealed that some pathologists were resistant to the idea of using PPE. If the pathologist or a morgue assistant chooses not to wear PPE, that certainly is their prerogative. In this event, the forensic identification specialist should set the standard. Insist on using the recommended equipment of a lab coat or disposable coveralls, goggles, particulate mask and latex or nitrile gloves. An air-purifying respirator with a HEPA filter (and possibly an organic vapor filter for the odors) is optional. A face shield can be worn in addition to goggles and will protect the face and neck from splashed materials. Definitely use a face shield if you have any open sores (dermatitis, wounds) or photography necessitates leaning down and over into the body cavity. If PPE is not made available to you, refuse to continue until the equipment (preferably disposable) is obtained.

Some people who work around the deceased seem to adjust to the unpleasant odors. However, most people never get used to it and seek ways to mask the odors. In the past, Vicks® or other mentholated petroleum products have been placed in the nose. NEVER put these materials in your nostrils. They will burn the interior lining of the nose. Additionally, odors become trapped in the material causing the unpleasant odors to linger after removal from the source. However, there are ways to mask such undesirable odors. You can wear a charcoal impregnated particulate mask (nuisance odor) or an air-purifying respirator with an organic vapor cartridge. Or place peppermint oil on the lining of the particulate mask. There are also new products being marketed that claim to mask unpleasant organic odors.

Maintain a separate, dedicated autopsy kit with supplies for collecting trace evidence and fingerprints. Limit supplies to only those items necessary. Do NOT use this kit at other scenes or transfer equipment back and forth to other kits. Prints obtained from deceased must be packaged in a plastic, heat-sealed pouch or in a plastic zipper lock bag with an evidence tape seal at the top. Deceased print cards are always considered contaminated with biological material. Non-disposable PPE and equipment is placed in a biohazard bag and labeled for later cleaning and disinfecting.

Wash hands, including fingers and under nails, and forearms with antimicrobial soap and water before leaving the morgue.

Clandestine Drug Laboratories

Clandestine drug laboratories pose the greatest risk of all crime scenes. They are inherently dangerous due to the possible presence of booby traps, unknown chemicals and ignorance of the "cookers". Many cookers who manufacture illicit drugs have absolutely no training in chemistry. Most possess a formulation (often obtained from a cellmate in jail) for the drug being manufactured and perhaps some basic warnings. Judging by the number of cookers who are suffocated by poisonous fumes, burned, maimed or dismembered in explosions, any safety warnings they had are not adequate enough! These cookers often create chemical concoctions for which there is no formula. Their ignorance helps create risk to the people who must "take down" the lab. Prior to entering a clandestine laboratory scene, officers will have made numerous observations regarding the presence of dead or dying foliage, dead animals or humans, and any signs of prior fire or explosions. These observations will often provide clues to the presence of gross chemical contamination, poisonous vapors or fumes and flammable chemicals.

Every agency involved in the working of clan labs should have established written policies on the approach and take down of the lab site. There was a time when there were no such written policies and we just tried to get out with our life and health. When I first worked clan labs, we went in with no protective equipment other than gloves. Our primary concern was to protect the latent print evidence! We wore our personal clothing, walked in spilled chemicals and breathed all sorts of chemical fumes. After 4 or 5 hours of inhalation exposures, a person without a great sense of humor got pretty surly. Upon completion of working the scene, we would get into the department's vehicle, contamination and all, and drive back to headquarters higher than a kite and sporting a killer headache. We have come a long way since those days. With the information and assistance available today, there is no excuse for haphazard takedowns.

A wealth of valuable information on Clandestine Drug Laboratory procedures is located in the California Department of Justice, Bureau of Narcotic Enforcement's *Clandestine Laboratory Safety Certification Training Manual*. Another source document is the *Clandestine Laboratory Manual of Instruction and Procedure* (CLMIP). This document was produced as a joint effort between the California Department of Justice's Bureau of Narcotic Enforcement and Bureau of Forensic Services. Such an endeavor was undertaken after years of lab takedowns without the advantage of environmental monitoring and personal protective equipment. As we developed knowledge, we developed procedures. They were long overdue, desperately needed and are made available to other agencies upon request. Some of that information is in the following material.

On Site Safety Officer/Case Agent

Naturally, every lab will have an investigating officer assigned as the case agent with the primary responsibility for the scene. Additionally, every scene must have an individual assigned as an on-site Safety Officer . The on-site Safety Officer must be trained in First Aid and CPR. The case agent and Safety Officer can be one and the same but this is not recommended. There are so many responsibilities in each role that involvement in one role can serve as a distraction from the other role. The case agent and on-site Safety Officer must also be trained in hazard evaluation and assessment; the stages of take down (Entry team, Assessment Team, Processing team and Disposal team), field air monitoring procedures and equipment, and the use of engineering controls at the scene. Additionally, both must be knowledgeable in proper use of personal protective equipment, hazard control and site control. These individuals should always be in close communication with each other and the on site Chemist or Criminalist to discuss the scene and any change in events. The only type of clandestine lab that should ever be approached without all the above mentioned considerations is the incidental lab. This is a lab which is discovered incidental to some other law enforcement action such as a vehicle stop, serving an unrelated warrant, a fire, or a citizen complaint. All other clandestine lab investigations should have a planning phase, entry phase, pre-assessment and/or assessment phase, as well as processing, disposal and post warning phases.

Medical Monitoring

Prior to any forensic identification specialist being assigned to work clandestine drug laboratories, he or she should be placed in a medical monitoring program (OSHA 29 CFR 1910.120). This program establishes a baseline physical for all clan lab personnel. It includes an individual's occupational and medical history, a physical examination, blood chemistry, urinalysis, pulmonary function and spirometry testing and may include a stress treadmill exercise test. These examinations ascertain any preexisting medical conditions (or problems which may be aggravated), lung function for wearing respirators and liver function. The program must be started prior to assignment and thereafter the examinations performed at least every twelve (12) months. An examination must be completed at termination of employment or reassignment to other job duties outside the area of clandestine lab responses. The employer retains these records in the event a medical condition should develop, to identify early changes from injury or overexposure or should an exposure event occur at a clan lab scene.

Forensic Identification Specialist Responsibilities

While the clandestine laboratory crime scene is a complex scene requiring training, knowledge and cooperation; the responsibilities of the forensic identification specialist are very specific and somewhat limited. Trained, sworn officers take responsibility for all pre-raid planning and activities. Additionally, they handle the actual entry and arrest of suspects. The Chemist or Criminalist should be involved in the assessment phase at the scene and will usually begin the deactivation of an operational lab. Some narcotics officers have adequate experience to perform this task but forensic personnel are most qualified to deal with a chemical environment. There is never a reason for the identification specialists to be involved in the take down (unless they are sworn personnel) or the assessment and any necessary deactivation of an operational lab (unless they are a trained chemist). Identification specialists are on scene as members of the processing team to evaluate, collect and process evidence for latent impressions. The on site Safety Officer is responsible for maintaining the integrity of the site in regard to various individuals being in established control areas. Let me reiterate this point. No matter how curious you may be or how many clan lab scenes you have worked or how well you know the case agent, you should never enter the scene unless you are cleared to enter and begin the processing phase.

Additional Personnel

The local fire department should be notified and on stand-by for an operational clandestine laboratory. They are a good source of additional SCBAs and spark proof fans for ventilation. In the event of an explosion or fire, you will want them on scene to render assistance and fire suppression. Additionally, officers may want to notify local health department personnel of possible contamination. There may be other personnel present for a variety of reasons. Unfortunately, clan labs draw interest and onlookers like bees to honey. This makes it imperative that site control be established and enforced. Other law enforcement personnel may include city, county, state and federal narcotics officers, traffic control officers, animal control officers, Alcohol, Tobacco and Firearms agents (inventorying illegal firearms), Secret Service agents (inventorying counterfeit money), Internal Revenue Service agents exploring asset seizure and forfeiture issues and licensed waste haulers. And the list can go on to include stand-by helicopter pilots, paramedics and ambulance personnel, as well as city or county officials who feel it is their responsibility to "be there". Often time, police officers not involved in the clan lab investigation will show up at the scene due to curiosity. They may bring friends or family with them in hopes of showing them a drug lab. While the temptation may be great to accommodate such ones in the name of public relations or a spirit of cooperation, unauthorized persons should never be allowed beyond the area of the Support Zone.

Emergency Equipment

There are essential pieces of emergency equipment that should be present at all clan lab scenes. Emergency equipment is provided by the narcotics officers and is usually housed in a clandestine laboratory response vehicle. Such equipment includes an emergency eyewash (capable of a 15 minute flow of water) and an emergency shower. There must be a First Aid kit and type A, B and C fire extinguishers readily available. Additionally, there should be a complete collection of Material Safety Data Sheets for any and all anticipated chemicals that could be found at the scene. The collection is based upon chemicals known for manufacturing various precursors and illicit drug products. Potable water must always be available at any scene.

Emergency Telephone Numbers

Part of the planning phase of the investigation is to obtain the telephone number and address of the nearest medical facility. Other required numbers are for the local fire department, ambulance service and Poison Center.

Emergency Evacuation

Evacuation routes should be determined prior to any personnel entering the contaminated area. Personnel working within the contaminated area should all be informed of the established evacuation route to take in the eventuality this becomes necessary.

Work Zones

Personnel NOT ACTIVELY involved in processing should be in the Support Zone. This includes identification specialists taking a break or rest period. Clandestine drug laboratory scenes should have established zones. The

Contaminated Zone (Hot Zone) will encompass the operational lab or area of the scene that is contaminated. The Contamination Reduction Zone (Warm Zone) is the barrier zone between contamination and non-contamination. This is the area where decontamination stations are established and used upon leaving the Hot Zone. The Support Zone (Cold Zone) is the area where all support personnel and operations are located. There should never be any potential for contamination occurring in this zone. The intent behind establishing zones is to limit contamination and keep it at the lab site.

People should never be allowed to enter the Contamination Zone unless they have received proper and adequate training (generally a minimum of 40 hours). (The decontamination area must have been established and set up prior to anyone entering this zone.) All personnel must be suited in all required PPE. Inspect your PPE before donning it and entering this zone. No food, drink or tobacco is allowed in the hot zone. Working in this zone requires a continuous re-evaluation of the scene. If you are working in the hot zone and see fire or smell chemical odors, get out and report it to the Safety Officer, Chemist/Criminalist or case agent immediately. (You may have experienced "break through" with your air-purifying respirator if you smell chemical odors and need to change the cartridge, but it never hurts to inform another person of your observations.)

The Contamination Reduction Zone limits the spread of contaminated material. This zone is set up first and is located upwind of the lab site. Monitoring equipment such as gas meters, drager tubes, combustible gas indicators, and/or oxygen deficiency meters are used to establish this area. There should be a checkpoint for entry into the warm zone. The same level of PPE or one level below is required in this zone. Everyone should review the decontamination procedures before using the decontamination materials. The narcotics agents at the scene usually provide such materials. Decontamination materials include laundry detergent and water for washing; fresh water for rinsing; scrub brushes, a respirator decontamination kit and paper towels. All used decontamination solutions must be removed and disposed of by the hazardous waste hauler. When removing contaminated equipment, start by removing the most contaminated items first and the less contaminated items last. So, start by removing and disposing of any boot covers, tape and outer gloves. Then remove and dispose of protective suit. Remove respirator face piece, followed with removal and disposal of inner gloves. Always wash your face and hands prior to leaving the scene.

The Support Zone provides a safe area for everyone who is not in the Contamination or Contamination Reduction Zones. This zone is established upwind and should include the command post and all vehicles. Nothing is allowed in this area from the other areas unless it is decontaminated or properly packaged. Such items include evidence being removed for return to the laboratory, latent print lift cards and samples of chemicals. This is the only area where eating, drinking or smoking is allowed. Rest breaks are taken here if an individual properly decontaminates prior to entry.

Personal Protective Equipment

At a very minimum, always wear protective clothing (Tyvek®, etc.), nitrile or neoprene gloves and eye protection. Respirators may be necessary. The selection of PPE should always be based on the hazard level of the clandestine laboratory. Clan labs are classified into four categories: Level A, Operational Laboratory, Investigative Laboratory and Incidental Laboratory.

Level A is a scene requiring the highest level of personal protective equipment. The skin as well as the respiratory system must be protected. Laboratories that fall into this category are fentanyl, LSD, MPPP and MPTP. These are incredibly dangerous scenes that put all investigative personnel at risk and can present great hazards to the community. Most agencies do not have clan lab teams prepared to deal with these labs. If such a team is not available, department supervisors should call their county hazardous materials team to request assistance in sampling evidence and processing the scene. Forensic Identification Specialists should never enter Level A scenes. They require donning fully encapsulating suits ("moon suits") and SCBA or Air supplied respirators.

Operational Laboratories are those which are active or cooking product. Personnel entering an operational lab must wear Level B personal protective equipment until the Safety Officer determines it is safe to downgrade to a lower level of PPE. These laboratories pose serious respiratory hazards as well as increased risk of fire or an explosion. By-products of cooking can include highly toxic gases such as phosphine or phosgene, which can be fatal if inhaled. Any ongoing chemical reaction can pose serious fire or explosion hazards. These reactions are often out of control and additional heating or sudden cooling can make the concoction unstable. Any cooking lab will probably be replete with flammable solvents such as ether and acetone.

An Investigative laboratory is one discovered through the investigative process. This situation allows the agents to develop information on the status of the lab; whether it is operational or non-operational (all materials are boxed up). With this available information, including knowledge of the type of chemicals present at the scene, the Safety Officer and case agent can determine the appropriate level of PPE. An investigative lab will require either Level B or Level C protection. These labs, like the operational laboratory, pose serious respiratory hazards as well as increased risk of fire or explosion.

The Incidental Laboratory is one located incidental to an unrelated event. Such an event could be a vehicle stop, unclaimed property at a storage facility or discovered while serving a search warrant. The type of chemicals present, the reliability of any chemical containers and the condition of the scene or storage site determine the level of protection (PPE).

The determination of the level of personal protective equipment required for working the scene is all part of the assessment phase. Assumptions should never be made about the safety of the lab environment. Decisions are based upon the observations made at the scene and monitoring for hazardous gases or oxygen depletion. Based on this cumulative information, a decision is made for required PPE. The level of protection can be downgraded if conditions at the lab change due to factors such as ventilation and/or deactivation of the chemical reaction. There are four basic PPE levels of protection.

Level A is the highest skin, eye and respiratory protection. This means wearing a fully encapsulating, chemical protective body suit, coveralls and Nomex™ (a fire retardant material). Respiratory protection is provided by a positive pressure, full facepiece SCBA. Additionally, two pair of chemical-resistant gloves is worn. The equipment is completed with the use of chemical-resistant boots with steel toe and shank. This level is used in fentanyl, LSD, MPPP and MPTP labs. Few agencies are prepared to handle this type of event and will need assistance from a HAZMAT team or waste hauler.

Level B requires the highest respiratory protection with the use of an SCBA or air-supplied respirator. There is a reduced level of skin protection. This level is used in operational and some investigative labs. Personal protective equipment required is a positive pressure, full facepiece SCBA; hooded, chemical-resistant clothing such as Saranex®; nitrile or neoprene chemical-resistant outer gloves; nitrile, latex or surgical type vinyl chemical resistant-inner gloves; chemical resistant, steel toe and shank boots; and outer, chemical-resistant, disposable boot covers. A Nomex garment can be worn underneath the chemical-resistant clothing.

Level C requires a lesser respiratory protection and reduced skin protection. This level of protection is worn in some investigative labs and with boxed labs. The required equipment includes a full facepiece air purifying respirator with canister; hooded, chemical-resistant clothing such as Saranex®, nitrile or neoprene chemical-resistant outer gloves; nitrile, latex or surgical type vinyl chemical-resistant inner gloves; chemical-resistant, steel toe and shank boots; and outer, chemical-resistant, disposable boot covers. Additionally, a NIOSH approved escape SCBA that provides 5 minutes of air must also be carried into the scene.

Level D requires minimum protection due to no known hazard. At a minimum an individual should wear long sleeves. Gloves and safety glasses are optional. However, forensic identification specialists will always wear gloves while processing for latent impressions to maintain the integrity of the evidence. No respiratory equipment is required. If a hazard develops or is later detected, this level could be upgraded to a higher level.

The above mentioned personal protective equipment provides state of the art protection based on the knowledge and materials of today. However, none of it is perfect. Nomex™ is a fire retardant material but is not fireproof. It prevents ignition of any clothing worn under it. However, never wear nylon undergarments to a lab as they will melt and stick to your skin in a fire. Nomex™ protects against flash explosions and allows for escape. Nomex™ does not provide any protection from chemicals and is too bulky to be worn under chemical gloves.

All chemical-resistant suits such as Tyvek® and Saranex® are disposable. While affording protection to the skin, they also have their negative aspects. Saranex® suits are like a Tyvek® suit wrapped in Saran wrap or plastic. While this provides a resistance to chemicals, it also induces heat stress. Imagine wrapping your body in Saran wrap on a hot day and you can relate to the problem. Additionally, the wrists and ankles are typically sealed with duct tape to prevent any chemicals from running into the sleeve or cuff. Cooling vests can be worn under the suit if ambient temperatures are 80° F or higher. These vests are packed with ice and will last about an hour but require a source and supply for ice.

Any gloves worn at the scene should first be blown into to detect any flaw in the material. Outer gloves are typically made of a chemical-resistant material called nitrile or neoprene. They are usually green in color or may be black. Gloves worn for inner protection are usually made of a lighter nitrile, latex or vinyl. (These are the types of gloves used by surgeons.) Remember that latex may present latex sensitivity problems. Inner gloves are worn in the event there is some limited exposure to chemicals such as touching the outer gloves upon removal. They do not protect against serious chemical contact. Their essential role is for removal of other personal protective equipment. If your outer gloves become obviously contaminated with chemical material, wipe them off with rags or paper towels. Remember that all glove material is designed to provide a protective barrier over a given period of time so they do degrade over time. Periodically inspect your gloves during processing to ensure that they still have integrity.

All boots worn to clan labs should have steel toe and shank. While Goretex™ provides good protection from water and dampness, it provides no protection from chemicals. Neoprene is a better choice of material for working labs. Disposable booties worn over neoprene boots can create trip and slip hazards. They do not have enough material strength and integrity to hold up if walking over rough terrain. They will break apart and will have to be replaced.

Eye and face protection must meet ANSI Standard Z 87. Sunglasses do not meet the specifications and are unacceptable for use as personal protective equipment. Safety glasses with side shields provide the best protection for the eyes and should always be worn where chemicals are present. If wearing a full-face respirator, remember that contact lenses are not allowed. While this may seem unreasonable and problematic, it is the standard.

Personal clothing should never be worn to clandestine laboratory scenes. Law enforcement agencies have an obligation to provide field clothing and outer disposable protective clothing such as Tyvek® and Saranex®. All scene photographers should wear the same PPE as Chemists or Criminalists if the scene is located in a structure. If the scene is outdoors, the photographer should don the same PPE as the latent print specialists.

The decisions on use of personal protective equipment are based on present knowledge and past experience, as well as good methodology. However; there are still varying opinions on "who" should be required to wear "what". Should narcotics officers be required to wear full Level B protective equipment into a clan lab to arrest the suspects? Obviously, the PPE could pose a greater risk to the officers than the ambient environment. By the same token, should forensic identification specialists be required to enter a clan lab and perform processing duties in Level B protective equipment? Again, I think not! If a scene presents hazards so great that Level B protection is required, then it is too hazardous for the identification people. What is to be gained by suiting identification specialists in SCBAs to do their job? Visibility is limited as is the time allowed by the air tanks. SCBAs introduce a fatigue factor as well. If the job can be done with a different, less stressful approach, pursue that course of action. **I believe that forensic identification specialists should never be placed in a position to need to don equipment above Level C at clan labs**. The agents and Chemist/Criminalist must access the scene to deactivate the lab, monitor the lab, begin ventilation and take photographs. However, any items for latent print processing can be removed from the interior and brought outside to the identification personnel. If moving items (like full reaction flasks) to the outside is not possible, then the lab should be stabilized through ventilation and the identification people given access with Level C protection. We always want to move to the least hazardous scenario. **If an air-purifying respirator is not capable of providing the necessary protection against known contaminants, the scene is too dangerous for latent print processing.** Now, that is according to the "Book of Nancy"!

Safety Protocols

While the following safety protocols are intended for the latent print processing team, they apply to everyone at the scene. The risks are high and one slip up can result in tragedy. Please take these protocols seriously.

- **Most important: Trust your instincts. If you smell something you feel you shouldn't or if you become uncomfortable with the progression of events then GET OUT!!!** You always have the right to remove yourself from the Contamination Zone of a clan lab scene if you feel your health or life is at risk. Get out and then explain your concerns to the Safety Officer or chemist. NEVER go back in unless you are totally comfortable with the situation. Don't be frivolous because you will have to explain to your supervisor.

- Do NOT eat, drink, smoke or apply cosmetics or insert contact lenses at a clan lab scene unless you have fully decontaminated and are in the Support Zone.

- NEVER eat food found at the scene! (It seems obvious but I observed a chemist eat snack foods laying around a clan lab where chemical contamination was layered and encrusted on most surfaces.)

- Do NOT open refrigerators or cupboards until cleared by the Chemist/Criminalist. These areas may be booby-trapped. Opening and closing refrigerator doors can create a spark resulting in an explosion.

- Do NOT turn any light switches on or off at the scene. This could result in an explosion.

- Do NOT touch anything that has not been pointed out to you for your attention. Booby traps are not uncommon at clan labs. They could be bombs, trip wires, rattlesnakes in cupboards, chemical traps, firearm traps, or acid baths to name a few. If you see anything suspicious, alert the Chemist/Criminalist immediately.

- Do NOT open or move containers containing chemicals or suspected chemicals.

- Do NOT sniff any containers. Not all hazardous chemicals have warning properties. Some hazardous chemical's permissible exposure limit is at the same level as its warning properties. In other words, once you actually smell it, you have received a possibly hazardous inhalation exposure. If the material is hazardous enough, the exposure could be fatal.

- Be ALERT to the presence of any chemicals or chemical mixtures during latent print processing. Bring these to the attention of the Chemist/Criminalist.

- Use the BUDDY SYSTEM while working clan labs. Make an effort to take notice of your colleagues. Pay special attention to any behavior that seems inappropriate for the situation or that particular individual.

- Use your powers of observation. If anything makes you uncomfortable or suspicious, bring it to the attention of the Safety Officer or Chemist/Criminalist.

- Do NOT process items of glassware, equipment or containers for latent prints that have visible contamination such as chemical residues or pump oil on the surface. Processing such items rarely results in usable prints and will result in contaminating your brush, powder and other equipment. You will now need to obtain a new brush to continue processing. One thing for certain is that any resulting latent lift cards will be seriously contaminated.

- All latent print processing should be performed in an outside environment if possible. Evidence from inside should be moved to the outside to a secure and protected area.

- Fingerprint materials such as brushes, tapes, powders, etc. should be discarded with other hazardous waste at the end of processing. The waste hauler will remove all contaminated equipment and waste from the site.

- Prepackaged latent print kits are highly recommended and can be prepared at headquarters prior to an assignment. Place a couple rolls of tape, a container of powder, supply of lift cards, pen, pencil, marker and two brushes into a Zipper Lock bag. Use these supplies to process the clan lab. At the end of processing, the bag goes with the waste hauler.

- Developed latent lift cards should be placed in a plastic pouch and heat-sealed or put in a Zipper Lock bag and a Hazard Warning Label affixed to the outside. Affix an additional label on sealed lift card pouches or bags that reads "Clan Lab". Remember that these lift cards are considered contaminated and should never be handled without gloves.

- Photographers must take special care in use of photographic equipment not to ignite gases present at the scene.

- If you receive a potentially harmful exposure of any kind or are injured, report it to the Safety Officer immediately. You should be removed from the scene and immediately taken to a medical clinic or hospital for examination. Be sure to follow up with a written report of the incident and submit any necessary forms. Now having said this, let me clarify. Just smelling chemical odors is probably not deleterious to your health and can be expected in a clan lab environment. However, if you can't breathe, your eyes burn or your lungs burn, you begin to cough or vomit, feel dizzy, faint or nauseated, then you have likely received a potentially harmful exposure. It is time to get out and get help.

Decontamination

As with all other aspects of working clandestine drug laboratories, there is a system to decontamination. All decontamination takes place in the Contamination Reduction Zone (Warm Zone). Equipment and water will be available and in place for accomplishing this effort. A series of stations are established for each step in decontamination. Assuming that Level C protective equipment was used, the following steps are taken.

Deposit any supplies or equipment (such as latent print kits) used on site onto plastic cloths or into marked, plastic lined containers. Scrub outer boots and outer gloves with decontamination solution or detergent water. Rinse off using copious amount of water. Remove tape around boots and gloves and deposit in plastic lined container. Remove boot covers and outer gloves, deposit in container with plastic liner. Wash splash suit, gloves and safety boots. Scrub with long handled brush and decontamination solution. Rinse off decontamination solution using water. Remove safety boots and deposit in plastic lined container. If possible, seek assistance in removing chemical splash suit and place it in the plastic lined container. Wash inner gloves with decontamination solution and rinse with water. Remove face piece of respirator. Avoid touching the face with fingers. The face piece is deposited in a container with a plastic liner. (If you have your own assigned respirator, you may wish to decontaminate it yourself using the decontamination kit.) Remove inner gloves and deposit in lined container. Thoroughly wash the face and hands. Shower as soon as possible.

The above procedures may be modified depending upon the scene and levels of possible contamination. At grossly contaminated scenes, showers should be taken at the scene and any perspiration soaked clothing placed in plastic bags. Definitely shower on site if highly toxic, skin corrosive or skin absorbable materials are known or suspected to be present. Put on clean clothes before leaving the scene. At a minimum, always wash hands and face if a shower is not present.

Chemical Spills

Chemical spills can occur at a clandestine laboratory scene. Moving chemicals whether in original containers or reaction flasks always presents a potential spill hazard. If a spill occurs, personnel wearing the necessary PPE can attempt to contain the spill using a Solid-a-Sorb or equivalent material. The site Safety Officer has responsibility for ensuring that spill materials are at the scene. In the event of an uncontrolled spill, the local health department should be notified as soon as possible. While the forensic identification specialist (if properly suited up in the appropriate PPE) can render assistance in the event of a chemical spill; dealing with the spill is the responsibility of the site Safety Officer and/or Chemist/Criminalist.

Hazardous Waste

Hazardous waste is an immense topic. At clandestine drug laboratory scenes, this waste is dealt with at the direction of the case agent and on site Safety Officer. Licensed waste haulers document and remove all hazardous wastes from the scene. Forensic identification specialists need to be aware of a couple of points. Containers for hazardous waste should be well marked at the scene leaving no doubt as to where to place items for disposal. All removed disposable garments are hazardous waste. All inexpensive sampling equipment and latent print supplies used for processing are hazardous waste. Decontamination solutions and water used in decontamination of equipment, respirators and personnel is hazardous waste. All these items are released to the licensed waste hauler for removal from the site. The best rule to keep in mind is this: When in doubt, throw it out!!!

Disaster Scenes

Disasters can range from earthquakes and landslides or floods to airplane and train crashes and now, acts of terrorism. Every site poses special hazards. Personal protective equipment is an absolute MUST! Each scene will dictate which equipment to select. All scenes will require protective clothing, goggles and gloves due to the potentially infectious materials. Most will require rubber foot wear. Some such as bombing sites and earthquake sites will require hard hats. Many will be so unpleasant with the stench of decaying flesh that, at a minimum, an air-purifying respirator with an organic vapor cartridge is needed. And, in the worst case scenario, self-contained breathing apparatus is required.

Constant hand washing is an absolute necessity. The amount of biological material at these types of scenes can be overwhelming. Crime scene people who worked the first bombing of the Trade Towers and the Oklahoma City building all wore state-of-the-art protective equipment. Many used SCBAs to do their search for survivors and evidence. And yet, according to some colleagues with the FBI, most everyone who worked those sites got sick afterward. And now we have seen it again at the destruction of the Trade Towers in New York City last year. The people who worked that scene day after day searching for survivors were exposed to raw sewage as well as human and animal remains. Yes, they too got sick. (I truly cringe when I see television coverage including the area called the "bath tub" that is full of water and located at the center of ground zero.) All buildings have extensive plumbing systems that when bombed into an unusable arrangement, spill sewage into the scene. That cesspool of raw sewage breeds organisms at an incredible rate. Everyone at the scene is eventually exposed to these bacteria due to the saturation level of material. The possibility of contamination from these materials increases with the concentrations. The potential for exposure to bloodborne pathogens increases when human remains are in an advanced stage of decomposition. Admittedly, washing hands and other exposed skin may not prevent an exposure in such a bacterial laden environment. It may however, reduce the exposure significantly.

Disaster scenes involving trains and airplanes also present special problems. There is often diesel fuel or airplane fuel and oil at the site. These fuels are all toxic and serious irritants to skin. There may be other chemicals present (from transport or in the environment) such as pesticides, fertilizers or industrial wastes. There may be serious fire hazards. If a train or airplane has landed in water, the hazards increase. Water containing human remains breeds a bacteria-rich environment that is also fouled with a fuel and oil mixture. Anyone working in such a watery environment can expect to get chemical burns on any exposed skin and may get sick. Unfortunately, there is no preventative measure that can be taken that will ensure not getting sick. However, using every piece of PPE available and washing all exposed skin and hands at every opportunity will help decrease the exposures. Lastly, decontamination procedures must be strictly followed.

Immediate decontamination of any non-disposable equipment will also assist in the effort to decrease exposure events. A disaster site should have a decontamination zone the same as a clandestine drug laboratory. If there is gross contamination, a Hazardous Materials Response Team should be requested for decontamination. Any one coming in contact with possibly contaminated equipment should wear rubber gloves. Any contaminated equipment should be sprayed down with a bleach solution and then hosed off after 3 to 5 minutes. As soon as possible, team members who have worked the site should shower and thoroughly scrub skin and scalp with an anti-bacterial soap. We are on a learning curve with these types of scenes and building knowledge and developing protocols is an ongoing process.

If you work one of these scenes and do get sick (usually influenza type symptoms of fever, headache, etc.), report it to a supervisor and complete any necessary paperwork. See a physician as soon as possible and tell him/her everything you know about what was present at the scene. There are diseases such as meningitis that can result from bacterial or viral overloads [13] and a physician needs this information to make an accurate diagnosis.

Exhumations

Exhumations, often mistakenly referred to as "body digs", do not usually involve forensic identification specialists. However, there is that rare opportunity that may come along to take part in this type of scene. In reality, any individual involved in an exhumation of a clandestine gravesite should be properly trained prior to the event. There are classes and workshops available that prepare a specialist for this type of scene.

In the not too recent past, a body exhumation often resembled a construction site. A typical scene would be complete with bulldozers and backhoes and an accompaniment of various individuals trampling the scene. As the forensic community looked more to the archeological community, they realized they were losing or destroying valuable clues, evidence and information with such a gross handling of the scene. These sites are now handled very methodically with the same protocols and procedures afforded archeological digs. Many high tech tools and instruments such as ground penetrating radar (GPR) and global positioning satellite (GPS) are brought into play to search and document the location of the remains and site. Scene parameters are set and secured. A dirt pedestal is dug around the remains allowing an area wide enough to include evidence other than the remains. Soil covering the remains is removed very carefully by the spoonful rather than by the shovel load. Remains being removed may be in the skeletal form or in various stages of decomposition. All forms of trace evidence are sought using a variety of tools such as probes, spades, brushes and screen-bottomed boxes. The search includes retrieval of hairs, fibers, bullets and/or bullet fragments, plant material, insects and insect larvae, fabric or clothing, geological matter and items left behind by the perpetrator to name a few.

Safety considerations are the same as those involving any scene with dead bodies. There may be concerns regarding potentially infectious materials and bloodborne pathogens. There can be issues relating to the environment in regard to ticks or poison ivy, oak or sumac. Every scene presents its own unique set of concerns. Personal protective equipment should be selected based on the elements present at the scene. Certainly, at a minimum, gloves and protective clothing should be worn. Rubber boots and goggles may also be desirable. Go prepared (or loaded for bear!) for any eventuality. The crime scene vehicle should always be equipped with any necessary safety equipment.

Homicide/Suicide Scenes

These scenes often contain potentially infectious materials. Always apply universal precautions. Use all recommended personal protective equipment. Consider all situations presented by the scene in selecting PPE, making processing decisions and completing a thorough hazard evaluation.

Wear goggles and dust/mist (particulate) respirators when removing portions of walls. Wear disposable head covers if ceilings are blood spattered. Disposable, contaminated materials such as paper coats, masks, gloves, and shoe or head covers should be double bagged and labeled as a biohazard. Non-disposable and non-evidential contaminated items such as clothing, air-purifying respirators and goggles are placed in a biohazard bag. Clothing being cleaned by a contract linen service should be placed in a biohazard bag for transport to the cleaners.

Non-disposable PPE should be disinfected for later use. This can be accomplished after returning to the laboratory. If PIMs are present at the scene, evidential items must be properly packaged to preserve latent prints or other trace evidence while providing a protective barrier. Place a biohazard label on the outside of the evidence packaging. NEVER attempt to recap, crimp or break a needle. Place needles or sharp objects in a puncture resistant container and affix a biohazard label.

The best protection from PIMs is washing. When washing hands, be sure to get soap and water over all skin surfaces, including between the fingers and under the nails. Wash your hands and forearms before taking a break (after glove removal) and before leaving the scene.

Report any exposure event to a supervisor as soon as possible and take all recommended post exposure steps.

Suspects at Large

A bulletproof vest may be worn at scenes where suspects are still at large and believed to be armed. Such individuals should always be considered dangerous. Unfortunately, these vests will not protect an individual from stab wounds from knives, ice picks or many other sharp objects. These vests should be made available to any individual requesting one if they are working at a scene where the apprehension of the suspects has not been accomplished.

Individuals who are not authorized and trained to carry firearms must never be left alone at a scene when suspects are at large! This has happened to forensic identification specialists in past years at clan labs involving Hells Angels! A sworn officer should always be posted at the scene to maintain scene security and provide protection for non-sworn personnel.

Underwater Scenes

Most forensic identification specialists will not be involved in an underwater crime scene. The nature of the scene requires that those who are involved are part of a very special team of highly trained individuals. The fact that team members are diving with self-contained underwater breathing apparatus (SCUBA) means that safety protocols are in place for the diving function. Each team member must have a clear understanding of the conditions and procedures involved in such an operation. This section will set out a few basic guidelines regarding being involved as a member of such a diving team.

Basic Protocols

The most important rule is that no team member should ever coerce another member into attempting any feat or performing any task that he or she either is not qualified for or does not feel comfortable to undertake. Each member must be the final judge as to his or her ability and capabilities of their equipment. Never should a member attempt a task that entails an unacceptable measure of risk. An unacceptable risk is any feat or act that fails to provide a margin of safety through a backup system capable of aborting the attempt and retrieving the participants. [14]

Diving is a team effort that requires a Team Leader and Chief of Operations. One individual can fulfill both assignments. However, most operations have different individuals in each role. The Team Leader has absolute authority over the events at the scene unless the Chief of Operations takes charge of the mission upon arrival. All members of the team take direction from one of these two individuals. There should never be any question as to who has responsibility and authority to make decisions at the scene.

A Safety Officer (SO) must be present at each training event and diving scene. This individual has full responsibility to take an aggressive approach on safety in a manner to ensure that that no one gets hurt. No scene can ever be made totally safe, but the SO must demand that all team members follow appropriate safety procedures, and ensure that all equipment is handled in a safe manner. This means that the Safety Officer also has the ultimate authority in matters directly involving safety and can suspend or terminate the operation in the event of unsafe practices and/or conditions. (The Team Leader is the channel for such termination and must communicate freely with the Safety Officer.) A safety briefing should be held with the diving team prior to training or working the scene. Completion of any paperwork as a follow up to training or a scene is coordinated between the SO and Team Leader and serves as documentation in the event of an accident or injury.

The Safety Officer should evaluate the need for a stand-by medical team at training sessions and should supply a prepared plan for medical evacuation and treatment if there is a medical emergency. Again, communication can not be stressed too much. The SO must interact with the Team Leader at all times. Access must be given to the SO to all locations so any unsafe conditions can be reported to the Team Leader immediately. Lastly, the SO should give a verbal report to the Team Leader on the safety aspects of the operation and prepare a written report in the event injuries or unsafe conditions were observed. Any report should focus not only on the concerns but also on preventative measures to take in the future.

Team members should only work at their classification level. The Team Leader or Chief of Operations should assign duties at the scene in accordance with your classification. Never accept an assignment you feel you can NOT handle based on your training, experience and certification. This should never really be an issue but it points up the fact that, ultimately, each person has a responsibility for her or his own safety. You always have a right of refusal to perform a task that you feel puts your health or life at risk.

Team members at the scene are usually divided into two groups, divers and shore personnel. There must always be at least a minimum of one person acting as shore personnel. The Team Leader or Chief of Operations can act in this capacity. All team members, with the exception of those wearing full dive gear, should wear a personal flotation device and helmets when in and around the water. This equipment ought to be donned upon arrival until completion of the scene.

(The Team Leader should have discretion on the removal of helmets by shore personnel.) There must always be a minimum of three divers. Divers enter the water in teams of two, employing the buddy system, watching each other for problems or difficulties. The third diver is a safety diver, suited up and ready in the event there is a problem. No diver should ever enter the water without authorization from the Team Leader. There are no exceptions to this rule.

Training

As previously mentioned, training as a diver is a basic and vital requirement for underwater scenes. Lessons taken for SCUBA diving on vacation in Hawaii does not qualify a person to dive at a scene! Training is an ongoing activity through the year. It is recommended that members attend a minimum of six training sessions per year (January through December). Of the six sessions, at least two must be practical shore or water training (hands-on training, open water or confined water exercises). [15] Additional training in relevant areas (first aid, CPR, etc.) is always recommended. All training must be properly documented with the instructor's name, title and description of training, date and location of training and the student's full name.

Safety Considerations

Experienced rescue divers acknowledge that adhering to certain guidelines tends to improve results, maintain a high level of safety, improve efficiency and make searching easier. Following are some of those guidelines: [16]

- Stay alert and maintain the proper attitude for effective searching during the task. Searching is hard work and can be boring, tedious and extremely fatiguing. If unable to search effectively due to fatigue, tedium or exertion, advise the Team Leader. If unable to maintain the necessary self-discipline for effective searching in less than ideal conditions (bad weather, cold, hot, tired, discouragement, etc.) participation as a diver should terminate. Other, less taxing, duties can be assigned at the scene.
- Use all your senses for searching. Use your eyes, nose and ears; but especially your head. Think through what you are doing and what problems the environment presents.
- Always be prepared to respond to the scene. Have the proper equipment and clothing with you. Have an equipment pack containing items such as

drinking water and high energy snacks, flashlight, plastic whistle, wool or nylon socks, parka for varying weather conditions, pants, shirt and shoes, sunglasses, sunscreen, hat, insect repellent and a first aid kit. Stay in touch with the condition of your equipment and be sure to always have your equipment pack adequately supplied.

- Wear socks and thermal protection at all times when wearing dry suits for diving. Otherwise, hypothermia can easily set in resulting in risk to the diver and safety diver.

- Know the names of your fellow team members and who has the authority to make assignments and decisions.

- At night, never shine your flashlight or headlamps into your eyes or those of another team member. The optimum visual condition for diving is eyes adjusted to the dark. It can take some time for the eyes to readjust to the dark again. If safety and effectiveness can be maintained, not using lights at all is preferred.

- The safety of team members is the primary concern at a scene and should supercede all other considerations and issues. Your safety is of primary concern followed by concern for the safety of your team members. If you place yourself in jeopardy, you also put your team members in jeopardy.

- Never run while on scene. Stay calm and collected.

Contamination/Decontamination

Diving may bring you into an environment containing hazardous materials. Such materials could be chemicals such as oil, fuel, pesticides, fertilizers and industrial waste; or biological in nature such as bloodborne pathogens. Rivers, sloughs, canals and lakes do usually contain some or all of these hazardous materials. Concentrations are normally low enough not be a cause for concern. There is a heightened possibility of serious exposures or contamination with increases in concentrations of the material. This can be a result of low water circulation from low water flows or eddies and currents do not disperse contaminants. A dead body in an advanced stage of decomposition increases the potential for exposure to bloodborne pathogens. [17]

Were there is a potential for contamination from a hazardous material, the following procedures are strongly recommended: [18]

- Divers should only dive in a dry suit with a full-face mask. (Socks and thermal protection must be worn at all times when wearing dry suits.) No wet suits or half-face masks are allowed because they allow contaminated water access to skin, mouth and ears.

- Line tenders and anyone coming in contact with wet equipment should always wear rubber gloves.

- The Team Leader and Safety Personnel must inspect each diver and the safety diver prior to their entering the water.

- Where there is a known seepage of chemicals, such as at the site of an airplane crash, divers should enter the water upstream if possible.

- Upon exiting the water, divers must be washed down prior to breaking the seal on their facemask or dry suit. If oil, gas or diesel is present, the diver must be scrubbed down with a soap solution and washed off again. If biological hazards are present, the diver must be sprayed down with a bleach solution and then hosed off after 3 to 5 minutes.

- Decontaminate all wet equipment by washing down and scrubbing with soap and/or bleach before placing in a vehicle.

- A scene report should note that divers were washed down, and detail what was used, the duration of the wash down, and what chemical and/or biological substance was present, if known. Such documentation is imperative should a diver become sick, develop a rash, or have some other possibly related complaint.

- As soon as possible, the diver(s) should shower and thoroughly scrub skin and scalp with an anti-bacterial soap.

- In the event of gross contamination, personnel should evacuate upwind a minimum of 250 feet to prevent further exposure. Potentially contaminated equipment is left behind until such time as a HAZMAT team releases it back to the agency or deems the area safe. [19]

It is vital to scene and personnel safety that the lines of communication are kept open at all times via the Team Leader or Chief of Operations. Any team member who is uncomfortable with the ambient conditions at the scene should be able to request that the above procedures in whole or in part be activated.

I have presented a quantity of material here on crime scene safety. However, due to the enormity of the topic, every possible scenario can not be covered any more than it can be anticipated in the field. The guidelines and protocols, along with the accompanying rationale, provide a good basis for protection from hazardous events or exposures. All things said and presented, it still all comes down to one bottom line. Safety begins with you. You have an obligation to yourself and your colleagues at the scene to approach all aspects of the scene in the safest manner possible. You always have the right of refusal to perform any task that you feel puts you at risk. Always choose to error on the side of safety.

Nancy Masters

23
Evidence Vault/ Property Room Safety

The exact same elements of a safety program developed for the chemical laboratory and/or crime scenes apply to the police facility evidence vault and property room. This is one of the most important areas in a law enforcement facility and yet it is often relegated to some unremarkable area of the building. While any area used for the custodial protection, maintenance and processing of evidence or recovered property should be in a discreet place; the actual location often seems an afterthought. Some property rooms are nothing more than a storage room or cubbyhole made available because other personnel or functions have vacated that section of the building. It is not uncommon for such rooms to be located in the darkest, dankest and least ventilated area of the structure. These are the very factors that create an unhealthy and unsafe work environment for the people who must daily function in these surroundings. There are a wealth of issues regarding the proper construction of such facilities including appropriate building materials; security, key and lock systems; shelving systems and configurations; separate vaults for drugs, firearms, currency and hazardous materials; proper and adequate ventilation; safety sinks and eyewashes; blood drying rooms or cabinets; and alarm systems. These are only a few of the issues that need serious consideration and points to the fact that an in-depth survey should be made before designating any area of a building for such purposes. An excellent source of information for such an endeavor is provided in the book written by Joseph T. Latta [1]. This book can be obtained through the California Association of Property and Evidence (CAPE).

Safety in the evidence vault or property room is an issue for two reasons. First, problems arise around the structural issues of facility materials composition, location, ventilation and lighting. Second is the evidence itself, and the "nature of the beast". Evidence from criminal cases rarely originates in the police facility (hopefully!). The items collected in a criminal matter are submitted to the facility from the outside environment. This means that any safety hazards associated with such items at the crime scene, whether chemical, physical or biological in nature, now pose the same hazards to personnel in the facility. Many of the safety issues are discussed in detail in other sections of the book. Personnel working in evidence vaults and/or property rooms are encouraged to read the remainder of this book to obtain the detailed information on pertinent safety topics.

In previous sections, I have made the statement, "Safety begins with you." almost to *ad nauseam*. Having acknowledged this, I again reiterate the importance of each individual being willing to take a stand on the side of safety. The most significant aspect of any established safety program is the commitment made by each person to be "safety minded". At the core of this philosophy is the motivation and resolve to take responsibility for safety; for compliance to all rules and guidelines; and for hazard awareness. Additionally, a person must be determined to observe issues and events not only for her or his own welfare but also for the safety of other people. (Yes, we do have a moral obligation to be our brother's keeper.) This will sometimes require that you take action. And action is not always easy. It could entail changing our entire mindset or modifying our approach to the way we do our work. It could also require making a complaint (perhaps about a coworker), documenting events, contacting OSHA or testifying at a hearing or trial. Vigilance in safety issues can mean the difference between life and death. Do not allow co-workers to lull you into poor work practices or a lackadaisical attitude.

While evidence vaults and property rooms come in all sizes and configurations, there are basic safety issues applicable to all of them. The following discussions will detail the basic concerns that must be addressed by the administration of any department that facilitates the safe-keeping, storage or processing of evidence and recovered property. These issues include biological hazards, chemical hazards, firearms, explosives, narcotics, sharps, facility design and equipment, availability of personal protective equipment and housekeeping.

Every police agency must have a written safety program that addresses any safety issues confronting personnel working for that agency. Individuals must be trained on these issues upon initial assignment as well as given periodical updated training. The requirements established by the federal government are detailed in Section 2.

Biological Hazards

Biological hazards are presented in two ways. One concern comes from any organic materials or items brought into the agency. This includes items contaminated with blood, items consisting of or contaminated with flesh (animal or human) and any plant material such as marijuana. These biological products grow fungal spores as a process of decomposition. Blood grows these bacterial elements just as readily as marijuana. A by-product of this process of "stuff" growing on these materials is the development of mycotoxins, both endotoxins and exotoxins. People can and do develop sensitivities to such mycotoxins. The resulting allergic reaction may require medical attention. So, the bloody clothing or bedding from a crime scene presents serious biological concerns (not to mention the occasional bear's gall bladder, amputated digit or mummified fetus being stored in a property room somewhere in the country).

If organic materials must be retained in the facility, they must also be properly packaged to contain any mycotoxins. The first rule is not to accept any wet or semi-wet evidence unless you have the capability of drying it prior to packaging. This requires a separate drying room or cabinet with a negative pressure ventilation system. A negative pressure inside the drying area will result in air being drawn in from the outside when doors are opened. This is an important aspect of keeping contaminants in a specified area. The worst scenario is for contaminants to be drawn or blown outside the drying area when a door is opened. The negative pressure ventilation system is completed with an exhaust duct to the outside.

The second area of concern with biological materials comes from the hazards posed by Bloodborne Pathogens. An in-depth discussion is found in Section 5. While there are a number of diseases transmitted through blood or other body fluids with traces of blood, Human Immunodeficiency Virus (HIV), Hepatitis B Virus (HBV) and Hepatitis C Virus (HCV) pose the greatest risks. Always apply **Universal Precautions**. Whenever working around any material that contains blood or body fluids with visible traces of blood, assume that all human body fluids are infectious. If you are unable to determine the type of body fluid, consider it potentially infectious.

Human Immunodeficiency Virus is the virus most feared because exposure can result in AIDS and death. Since there is no vaccination for HIV, an exposure event resulting in an infection is deemed very serious. However, the risk of developing AIDS as result of any single exposure is Y2 of 1%. It is also noteworthy to remember that HIV is very short lived in an open-air, non-liquid environment (such as on a dry counter top). This means that if it is not in a moist environment where it is protected and can multiply, it dies. Risks of an exposure event to HIV should and must be taken seriously, however there are greater risks posed by hepatitis.

Hepatitis B Virus is contracted much easier than HIV. It survives for long periods of time in an open-air, non-liquid environment. Consequently, HBV can be contracted as result of an exposure to dried blood particulate. An exposure event resulting in an infection can result in chronic hepatitis, liver cancer and death. The risk of developing a Hepatitis B infection following a needlestick or open cut-type exposure to blood is directly proportional to the probability that the blood is infected with HBV. The other most pertinent factors involved in the likelihood of infection are related to the immunity status of the individual and the means of transmission of the virus into an individual's system. People who receive a blood transfusion of HBV tainted blood are certainly more likely to develop the disease than people who get a particle of infected dried blood on an area of dermatitis on their skin.

Fortunately for those who work in law enforcement, a vaccination is available for HBV. The HBV vaccination is also effective against HDV. The vaccination is 100% effective when given prior to any exposure event and antibodies develop. (The employer must offer and pay for this vaccination.) The process of developing antibodies is called "seroconversion". Some people do not show signs of seroconversion. One reason may be the need for a booster. The other reason is that some people are genetically protected. They may not have the receptors that allow the infection to occur. The vaccination is a series of three (3) injections. One to three months after the last injection, a blood test is performed to test for antibodies. If no antibodies are expressed, a person may get the series a second time. Ten (10) percent of the population do not seroconvert after the first series. Of that 10%, half will show seroconversion after taking the series a second time. Five (5) percent of individuals do not seroconvert after both series and will never convert. These people are considered to have a natural immunity. A common concern revolves around the effective life of the vaccination. At this time, there is no indication that the vaccination is effective only for a limited period of time. This is an issue between the individual and his or her physician. If in doubt, a blood test can be administered to determine whether antibodies are still present.

What if an exposure event occurs and the affected person has not had the vaccination? The vaccination can still be administered but is only 70 – 88% effective. For this reason, all medical evidence indicates that receiving the vaccination prior to any potential exposure event is the best possible methodology. This exemplifies one situation in which the most effective approach to the safety issue is prevention.

The hepatitis virus is tenacious and has mutated over the years. This has resulted in a serious rise in cases of Hepatitis C Virus. HCV was once referred to as Non-A, Non-B hepatitis. This virus is contracted in the same ways as HIV and HBV. It is supposedly more difficult to contract and yet, it is more prevalent in the general population. This reality has puzzled the research community. (Four times more people are infected with HCV than HIV.) It is often referred to as "the silent virus" because it lays inactive in the liver and may not express itself for decades. Approximately only 5 percent of individuals know that they are infected. Of those people infected, 15% will fight the disease off through their immune response. Eighty (80) percent will become chronically sick with liver problems. Five (5) percent die of cirrhosis of the liver or liver cancer. While rumors abound, there is currently no vaccine for HCV. And the virus has continued to mutate to HDV (covered by the HBV vaccination), and HEV (no vaccination but few cases in the United States as of 2001). This process of mutation will no doubt continue over time.

The key factor to being infected with a bloodborne pathogen is an exposure event. It is important to understand what defines an exposure event. An exposure in the work environment occurs by inoculation, mucous membrane or non-intact skin contact with infected blood, blood components or blood products. So, an exposure event can be as result of sticking yourself with a needle or bloody knife, getting wet blood into an open wound or getting dried blood particulate in your eye. Exposure "does *not* mean handling a vial of blood or transporting a sealed, non-contaminated, properly packaged, piece of evidence." [2]

The federal standard regulating requirements on employers is 29 CFR 1910.1030. The elements of the standard detail the need for a Written Exposure Control Plan, Engineering Controls, Work Practices, Personal Protective Equipment (PPE), Housekeeping and the HBV Vaccination.

The Written Exposure Control Plan details the department's hazard communication policy, a determination of employee risk for exposure, and procedures for dealing with exposures and vaccinations.

Engineering Controls are physical or mechanical systems in place to eliminate hazards at their source. This includes puncture resistant sharps containers for the disposal of any sharp items such as needles, broken glass or razor blades. Another engineering control is having proper evidence packaging materials on hand at all times. Evidence is sometimes submitted in inadequate packaging and must be either repackaged or placed in additional packaging. Such packaging includes puncture resistant sharps containers and bags and pouches that can be heat or otherwise sealed. Additionally, a supply of biohazard waste bags must be available for use to discard bio-hazardous materials or submit departmental laundry items to a professional cleaning service. Every evidence vault and property room should have a supply of biohazard labels so a label can be affixed to the outside of any packaging containing potentially infectious items.

Facility Design is at the core of prevention of potential safety problems. Every police facility should have a separate area, bunker, building or portable containment structure for storing hazardous materials. Hazardous materials include all flammables such as fuels (gasoline, kerosene, Coleman fuel), chemicals from arson or clandestine drug lab scenes, automobile batteries, and any fireworks. Items of this nature should never be stored in the facility proper. They pose too many potentials for contamination, fire or explosion. Every property room should be equipped with a hand sink for hand washing and eyewash capable of producing a 15-minute flow of water. Personnel working in evidence vaults or property storage areas must be able to wash their hands and arms or flush their eyes in the event of a contamination incident. A separate blood drying room or cabinet is necessity for dealing with potentially infectious materials. A refrigerator and freezer are needed for storing biological property such as blood and urine samples, rape kits and bloodstained evidence. There must be adequate lighting, ventilation, and shelving as well as back up systems in the event of power failure.

Work Practices include a series of protocols designed to protect workers from exposure and contamination events. Some basic protocols follow.

Safety Protocols

- Wash hands, fingers and wrist areas with soap and water after removing gloves, at end of shift, before and after using the restroom, before eating or drinking, applying cosmetics or inserting contact lenses, or any time suspected contaminated items or surfaces are touched. This is one of the very best safety strategies to prevent hazardous exposures.

- Wear proper attire when handling evidence. Personal clothing is the poorest choice. Protective clothing should be provided for use.

- Never wear contaminated personal protective clothing such as jumpsuits, aprons, lab coats or overalls into other work areas. Always remove such clothing before leaving the evidence area to access other locations such as hallways and offices, restrooms, break rooms or the cafeteria.

- Never touch your face or other unprotected areas of skin with contaminated hands or personal protective equipment.

- Avoid placing pencils or pens in your mouth. They may be contaminated.

- Avoid handling the telephone with gloved hands. Contaminated gloves merely transfer contamination to the telephone. Even if you have just donned a new pair of gloves and the phone rings, remove the gloves to answer.

- Use proper waste disposal. Contaminated items of protective equipment or waste from housekeeping efforts should always be placed in clearly marked containers lined with plastic bags. Licensed hazardous waste haulers are used to periodically remove chemical and bio-hazardous wastes for legal disposal.

- Dispose of sharps in a manner that minimizes the potential for injury. Never try to bend, break or snip hypodermic needles. If dealing with broken glass, use tongs to pick it up or scoop up with a dustpan. Use tweezers to pick up needles and razors. All sharps are placed in a clearly marked sharps container for disposal. Do not overfill these containers.

- If inventorying contents of a purse or backpack turn it upside down and dump it out on the counter. Never reach into such an enclosed container. This is a needlestick injury waiting to happen.

- Never eat, drink or smoke in the evidence storage facility. Never apply cosmetics or insert contact lenses while in this area. These are common modes of transmission of contamination.

- Never place drinks, lunches, snacks or other consumables in the storage facility refrigerator. To do so is to set yourself up for a dose of contamination. Management must be firm on this issue.

Personal Protective Equipment (PPE)

PPE is equipment provided by the employer used to create a barrier between the wearer and materials that may cause injury. Most of this equipment is disposable in nature and intended for only one wearing. Personnel working in the evidence vault or property storage facility should be provided the following PPE.

Protective clothing includes such items as jumpsuits, lab coats, overalls or aprons. This should be worn over personal clothing to protect street clothes from becoming contaminated. Additional items to keep on hand are boot or shoe covers and hair covers. These are recommended if working around potentially infectious materials where particulate can get on the floor or in your hair.

Gloves are one of the most common items of PPE. The primary difficulty other than getting a size that fits is getting gloves made of the correct material. Gloves are made from a number of different materials. Each is designed for a specific purpose and will degrade over a reasonably predictable amount of time due to an exposure to temperature, chemicals or UV light. The most commonly used gloves in the property facility are latex or vinyl, nitrile and neoprene. Latex (also known as surgical gloves) is worn when handling potentially infectious materials. It is meant to be disposable after one use. Latex, however, has negative aspects to it. The most serious problem is one of latex sensitivity.

Latex sensitivity can develop without warning. Individuals who have never had problems with latex materials can be suddenly compromised. People exposed to latex gloves (and other products containing natural rubber latex) may develop allergic reactions including skin rashes, hives, nasal, sinus or eye symptoms, asthma and even shock. If you choose latex gloves, use powder-free gloves with reduced protein content. (The allergy-causing proteins or antigens are the problem.) Learn to recognize symptoms of latex allergy: skin rashes; flushing; itching; nasal, eye, or sinus symptoms. Some people know they have this sensitivity and use other gloves. But for others, the sensitivity comes on suddenly and unexpectedly. Be aware that once a latex sensitivity rears its ugly head, you can never come in contact with latex materials again. If you develop symptoms of latex allergy, avoid direct contact with latex gloves and products until you can see a physician experienced in treating latex allergy. If you have latex allergy, consult your physician regarding taking precautions. These may include: avoiding contact with latex gloves and products; avoiding areas where you might inhale the powder from the latex gloves worn by others; telling your employer, physicians, nurses, and dentists that you have latex allergy; and wearing a medical alert bracelet. Take advantage of all latex allergy education and any training provided by your employer. [3]

Another problem with latex is the fact that if it gets a pinhole in it, it self seals. Before donning a pair of latex gloves, blow into them to determine the integrity of the glove. Latex also degrades when left too long on the shelf; or when exposed to heat or UV light. In lieu of wearing latex gloves, some people prefer vinyl gloves. Vinyl gloves are worn under the same circumstances as latex. They do not provide protection against solvents, acids or other corrosive chemicals. This is a disposable, one-use glove. And do not let anyone tell you that simply wearing two pair of gloves will afford you adequate protection. This is fallacious thinking. If two pair of gloves is safer than one, why not don eight or ten pairs. A better safety strategy is to wear a better, less impervious glove such as nitrile.

For protection against chemicals, choose a glove manufactured of nitrile or neoprene. Nitrile gloves can be worn rather than latex or vinyl. These gloves are readily available, inexpensive and thin, which allows for a sense of dexterity. One distinct advantage to nitrile is that if the glove is flawed, it will rip or tear when donned. This is a good alert to the fact you have a flawed glove. This is a disposable, one-use glove.

Neoprene is the heaviest glove material and should be worn if handling any solvents, acids or other corrosives. It is the most appropriate chemically impervious glove for use in the evidence vault or property room. If moving or shelving fuels, drug lab chemicals or an automobile battery, always wear neoprene gloves. These gloves can be washed with soap and water and worn again.

Eye Protection is a must if handling, moving or shelving any chemicals or items that could be contaminated with blood or other potentially infectious materials or *Aspergillus*. At a minimum, wear safety glasses equipped with side shields. A better choice for total protection of the eyes is chemical splash goggles. These are made to fully surround the eye to eliminate any material getting into this area. Some people prefer to wear a face shield to protect all the exposed skin on the face. A face shield, however, should never take the place of safety glasses or goggles; but rather is worn in addition to eye protection. A face shield will also help protect the nose from direct exposure to particulate matter, but a better choice is a particulate mask.

Respiratory Protection in the evidence vault or property room will usually involve wearing a dust/mist particulate mask. These are often called "painter's masks" but do not purchase painter's masks for use in the property room. Since there is a potential for inhalation exposures to dried blood particulate or mold spores, always purchase masks made to filter toxic dusts. People who must wear glasses generally have problems with their mask fogging up due to moisture in exhaled breaths. A valved particulate mask can be worn in place of a non-valved mask. This type of particulate mask has a small exhalation valve in the middle of the mask allowing the exhaled breath to be directed out and down away from the eyes. Particulate masks, valved or not, are disposable and intended for one-time use. Some people are especially concerned about mold spores, such as *Aspergillus*, and want the reassurance that their mask will filter out these spores. Such a mask must contain a High Efficiency Particulate Filter (HEPA). These masks are more expensive and usually are disposable (one-time use) but they do offer considerably more protection. Never wear a disposable mask more than once or pass it around for others to use. Considered any used mask contaminated and toss it into the waste bin.

If your department supplies you with a half-face respirator, then there must be a written respiratory program (WRP) in place. For further information on Personal Protective Equipment and Respiratory Protection, see Section 8.

Housekeeping

Housekeeping is an extremely important part of maintaining the evidence vault or the property room. It is also one of the most unpopular tasks that must be performed routinely. No one likes to be stuck with doing the cleaning. However, a system must be in place to ensure that a program of disinfecting the necessary work areas is accomplished. The bottom line: it is a part of the job duties and responsibility of all property room personnel to clean the area. (It would be inappropriate to expect the janitorial staff to perform this task. They are not properly trained and it creates security issues.) When should this cleaning task be performed?

Disinfect the work counter of the blood drying room and the property intake station whenever contamination is suspected, when changing station operators or at the end of each shift. Always use the appropriate PPE while performing decontamination. At a minimum, use protective clothing, gloves and eye protection. A very effective disinfecting solution is a mixture of one or two cups of liquid bleach to one gallon of water.

Part of the safety strategy in housekeeping is to isolate hazards as much as reasonably possible. Use marked containers for regulated waste. This includes containers for biological waste and chemical waste. Dispose of Sharps in a puncture resistant container that can be closed. Never overfill these containers as it sets the next individual up for a cut or puncture wound when they reach into it. Use PPE when handling contaminated items or even if you suspect an item is contaminated.

Protect surfaces that may become contaminated by covering with newspaper or butcher paper. Dispose of this covering and replace whenever the area is contaminated. Such areas are any counters in the blood drying room and the intake counter in the property room.

Routes of Exposure

Everyone must have a fundamental understanding of how we can get exposed to materials that pose health and safety hazards. For a detailed discussion, see Section 6. Be aware that there are four avenues that provide entry of foreign materials into our body. Absorption exposures occur by material getting on the skin, mucous membranes or into cuts and abrasions on the skin. Inhalation exposures result from breathing foreign materials in through the nose and mouth. Ingestion exposures result from foreign material getting into our mouth while eating, drinking, smoking or applying cosmetics. If proper work practices and safety protocols are followed, an ingestion exposure should never occur. Lastly, Injection exposures occur as result of a poke or stick injury by a sharp or pointed item that is contaminated. Needles, broken glass, knives and razors are just a few of the items that pose this hazard.

Again, while a person may receive an exposure this does not mean that it is a hazardous exposure. A sharp object may stick you, but it may not be contaminated with a harmful substance. When pumping gasoline into our vehicle, we usually smell the gasoline fumes. This constitutes an inhalation exposure. But is it a harmful exposure? No, because the amount of fumes and vapors inhaled are within the acceptable limits for that material. So, do not panic if an exposure occurs but report it immediately to your supervisor and follow up with any reports or visits to a physician.

Storing hypodermic needles in an evidence facility poses serious risks to personnel. Of all potential exposures to materials in the evidence vault or property room, a percutaneous puncture with a needle can lead to the very worst health and life threatening results. Let me submit to all property room supervisors a radical proposition. Stop storing hypodermic needles! A random (unscientific) survey of thousands of people who work in property rooms revealed that less than 1% per year ever check a hypodermic needle out to go to court. So why do we continue to keep this dangerous apparatus in the workplace? As yet, no one has given a satisfactory answer to this question. Rather than storing needles, document them and send them for destruction as hazardous sharps. The problem can be simply resolved with a form, a photograph and a disposable sharps container. Still not convinced? Consider the fact that most city, county and state crime laboratories do **not** accept needles into evidence. The same logic applies to needles as to quantities of marijuana, clandestine drug laboratory chemicals and explosives. All these materials pose serious health or safety hazards in the evidence storage facility that are unnecessary and totally unacceptable. Good written and photographic documentation should meet all legal requirements. Educate your administrators and district attorneys.

Chemical Hazards

Chemicals in the work place can create fire, reactive, physical and toxicity hazards. (For more information on chemical hazards see Section 4.) Chemicals should never be stored in the evidence vault or main property room. These items should always be stored in a separately ventilated and temperature controlled structure.

Chemicals that are flammable or combustible pose fire hazards. Once vapors or fumes escape the container and accumulate in a room; an explosive air mixture is created that can explode with a small spark. This will result in a fire. Any flammable chemicals must be stored in a well-sealed container and labeled as "Flammable".

Reactive chemicals are those that are not compatible with some other chemical. If they come into contact with each other, an explosion will result. Reactive chemicals can be unstable in one situation or another. A good example is pure sodium, which is packed in a metal can in oil. It is very unstable when it comes in contact with water. A very small amount thrown into a pail of water creates a terrific explosion. Reactive chemicals must be properly labeled.

Chemicals that will burn through or destroy human flesh upon contact cause physical hazards. This includes corrosive chemicals which are either an acid or alkaline. If handling corrosive chemicals, or automobile batteries, be sure to wear neoprene gloves. A strong acid that comes in contact with the skin will burn until it reaches the bone. This type of injury may take many months to heal and is very miserable.

Toxicity hazards come from any number of chemicals. These hazards are categorized into four types. The first is poisons. Many chemicals are poisonous by nature and pose a threat to health and life. The second type is a carcinogen. These chemicals cause cancer. Cancer generally results after a repeated number of exposures to a carcinogen over a period of time. (There are no documented cases of anyone developing lung cancer after smoking their first pack of cigarettes.) Very few carcinogens can cause an immediate effect upon the body. The one carcinogen that can have an immediate effect, based on a substantial exposure, is radiation. This will not be a concern in the property room unless radioactive material has been submitted as evidence in a case. If an officer ever tries to submit such evidence, refuse it! The third type of toxic material is mutagens. These are materials that cause a permanent change in an individual's DNA. And lastly, are terotogens. These are chemicals that change the DNA in a developing fetus in the uterus. An example of this is thalidomide. Women were given thalidomide back in the 1960's as a sedative to help them with morning sickness. No one realized the dangers of this chemical until thousands of babies were born with severely malformed limbs or no limbs at all. They, in fact, were referred to as "thalidomide babies".

One way to deal with the inherent hazards presented by various chemicals is using a system for storing them. Like chemicals are stored together; flammables with other flammables, acids with acids, and bases with bases. Chemicals that have known incompatibilities are always segregated and stored away from all other chemicals. Chemicals that pose no known flammable, corrosive or incompatibility hazards can be stored together.

Chemicals can present more than one hazard. Kerosene is both flammable and toxic. Sulfuric acid is both extremely corrosive and toxic. Try to educate yourself regarding any chemicals in your work area. How can you know the hazards of chemicals in your work area? By asking questions and consulting Material Safety Data Sheets (MSDS). Chemicals under submission are not going to come with an MSDS but these can be obtained online or from a library. When in doubt about chemicals, refuse to handle them. Call a Chemist or Criminalist with your local crime laboratory to render assistance. If an error is to be made, always error on the side of safety.

Narcotics

Narcotics taken into custody for storage present some of the problems mentioned in the chemical hazard section. Narcotics include cocaine and its derivatives, heroin, PCP, MPPP, MDA and MDDA or other designer drugs, LSD, methamphetamine, morphine and its derivatives. Always wear appropriate PPE when handling any narcotics. Any of these drugs in the dry form must be packaged in 4 mil (at a minimum) thick polyethylene bags and heat-sealed. Avoid inhaling the dust from cocaine and methamphetamine or getting it on your skin. Liquid LSD or PCP (or other designer drugs) must be packaged in a barrier proof vial. The vial is then placed in a 4-mil thick polyethylene bag and heat-sealed.

Never get liquid LSD or PCP on your bare skin. This can not be overemphasized. An area the size of a dime of LSD on bare skin can mean death. Narcotics should never really come to the property room in inappropriate packaging. If you are in doubt or in trouble, call for a Chemist or Criminalist from your nearest crime laboratory to render assistance.

Marijuana presents its own host of issues. Read section 21 on *Aspergillus* for a discussion of all the issues. In fact, property room personnel all across the United States are suffering from mold contamination. If you can smell marijuana when you walk into the property room and then experience headaches, you may have a problem. Some have even experienced Aspergillus pneumonia. This is preventable. Bottom line: why are police departments storing massive quantities of marijuana? They do not store massive quantities of clandestine drug lab chemicals because we have learned of their hazardous nature. Why not photograph and document the marijuana and destroy all but that amount required by law to adjudicate the case. Transporting bushels of dope into our courtrooms promotes the spread of contamination to that environment.

Narcotics should be stored in a separate designated vault and not in the main storage area. This vault should have a negative pressure ventilation system. Any filters in the H-VAC system must be routinely replaced or cleaned if marijuana is stored in the vault. Additionally, wherever marijuana is stored there may be special consideration given to building materials. Any selected building materials should not provide a matrix for the propagation of mold spores. Never cover the floor of the evidence vault with carpet but use flooring that can be decontaminated. Walls may also require periodic decontamination with a bleach solution.

Explosives

Explosives never, under any circumstances, belong in the evidence vault or property room. Explosives include dynamite, plastic explosives, pipe and letter bombs, black powder, railroad flares, blasting caps, rockets, hand grenades, artillery shells or unexploded money packs from banks. If any of these items are brought to you for submission, refuse to accept it. Photograph the item for documentation and have it removed from the facility. Call the Fire Department, the Bomb Squad, Alcohol, Tobacco and Firearms or a Chemist or Criminalist.

Another item that falls into the category of explosives but is often accepted into property rooms is fireworks. Preferably, these should not be accepted into evidence. They can be very unstable and do a tremendous amount of damage. One West Coast police department suffered an incredible amount of damage when stored fireworks exploded and the ensuing fire incapacitated their 911 system. However, if the powers that be absolutely insist that you store fireworks, pack them in metal drums in a substantial packing material. (There are issues with using metal storage drums but they are the strongest containment material available.) Place the packed drums in the separate hazardous materials storage area away from the main property or evidence area.

Firearms

Discharged firearms injure an alarming number of property room personnel every year. While discussing this in a class and relating how an individual from a past class had been shot in the leg; a woman revealed that she had been shot in the head by a pellet pistol. Not only is this almost unbelievable but it is totally unacceptable. Firearms must be rendered safe prior to submission into evidence.

If a loaded weapon is discovered, insist that the submitting officer or the supervisor remove it from the area. Do not touch it unless you are considered a firearms expert by your department. If no officer is available, call the Range Master, a Criminalist or other qualified help. Once unloaded and any magazine removed, the safety must be activated and a plastic tie placed in the action of the weapon. Officers must be discouraged from leaving loaded firearms in the night drop box. If they are called back before the next shift and required to render them safe, this habit will soon be changed.

In the event a firearm must be stored in a loaded condition, place a metal trigger lock to the firing mechanism and tag it. Personally, as a forensic identification specialist who has handled any number of firearms in criminal cases, I can think of very few reasons why this should ever be necessary. Discourage it. The location of ammunition in a firearm is easily documented. Do not accept loaded firearms.

When releasing firearms from evidence or property storage to the owner; always place a plastic tie in the action of the weapon. This preventative measure will prevent the owner from loading the weapon on site.

Firearms and all ammunition should be stored in a separate, secure vault apart from other property or evidence. Ammunition that looks corroded or is suspected of being old and possibly unstable should be considered hazardous and removed from the facility.

Lastly, but most important, never point a weapon at any person unless you are prepared to cause a death. As statistics on accidental shooting deaths reveal, "unloaded" firearms do discharge. Always know what is down range of the barrel. If a co-worker has the habit of waving firearms around indiscriminately while processing them, have a tactful but pointed discussion with them. Problems of this nature that do not stop must be reported to a supervisor. This is when being "safety minded" can get sticky but something must be done to avoid the worst of possible events.

Lighting

When vacated areas are made available for evidence or property storage or the selected area is not initially designed for this function, lighting is often an afterthought. Simply being able to see into a room or area is not adequate for the evidence or property maintenance task. The amount and nature of light provided in the work area can greatly influence the amount of work being accomplished. Glare, too much, or too little light can have negative consequences on the people in that environment. Improper, inadequate or poor lighting can create tripping or falling hazards. Such lighting can also result in the inability to properly identify an article being handled or to recognize hazards such as broken glass or spilled materials. The effect of fluorescent versus incandescent bulbs is an important consideration. Fluorescent lights, in addition to being more energy efficient, are cooler and give better visibility.

All lighting fixtures must meet electrical codes. Plastic shields should protect fluorescent and incandescent bulbs unless the shielding would result in a hazard. Lighting should not be patterned in a manner that provides adequate visibility in some areas while other others are essentially in the dark. This situation may occur as result of the location of lights in relation to shelving. Good lighting requires some preplanning based on the storage facility size and configuration.

Any evidence or property storage facility must have a battery-operated emergency lighting system. In the event there is a power failure, people must be provided a safe exit from an otherwise totally dark area. These are basic requirements and considerations. Local building and/or health codes may include additional requirements.

Shelving

Storage systems are available in any number of types, styles and arrangements. This can include bins, drop boxes, temporary lockers, files, cabinets, shelves and permanent lockers. While all these systems have their place, the selected type of shelving is often dictated by the size of the facility, the volume and type of evidence and property processed and the configuration of the available physical space. For medium or larger facilities, mobile filing shelves are desirable. These shelves are the most space efficient as they are installed on tracks or rails. Each bank of shelves is moveable and compress together in a manner that exposes only the necessary shelving area. "A high density mobile filing system with adjustable shelving can increase storage capacity by 80 percent and save up to 72 percent of floor space. This is an economical alternative to major renovation or expansion." [4] These shelving systems are very good but do create lighting problems. Lights must be positioned in a manner that dark areas do not result from the movement of the files.

Whatever shelving system is installed, it must be assessable to all personnel. If items are located on a high top shelf, then an adequate ladder system must be available. Step ladders such as ones used by the homeowner are never acceptable. Some facilities are so large that personnel use forklifts to place and remove property located on the higher shelves. All these arrangements are acceptable as long as personnel receive proper training in using them as well as proper lifting techniques. And lastly, property should never be stacked. This can damage items in a manner that compromises the integrity of the evidence and can make retrieval difficult and hazardous.

Ventilation

Ventilation is probably the greatest issue of concern to property room personnel. Since many property storage areas are not specifically designed for that function, the ventilation is extremely inadequate. The cost of installing a ventilation system that is adequate and appropriate for the separate evidence and property storage areas is not inexpensive. However, a ventilation system properly configured need only be built one time and only requires periodic maintenance. Good ventilation is a necessity for the health and well being of personnel who work in the evidence vaults or property storage facility. Unfortunately, ventilation systems are often inadequate and complaints of illness abound across the nation.

The ventilation system for these facilities are complex in that one system may not be adequate for all the areas. The general property storage area must have a ventilation system separate from the remainder of the building. Air from the property area should never be circulated into other areas of the building. Blood drying rooms must be equipped with negative pressure airflow to prevent contaminants being drawn out from the room (when doors are opened) into other general areas. These rooms should be equipped with a HEPA filter. (This also applies to blood drying cabinets.) Rooms or areas where drug vaults and flammable liquids are maintained should have negative pressure systems with constant exhaust ventilation. No air should re-circulate in these zones. This is especially important if a quantity of marijuana is being stored where *Aspergillus* spores could begin to proliferate.

Unfortunately, there is no national standard for ventilation. OSHA basically takes the position that a ventilation system is adequate if it functions according to the manufacturer's specifications. While this may sound satisfactory, it leaves a lot of folks working in environments where unpleasant odors abound and headaches and sinus problems are the norm. This creates very poor employee morale and lost work hours due to illness. Additionally, should the employee ever be able to prove the health problems relate to the environment and ventilation problems, the department will be liable for any resulting medical expenses and disabilities. If an administrator or supervisor suspects problems related to ventilation, an industrial hygienist should be hired to perform air-monitoring tests. Not uncommonly, air quality problems begin in the evidence and property area but eventually become a problem in other areas of the building. When inadequately or defectively configured ventilation systems are coupled with a building constructed so tight that is can not *breathe*, "sick building" syndrome results and personnel from all areas of the structure are negatively affected.

As a general guideline, ventilation systems should accommodate a minimum of seven (7) room air changes per hour. Some systems are designed to provide room air changes based upon the size of the area and the number of persons working in that given area. Regardless of the system in place, it must be adequate for the health of all persons who work in the building.

People working in the evidence vaults and property storage areas of law enforcement agencies are as negatively impacted by safety issues as personnel working crime scenes or processing evidence in the laboratory. It is imperative for management to realize that maintenance of evidence and property is not an insignificant ancillary function to enforcing the law and protecting the community. Just as protection is afforded the officers on the street, people inside the facility providing support functions must also be afforded protection and consideration. This is a process of education, evaluation and hazard awareness. Spread the message.

References

1. Introduction

[1] Shaw, Lynette and Sichel, Herbert S., "Accident Proneness - Fact and Fiction," and Allison, William W., "Accident Prone Theory Can Affect Safety Performance", *Directions in Safety*, Ted S. Ferry and D.A.Weaver, Charles C. Thomas: Springfield, Illinois, 1976: 7, 312-319.

[2] *Directions in Safety*, Miller, Charles O., Why "Systems Safety": 69.

[3] Personal communication from Thomas Valentine, Safety Coordinator, Bureau of Forensic Services, California Department of Justice.

[4] *Directions in Safety*, Greenberg, Leo, Why Safety: 99.

[5] Business and Legal Reports, Inc., *A Pocket Guide to MSDSs and Labels*, 1990.

[6] *Directions in Safety*, Griep, D.J., Propaganda and Alternative Countermeasures for Road Safety: 81.

[7] *Directions in Safety*, Zeller, Archard F., The Limitations of Man: 212.

[8] Employee Rights granted by the U.S. Occupational Safety and Health Act, Public Law 91-596.

[9] *Directions in Safety*, Greenberg, Leo, Why Safety: 105.

[10] Personal communication from Angie Hernandez, United States Department of Labor, Occupational Safety and Health Administration, North Chicago Office, Illinois.

2. Written Policies

[1] *29 Code of Federal Regulations* (CFR) 1920.1200

[2] *29 Code of Federal Regulations* (CFR) 1920.1200

[3] Stricoff, R. Scott and Walters, Douglas B., *Laboratory Health and Safety Handbook - A Guide for the Preparation of a Chemical Hygiene Plan*, John Wiley and Sons, Inc.: New York, 1990: 35.

3. Material Safety Data Sheets

[1] 29 CFR 1910,1200 (b)(4)(i).

[2] 29 CFR 1910.1200 (b)(4)(ii).

[3] 29 CFR 1920.1200 (b)(4)(iii).

[4] 29 CFR 1920.1200 (b)(4)(iv).

[5] 29 CFR 1920.1200 (b)(5)(i).

[6] 29 CFR 1920.1200 (b)(5)(ii).

[7] 29 CFR 1920.1200 (b)(5)(v).

[8] *Webster's New World Dictionary of the American Language*, 2nd Ed., World Publishing Company: New York, 1972.

[9] 29 CFR 1920.1200 (g)(2)(iv).

4. Chemical Hazards

[1] Rose, Susan L., *Clinical Laboratory Safety*, J. B. Lippincott Company: Philadelphia, 1984: 49.

[2] *Clinical Laboratory Safety*: 51.

[3] Personal communications from John Murdock, per Contra Costa County, California, Criminalistics Laboratory Safety Policies; and Steere, Norman V. Ed. *Handbook of Laboratory Safety*, 2nd Edition. The Chemical Rubber Company: Cleveland, Ohio, 1971: 296-7.

[4] *Clinical Laboratory Safety*: 54.

[5] *Clinical Laboratory Safety*: 58.

[6] *Clinical Laboratory Safety*: 70.

[7] *Clinical Laboratory Safety*: 76.

[8] *Clinical Laboratory Safety*: 59.

[9] *Clinical Laboratory Safety*: 59.

[10] *Clinical Laboratory Safety*: 59.

[11] *Risk Analysis and Authoritative Misinformation*. Today's Chemist At Work, October 1992: 23.

[12] *Clinical Laboratory Safety*: 71.

[13] *Clinical Laboratory Safety*: 71-72.

[14] *Clinical Laboratory Safety*: 71.

5. Biological Hazards

[1] Plog, Barbara A. Ed. *Fundementals of Industrial Hygiene*, 3rd Edition, National Safety Council: 7.

[2] 29 CFR 1910.1030 and 29 CFR 1910.1030 (d)(1).

[3] *Federal Register*, Vol. 54, No. 102, Tuesday, May 30, 1989, Proposed Rules. Department of Labor, Occupational Safety and Health Administration, 29 CFR Part 1910, Occupational Exposure to Bloodborne Pathogens: 23048.

[4] *Hazard Communication Program for Infectious Biologicals*, California

Department of Justice, Office of the Attorney General, 1991: 5; and *Federal Register*: 23048.

[5] *Federal Register*: 23049.

[6] *Hazard Communication Program for Infectious Biologicals*: 8.

[7] *Hazard Communication Program for Infectious Biologicals*: 8; and *Federal Register*: 23052.

[8] *Guidelines for Prevention of Transmission of Human Immunodeficiency Virus and Hepatitis B Virus to Health-Care and Public Safety Workers*. A Response to P.L. 100-607 The Health Omnibus Programs Extension Act of 1988, U.S. Department of Health and Human Services, Centers for Disease Control, Atlanta, Georgia, February 1989: 2.

[9] *Hazard Communication Program for Infectious Biologicals*: 6.

[10] *Hazard Communication Program for Infectious Biologicals*: 6.

[11] *Hazard Communication Program for Infectious Biologicals*: 6.

[12] *Federal Register*: 23048.

[13] *Hazard Communication Program for Infectious Biologicals*: 6.

[14] *Hazard Communication Program for Infectious Biologicals*: 7.

[15] *Awake!* "AIDS - Unique in World History!", April 22, 1986, Watchtower Bible and Tract Society of New York, Inc., Brooklyn, New York: 3-4.

[16] *Watchtower*. "What Hope for the Dead?", October 15, 1989, Watchtower Bible and Tract Society of New York, Inc., Brooklyn, New York: 7.

[17] *Awake!* "AIDS A Global Killer", October 8, 1988, Watchtower Bible and Tract Society of New York, Inc., Brooklyn, New York: 6.

[18] *Awake!* "Watching the World. AIDS in the 1990's", February 22, 1990,

Watchtower Bible and Tract Society of New York, Inc., Brooklyn, New York: 28.

[19] *Awake!* "Our Immune System. A Miracle of Creation", November 22, 1990, Watchtower Bible and Tract Society of New York, Inc., Brooklyn, New York: 4, 8.

[20] Thomas, Clayton L. Ed. *Taber's Cyclopedic Medical Dictionary*, 16th Edition. F.A. Davis Company: Philadelphia, 1989: 1058.

[21] *Federal Register*: 23053.

[22] *Surgeon General's Report on Acquired Immunodeficiency Syndrome*, U.S. Department of Health and Human Services, 1987: 10.

[23] *Surgeon General's Report*: 11.

[24] *Federal Register*: 23053.

[25] *Federal Register*: 23054.

[26] *Federal Register*: 23053.

[27] *Hazard Communication Program for Infectious Biologicals*: 6.

[28] *Hazard Communication Program for Infectious Biologicals*: 7.

[29] *Hazard Communication Program for Infectious Biologicals*: 7; and Thomas. Valentine, California Department of Justice.

[30] *Federal Register*: 23060.

[31] *Federal Register*: 23060.

[32] *Taber's Cyclopedic Medical Dictionary*: 1725.

[33] *Federal Register*: 23061.

[34] *Federal Register*: 23061 and *Taber's Cyclopedic Medical Dictionary*:

1073.

[35] *Federal Register*: 23061 and *Taber's Cyclopedic Medical Dictionary*: 177.

[36] *Federal Register*: 23061 and *Taber's Cyclopedic Medical Dictionary*: 255.

[37] *Federal Register*: 23061 and *Taber's Cyclopedic Medical Dictionary*: 1016.

[38] *Taber's Cyclopedic Medical Dictionary*: 133.

[39] *Federal Register*: 23061.

[40] *Federal Register*: 23061 and *Taber's Cyclopedic Medical Dictionary*: 1579.

[41] *Federal Register*: 23061.

[42] *Federal Register*: 23061.

[43] "Safety Bulletin on Infectious Biologicals # 91-01", California Department of Justice, Office of the Attorney General, 1991: 1.

[44] *National Committee for Clinical Laboratory Standards*, Vol. 11, No. 15, September 1991: 17.

[45] *Guidelines for Prevention of Transmission of Human Immuno-deficiency Virus and Hepatitis B Virus to Health-Care and Public Safety Workers*: 8.

[46] *Guidelines for Prevention of Transmission of Human Immuno-deficiency Virus and Hepatitis B Virus to Health-Care and Public Safety Workers*: 8.

[47] *Guidelines for Prevention of Transmission of Human Immuno-deficiency Virus and Hepatitis B Virus to Health-Care and Public Safety Workers*: 7.

[48] *Guidelines for Prevention of Transmission of Human Immuno-*

deficiency Virus and Hepatitis B Virus to Health-Care and Public Safety Workers: 7.

6. Routes of Exposure

[1] Young, Jay A. Ed. *Improving Safety in the Chemical Laboratory: A Practical Guide*, John Wiley and Sons, Inc., New York, 1987: 116.

[2] *Improving Safety in the Chemical Laboratory: A Practical* Guide: 116-117.

[3] *Improving Safety in the Chemical Laboratory: A Practical Guide*: 117.

[4] Plog, Barbara A. Ed. *Fundamentals of Industrial Hygiene*, 3rd Edition, National Safety Council: 17.

[5] *Guide for Safety in the Chemical Laboratory*. The General Safety Committee of the Manufacturing Chemist's Association, Inc., D. Van Nostrand Company, Inc., New York, New York, 1954: 128.

[6] *Fundamentals of Industrial Hygiene*: 17

[7] Young, Jay A. Ed. *Improving Safety in the Chemical Laboratory: A Practical Guide*, John Wiley and Sons, Inc., New York, 1987: 118.

[8] 29 C.F.R. 1910.1450 Appendix C.

[9] *Fundamentals of Industrial Hygiene*: 17.

[10] *Guide for Safety in the Chemical Laboratory*: 128.

[11] *Fundamentals of Industrial Hygiene*: 17.

[12] *Improving Safety in the Chemical Laboratory: A Practical* Guide: 118.

[13] Personal communication from Jay Mark, California Department of Justice, per Bureau of Forensic Services Safety Policies.

[14] *Awake!* "Our Versatile Sense of Smell", July 22, 1993, *Awake!* "AIDS - Unique in World History!", April 22, 1986, Watchtower Bible and Tract

Society of New York, Inc., Brooklyn, New York: 24-25.

[15] *Awake!:* 24-25.

[16] Material Safety Data Sheet, From Genium Reference Collection, Genium Publishing Corporation, Schenectady, New York, No. 34, Ozone, August 1987.

[17] Personal communication from Patti Blume, Orange County Sheriff's Department, Santa Ana, California, per Forensic Services Safety Policies.

7. Ventilation Systems

[1] Material Safety Data Sheet From Genium's Reference Collection, Genium Publishing Corporation, Schenectady, New York, No. 34, Ozone, August 1987.

[2] Stricoff, R. Scott and Walters, Douglas B., *Laboratory Health and Safety Handbook - A Guide for the Preparation of a Chemical Hygiene Plan*, John Wiley and Sons, Inc.: New York, 1990: 118.

[3] 29 CFR 1910.1450 (c) (4) (g).

[4] *Chemical Hygiene Plan*. California Department of Justice, Bureau of Forensic Services, 1992.

8. Personal Protective Equipment

[1] 29 CFR 1910.132 Subpart 1.

[2] Furr, A. Keith Ed. *CRC Handbook of Laboratory Safety*, 3rd Edition. The Chemical Rubber Company: Boca Raton, Florida, 1990: 670.

[3] *CRC Handbook of Laboratory Safety*: 669-70.

[4] *CRC Handbook of Laboratory Safety*: 671.

[5] 29 CFR 1910.134 (e) (3).

[6] *CRC Handbook of Laboratory Safety*: 671.

[7] *CRC Handbook of Laboratory Safety*: 671.

[8] *CRC Handbook of Laboratory Safety*: 672-3.

[9] *CRC Handbook of Laboratory Safety*: 674.

[10] *CRC Handbook of Laboratory Safety*: 674.

[11] *CRC Handbook of Laboratory Safety*: 675.

[12] *CRC Handbook of Laboratory Safety*: 675-76.

[13] *CRC Handbook of Laboratory Safety*: 677.

[14] *CRC Handbook of Laboratory Safety*: 679.

[15] *Guidelines for the Selection of Chemical Protective Clothing*, 3rd. ed., Schwope, A. D., Costas, P. P., Jackson, J. O., Stull, J. O., and Weitzman, D. J., Eds., Arthur D. Little, Inc., U.S. Environmental Protection Agency, and U.S. Coastguard, American Conference of Governmental Industrial Hygienists, Cinncinnati, OH, 1987.

[16] *CRC Handbook of Laboratory Safety*: 679.

[17] *CRC Handbook of Laboratory Safety*: 680.

[18] *Chemical Hazard Appraisal and Recognition Planning*, "Protective Clothing", Office of the Attorney General, California Department of Justice, 1986: 9.

[19] *Chemical Hazard Appraisal and Recognition Planning*: 9.

[20] *Chemical Hazard Appraisal and Recognition Planning*: 9.

[21] *Chemical Hazard Appraisal and Recognition Planning*: 10.

[22] *Chemical Hazard Appraisal and Recognition Planning*: 5.

[23] *CRC Handbook of Laboratory Safety*: 679.

[24] *Chemical Hazard Appraisal and Recognition Planning*: 12.

[25] *CRC Handbook of Laboratory Safety*: 685.

[26] *CRC Handbook of Laboratory Safety*: 686.

[27] *CRC Handbook of Laboratory Safety*: 684.

9. Spraying Chemicals

[1] Personal communication from Jay Mark, California Department of Justice, per Bureau of Forensic Services Safety Policies.

[2] Thomas, Clayton L. Ed. *Taber's Cyclopedic Medical Dictionary*, 16th Edition. F.A. Davis Company: Philadelphia, 1989: 1268.

[3] Personal communication from Victor Reeve, California Department of Justice, Bureau of Forensic Services, California Criminalistics Institute.

[4] 29 C.F.R. 1910.134 (b) (10).

[5] 29 C.F.R. 1910.134 (b) (3).

10. Laboratory First Aid Kit

[1] Furr, A. Keith Ed. *CRC Handbook of Laboratory Safety*, 3rd Edition. The Chemical Rubber Company: Boca Raton, Florida, 1990: 686.

[2] *CRC Handbook of Laboratory Safety*: 686.

11. Mixing Chemicals

[1] Personal communication from Patti E. Blume, Orange County Sheriff-Coroner, Santa Ana, California.

[2] Bigbee, David, *The Law Enforcement Officer and AIDS*, 4th Edition. U.S. Department of Justice, Federal Bureau of Investigation Laboratory, Washington, D.C., 1991: 13.

[3] Personal communication from John Murdock, Contra Costa County Crime Laboratory, Martinez, California.

12. Deceased Casework

[1] H. Douceron, L. Deforges, R. Gherardi, A. Sobel, and P. Chariot, "Long-Lasting Postmortem Viability of Human Immunodeficiency Virus: A Potential Risk in Forensic Medicine Practice", *Forensic Science International*, 60, 1993: 61-66.

[2] Thomas, Clayton L. Ed. *Taber's Cyclopedic Medical Dictionary*, 16th Edition. F.A. Davis Company: Philadelphia, 1989: 1918.

[3] Personal communication from Marsha Bradford, Head Registered Nurse, Infection Control Department, University of California (Davis) Medical Center, Sacramento, California.

[4] Personal Communication from Thomas E. Valentine, Safety Coordinator, Bureau of Forensic Services, California Department of Justice, Sacramento, California.

[5] *Taber's Cyclopedic Medical Dictionary*: 1918.

[6] Personal communication from Dr. Robert Anthony, Head Pathologist, Sacramento County Coroner's Office, Sacramento, California.

[7] Personal Communication from Thomas E. Valentine, Safety Coordinator, Bureau of Forensic Services, California Department of Justice, Sacramento, California.

[8] Personal Communication from Marsha Bradford, Head Registered Nurse, Infection Control Department, University of California (Davis) Medical Center, Sacramento, California.

[9] *Taber's Cyclopedic Medical Dictionary*: 693.

[10] "Processing of Deceased Hands or Fingers" Memorandum, Bureau of Forensic Services, California Department of Justice, 1987.

[11] Personal Communication from Dr. Gary Stuart, Pathologist, Sacramento County Coroner's Office, Sacramento, California.

[12] Personal communication from Dr. Robert Anthony, Head Pathologist, Sacramento County Coroner's Office, Sacramento, California.

[13] Personal Communication from Marsha Bradford, Head Registered Nurse, Infection Control Department, University of California (Davis) Medical Center, Sacramento, California.

[14] *National Committee for Clinical Laboratory Standards*, Vol. 11, No. 15, September 1991: 17.

[15] Personal Communication from Marsha Bradford, Head Registered Nurse, Infection Control Department, University of California (Davis) Medical Center, Sacramento, California.

[16] Personal Communication from Steve Kubo, Safety Engineer, Environmental Health, University of California, Davis, California.

13. Confining Contamination

[1] 29 CFR 1910.1450 Appendix A. E. 4.

14. Labeling Containers

[1] 29 CFR 1910.1200 (a) (2).

[2] 29 CFR 1910.1200 (b).

[3] 29 CFR 1910.1200 (f).

[4] 29 CFR 1910.1200 (f) (9).

[5] 29 CFR 1910.1200 (c).

[6] 29 CFR 1910.1200 (d) (5) (ii).

[7] Rose, Susan L., *Clinical Laboratory Safety*, J. B. Lippincott Company: Philadelphia, 1984: 56 - 58; and *The MSDS Pocket Dictionary*, Genium

Publishing Corporation, Schenectady, New York, 1993: 34.

15. Electrical

[1] Personal communication from John A Juhala, Forensic Science Division, Michigan State Police, East Lansing, Michigan.

[2] *Chemical Hygiene Plan*, California Department of Justice, Division of Law Enforcement, Bureau of Forensic Services, 1993: 14 - 15.

16. Chemical Storage

[1] Young, Jay A. Ed. *Improving Safety in the Chemical Laboratory: A Practical Guide*, John Wiley and Sons, Inc., New York, 1987: 210.

[2] Masters, Nancy E. and Patti E. Blume, "An Overview of Laboratory Safety," *Journal of Forensic Identification*, Vol. 44, No. 1, 1994: 47.

[3] Personal Communication from Torrey Johnson, Criminalist, California Department of Justice, Division of Law Enforcement, Bureau of Forensic Services, Sacramento, California.

[4] *Improving Safety in the Chemical Laboratory: A Practical Guide*: 209.

[5] *Improving Safety in the Chemical Laboratory: A Practical Guide*: 216.

17. Spill Control and Waste Disposal

[1] Masters, Nancy E. and Patti E. Blume, "An Overview of Laboratory Safety", *Journal of Forensic Identification*, Vol. 44, No. 1, 1994: 48.

[2] Furr, A. Keith Ed. *CRC Handbook of Laboratory Safety*, 3rd Edition. The Chemical Rubber Company: Boca Raton, Florida, 1990: 449.

[3] Rose, Susan L., *Clinical Laboratory Safety*, J. B. Lippincott Company: Philadelphia, 1984: 98.

[4] *Chemical Hygiene Plan*, California Department of Justice, Division of Law Enforcement, Bureau of Forensic Services, 1993: 37 - 38.

[5] Young, Jay A. Ed. *Improving Safety in the Chemical Laboratory: A Practical Guide*, John Wiley and Sons, Inc., New York, 1987: 254.

[6] Personal communication from John A Juhala, Forensic Science Division, Michigan State Police, East Lansing, Michigan.

[7] 40 CFR 261.3

[8] Personal communication from John A Juhala, Forensic Science Division, Michigan State Police, East Lansing, Michigan.

[9] *Improving Safety in the Chemical Laboratory: A Practical Guide*: 258.

[10] *Improving Safety in the Chemical Laboratory: A Practical Guide*: 255.

18. Light Sources

[1] Dalrumple, B E, Duff J M and E R Menzel, "Inherent Fingerprint Luminescence - Detection by Laser," *Journal of Forensic Science*, Vol. 22, No. 1, 1977: 106 - 115.

[2] *Scene of Crime Handbook of Fingerprint Development Techniques*, Police Scientific Development Branch, Home Office, Derbeyshire, England, United Kingdom, 1993: 51 - 52.

[3] Personal Communication from David Crowe and David Moore, Questioned Document Examiners, California Department of Justice, Bureau of Forensic Services, Questioned Document Section, Sacramento, California.

[4] *Scene of Crime Handbook of Fingerprint Development Techniques*: 51.

[5] Chang, Insun, "Laser Safety", *Professional Safety*, November 1986: 51.

[6] Hardwick, S A, Kent, T and V G Sears, *Fingerprint Detection by Fluorescence Examination, A Guide to Operational Implementation*, Police Scientific Development Branch, Science and Technology Group, Home Office, Hertfordshire, United Kingdom, 1990: 7.

[7] *Fingerprint Detection by Fluorescence Examination, A Guide to Operational Implementation*: 7.

[8] *Fingerprint Detection by Fluorescence Examination, A Guide to Operational Implementation*: 7.

[9] Personal Communication from Martin Collins, Latent Print Supervisor, California Department of Justice, Bureau of Forensic Services, Latent Print Program, Sacramento, California.

[10] *Fingerprint Detection by Fluorescence Examination, A Guide to Operational Implementation*: 8.

[11] *Professional Safety*: 51, and Sliney, David and Myron Wolbarsht, *Safety with Lasers and Other Optical Sources, A Comprehensive Handbook*, Plenum Press, New York, 1980: 1.

[12] Hecht, Jeff, "Lasers Designed to Blind" (How an Eye Injury Feels), *New Scientist*, #1833, August 8, 1992: 27 - 31.

[13] *Safety with Lasers and Other Optical Sources, A Comprehensive Handbook*: 1 - 2.

[14] *Fingerprint Detection by Fluorescence Examination, A Guide to Operational Implementation*: 12 - 13.

[15] *Omnichrome Users Manual*, Omnichrome Corportion, Chino, California.

[16] *Fingerprint Detection by Fluorescence Examination, A Guide to Operational Implementation*: 51.

[17] *Safety with Lasers and Other Optical Sources, A Comprehensive Handbook*: 161.

[18] *Fingerprint Detection by Fluorescence Examination, A Guide to Operational Implementation*: 16.

[19] *Fingerprint Detection by Fluorescence Examination, A Guide to Operational Implementation*: 7.

[20] *Safety with Lasers and Other Optical Sources, A Comprehensive Handbook*: 693.

[21] *Fingerprint Detection by Fluorescence Examination, A Guide to Operational Implementation*: 43.

[22] *Fingerprint Detection by Fluorescence Examination, A Guide to Operational Implementation*: 43.

[23] *Fingerprint Detection by Fluorescence Examination, A Guide to Operational Implementation*: 16.

[24] *Fingerprint Detection by Fluorescence Examination, A Guide to Operational Implementation*: 15.

[25] *Safety with Lasers and Other Optical Sources, A Comprehensive Handbook*: 187.

[26] *Safety with Lasers and Other Optical Sources, A Comprehensive Handbook*: 3 - 4.

[27] *Safety with Lasers and Other Optical Sources, A Comprehensive Handbook*: 106.

[28] *Safety with Lasers and Other Optical Sources, A Comprehensive Handbook*: 5.

[29] *Fingerprint Detection by Fluorescence Examination, A Guide to Operational Implementation*: 16.

[30] *Scene of Crime Handbook of Fingerprint Development Techniques:* 81.

[31] *Scene of Crime Handbook of Fingerprint Development Techniques:* 81.

[32] Personal communication from Terry Kent, Police Scientific Development Branch, Science and Technology Group, Home Office, Sandridge, St. Albans, Hertfordshire, United Kingdom.

19. Training

[1] 29 CFR 1910.1200 (h) and *CRC Handbook of Laboratory Safety*: 375 - 376.

[2] *Guide to Developing Your Workplace Injury and Illness Prevention Program*, Cal/OSHA Consultation Service, State of California, Department of

Industrial Relations, Division of Occupational Safety and Health, January 1991: 12.

[3] *Bloodborne Pathogen Exposure Control Plan*, California Department of Justice, Bureau of Forensic Services, August 1993: 14.

[4] *Guide to Developing Your Workplace Injury and Illness Prevention Program*: 12.

[5] *Guide to Developing Your Workplace Injury and Illness Prevention Program*: 12.

[6] *Guide to Developing Your Workplace Injury and Illness Prevention Program*: 12.

[7] *Illness and Injury Prevention Program*, California Department of Justice, Bureau of Forensic Services, February 1994: 6.

[8] *Improving Safety in the Chemical Laboratory: A Practical Guide*: 30.

[9] Furr, A. Keith Ed. *CRC Handbook of Laboratory Safety*, 3rd Edition. The Chemical Rubber Company: Boca Raton, Florida, 1990: 377.

[10] *Chemical Hygiene Plan*, California Department of Justice, Division of Law Enforcement, Bureau of Forensic Services, 1993: 76.

20. Applications

[1] Masters, Nancy E. and Patti E. Blume, "An Overview of Laboratory Safety", *Journal of Forensic Identification*, Vol. 44, No. 1, 1994: 45.

21. Aspergillus

[1] "Howard Carter and the Curse of the Mummy. The rumor of an ancient curse didn't stop this archaeologist from opening the tumb of King Tut." Virtual Exploration Society. http://unmuseum.mus.pa.us/mummy.htm

[2] Arizona Department of Public Safety, Information Bulletin #85-01, dated 2/1/85

[3] Personal communication from Dr. Steve Kagen, skagen@allernet.com, June 1, 2000.

[4] *Aspergillosis* by Dr. Michael R. McGinnis. Medical Mycology Research Center, University of Texas Medical Branch at Galveston, Texas, USA, page 1.

[5] *Aspergillus* by Dr. Javier Vilar, Infectious Diseases, Manchester University, United Kingdom, Aspergillosis Website, pages 1-3.

[6] *Aspergillus.*

[7] *Aspergillus.*

[8] *Aspergillus.*

[9] *A Bioaerosol Investigation in the Evidence and Supply Area* by Mitchell L. Payes, Consulting Industrial Hygienist, January 14, 1989, page 15.

[10] *A Bioaerosol Investigation in the Evidence and Supply Area.*

[11] *How to Preserve Pot Potency* by The Bush Doctor, High Times, May 1993, page 3.

[12] *A Bioaerosol Investigation in the Evidence and Supply Area:* 4.

[13] *Hantavirus* by Dawn Viebrock and Mary Ann O'Garro, Grant County Health District, Washington, http://www.granthealth.org/hantavirus.htm, dated May 14, 2001.

[14] *Hantavirus Health Sheets, Questions and Answers about Hantavirus Pulmonary Syndrome*, http://www.granthealth.org;hantagchd.htm, dated July 1998.

[15] *Hantavirus.*

22. Crime Scene Safety

[1] NIOSH Alert, "Preventing Allergic Reactions to Natural Rubber Latex in the Workplace", 1997.

[2] *Taber's Cyclopedic Medical Dictionary:* 1057, and *Clandestine Laboratory Safety Certification Manual*, California Department of Justice, Bureau of Narcotic Enforcement, 1993.

[3] *Taber's Cyclopedic Medical Dictionary:* 375, and *Clandestine Laboratory Safety Certification Manual.*

[4] Personal Communication from Barbara Andersen, Project Coordinator, Valley Fever Center for Excellence, vfever@public.arl.arizona.edu, January 28, 2002.

[5] *Taber's Cyclopedic Medical Dictionary:* 375, and, *Clandestine Laboratory Safety Certification Manual.*

[6] Personal communication from Theo N. Kirkland, MD, Departments of Pathology and Medicine, University of California, San Diego School of Medicine, tkirkland@ucsd.edu, January 28, 2002.

[7] *Taber's Cyclopedic Medical Dictionary:* 1436-37, and *Clandestine Laboratory Safety Certification Manual.*

[8] *Awake!*. "What Makes Workplaces Dangerous", February 22, 2002, Watchtower Bible and Tract Society of New York, Inc., Brooklyn, New York: 6.

[9] *Manual of Fingerprint Development Techniques, A Guide to the Selection and Use of Processes for the Development of Latent Fingerprints*, 2nd Edition, Police Scientific Development Branch, Home Office, Sandridge, United Kingdom, 1998: Chapter 4, Section 6.2.2, page 6.

[10] *Taber's Cyclopedic Medical Dictionary:* 1394.

[11] "Use Your Head to Protect Your Head", *Lab Safety Saf-T News*, listmaster@labsafety.com, January 18, 2002.

[12] "Use Your Head to Protect Your Head", *Lab Safety Saf-T News.*

[13] *Taber's Cyclopedic Medical Dictionary:* 1104.

[14] *Policies and Procedures of the Drowning and Accident Rescue Team (DART)*, Sacramento County, Elk Grove, California, 1998: 1-3.

[15] *Policies and Procedures of the Drowning and Accident Rescue Team:* 4-1.

[16] *Policies and Procedures of the Drowning and Accident Rescue Team:* 5-1, 5-2.

[17] *Policies and Procedures of the Drowning and Accident Rescue Team:* 5-2.

[18] *Policies and Procedures of the Drowning and Accident Rescue Team:* 5-2, 5-3.

[19] *Policies and Procedures of the Drowning and Accident Rescue Team:* 5-3.

23. Evidence Vault/Property Room Safety

[1] Latta, Joseph T. and George E. Rush , *Evidence and Property Management*, Copperhouse Publishing Company, Nevada: 1998.
California Association of Property and Evidence: 1-800-449-4273

[2] *Evidence and Property Management:* 123.

[3] NIOSH Alert, "Preventing Allergic Reactions to Natural Rubber Latex in the Workplace", 1997.

[4] *Evidence and Property Management:* 35

Appendix A

EMPLOYEE RIGHTS

Granted by Occupational Safety and Health Act Public Law 91-596

1. To employment and place of employment free from recognized hazards that are likely to cause death or serious physical harm.

2. To petition the Secretary of Labor to commence the procedure for promulgating standards.

3. To file written objections to proposed rules and to request a public hearing on such objections.

4. To standards which most adequately and feasibly assure that no employees will suffer any impairment of health or functional capacity or diminished life expectancy, even if such employee has regular exposure to toxic or harmful materials.

5. To standards which prescribe, where necessary, the labeling of hazardous substances, protective equipment, and monitoring.

6. To medical examinations so as to determine whether exposure is adversely affecting health.

7. To have results of his medical examinations transmitted to an employee's physician.

8. To have emergency temporary standards declared when employees are exposed to grave danger.

9. To be notified of an employer's request for variance and to participate in the hearing called to evaluate the requester.

10. To representation of the National Advisory Committee on Occupational Safety and Health and on the Standard Setting Advisory Committees.

11. To receive same fee and mileage when testimony is required as in courts of the United States.

12. To have employers keep them informed of their rights under the act.

13. To observe the monitoring of harmful substances and to have access to records of monitoring.

14. To be notified when exposures to harmful substances exceed prescribed levels.

15. To have a representative accompany an OSHA inspector.

16. To request an OSHA inspection by giving notice to the secretary in writing and signed.

17. To be able to inform the inspector of alleged violations and to receive written explanation if no citation is issued and to receive an informal review thereof.

18. To have all citations posted at or near the scene of the violation.

19. To appeal to the Review Commission if abatement time is unreasonably long.

20. To oppose any appeal taken by an employer.

21. To protection against disciplinary or discriminatory action for exercising rights under the Act.

22. To request HHS-CDC determination of toxicity of any substance normally found in work place.

23. To request MSDS's from your employer.

24. To have right of access to all medical monitoring records.

Appendix B

TABLE OF INCOMPATIBLE CHEMICALS

Separate storage areas should be provided for "incompatible chemicals" that may react together and create a hazardous condition. Some examples of these incompatible chemicals are listed below.

Chemical	Do not store or mix with:
Acetaldehyde	Strong oxidizers, acids, bases, alcohol, ammonia, amines, phenols, ketones, hydrogen cyanide, hydrogen sulfide
Acetates	Nitrates, strong oxidizers, strong alkalies, strong acids
Acetic Acid	Chromic acid, nitric acid, hydroxyl compounds, ethylene glycol, perchloric acid, peroxides, permanganates
Acetic anhydride	Water, alcohols, strong oxidizers, chromic acid, amines, strong caustics
Acetone	Concentrated nitric acid and sulfuric acid mixtures
Acetylene	Chlorine, bromine, copper, fluorine, silver, mercury

Alkaline and alkaline earth metals, such as powered aluminum or magnesium, sodium, potassium, cesium, lithium, calcium	Water, carbon tetrachloride or other chlorinated hydrocarbons, carbon dioxide, the halogens or any free acid
Amines	Strong oxidizers, acids
Ammonia, anhydrous	Mercury (in manometers, for instance), chlorine, calcium, hypochlorite, iodine, bromine, hydrofluoric acid (anhydrous)
Ammonium nitrate	Acids, metal powders, flammable liquids, chlorates, nitrites, sulfur, finely divided organic or combustible materials
Aniline	Nitric acid, hydrogen peroxide
Benzyl chloride	Active metals: copper, aluminum, magnesium, iron, zinc, tin; strong oxidizers
Bromine	Ammonia, acetylene, butadiene, butane, methane, propane (or other petroleum gases), hydrogen, sodium carbide, turpentine, benzene, finely divided metals
Calcium carbide	Water, chlorine, bromine, copper, fluorine, silver, mercury
Carbon, activated	Calcium hypochlorite, all oxidizing agents
Carbon disulfide	Strong oxidizers, azides, organic amines, chemically active metals such as sodium, potassium, zinc
Chlorates	Ammonium salts, acids, metal powders, sulfur, finely divided organic or combustible materials
Chlorine	Ammonia, acetylene, butadiene, butane, methane,

	propane (or other petroleum gases), hydrogen, sodium carbide, turpentine, benzene, finely divided metals
Chlorides	Strong oxidizers, strong caustics, chemically active metals such as aluminum or magnesium powder, sodium, potassium
Chlorine dioxide	Ammonia, methane, phosphine, hydrogen sulfide
Chloroacetophenone	Water, steam
Chromic acid	Acetic acid, naphthalene, camphor, glycerine, turpentine, alcohol, flammable liquids in general, paper, or cellulose
Copper	Acetylene, hydrogen peroxide
Cumene hydroperoxide	Acids, organic or inorganic
Cyanides	Strong oxidizers, such as nitrates, chlorates, acids, and acid salts
Dimethyl formamide	Carbon tetrachloride, other halogenated compounds when in contact with iron, strong oxidizers, alkyl aluminiums
Dimethylsulfate	Strong oxidizers, ammonia solutions
Ethylenediamine	Strong acids, strong oxidizers, chlorinated organic compounds
Flammable liquids	Ammonium nitrate, chromic acid, hydrogen peroxide, nitric acid, sodium peroxide, the halogens
Fluorides	Strong acids
Fluorine	Isolate from everything
Formaldehyde	Strong oxidizers, strong alkalies, strong acids, phe-

	nols, urea
Formic acid	Strong oxidizers, strong caustics, concentrated sulfuric acid
Hydrocarbons (butane, propane, benzene, gasoline, turpentine, etc.)	Fluorine, chlorine, bromine, chromic acid, sodium peroxide
Hydrochloric acid	Most metals, alkali, or active metals
Hydrocyanic acid	Nitric acid, alkali
Hydrofluoric acid, anhydrous (Hydrogen fluoride)	Ammonia, aqueous or anhydrous
Hydrogen peroxide	Copper, chromium, iron, most metals or their salts, alcohols, acetone, organic materials, aniline, nitromethane, flammable liquids, combustible materials
Hydrogen sulfide	Fuming nitric acid, oxidizing gases
Iodine	Acetylene, ammonia (aqueous or anhydrous), hydrogen
Mercury	Acetylene, fulminic acid, ammonia
Nitric acid (concentrated)	Acetic acid, aniline, chromic acid, hydrocyanic acid, hydrogen sulfide, flammable liquids, flammable gases
Nitroparaffins	Inorganic bases
Oxalic acid	Silver, mercury
Oxygen	Oils, grease, hydrogen, flammable liquids, solids or gases

Perchloric acid	Acetic anhydride, bismuth and its alloys, alcohol, paper, wood, grease, oils, organic amines or antioxidants
Phenol	Strong oxidizers, calcium hypochlorite
Phosphoric acid	Strong caustics, most metals
Phosphorus (white)	Air, oxygen
Potassium	Carbon tetrachloride, carbon dioxide, water
Potassium chlorate	Sulfuric and other acids, ammonium salts, metal powders, sulfur, finely divided organic or combustible materials
Potassium perchlorate	Sulfuric and other acids, ammonium salts, metal powders, sulfur, finely divided organic or combustible materials
Potassium permanganate	Glycerine, ethylene glycol, benzaldehyde, sulfuric or any free acid
Silver	Acetylene, oxalic acid, tartaric acid, fulminic acid, ammonium compounds
Sodium	Carbon dioxide, carbon tetrachloride, and other chlorinated hydrocarbons, any free acid or halogen, water
Sodium nitrate	Ammonium nitrate and other ammonium salts
Sodium oxide	Water, any free acid
Sodium peroxide	Ethyl or methyl alcohol, glacial acetic acid, acetic anhydride, benzaldehyde, carbon disulfide, glycerine, ethylene glycol, ethyl acetate, methyl acetate, furfural

Sulfuric acid	Potassium chlorate, potassium perchlorate, potassium permanganate (or compounds with similar light metals, such as sodium, lithium)
Zirconium	Prohibit water, carbon tetrachloride

This list is not complete, nor are all incompatible substances shown.

Adapted from the *Dangerous Chemicals Code,* 1951, Bureau of Fire Prevention. City of Los Angeles Fire Department and the *NIOSH Pocket Guide to Chemical Hazards*, U.S. Department of Health and Human Services, 1985; and *Clinical Laboratory Safety,* Susan L. Rose, U.S. Department of Energy, J. B. Lippincott Company, New York, 1984.

APPENDIX C

Definitions - Flammables

Flash point of a liquid is the temperature at which it gives off vapors sufficient to form an ignitable mixture with the air near the surface of the liquid.

Flammable liquids are those having a flash point below 140° F.

Combustible liquids have a flash point at or above 140° F.

Liquefied compressed gases are flammable liquids with a vapor pressure above forty pounds per square inch absolute at 100° F.

Ignition temperature (auto ignition temperature) of a substance is the minimum temperature required to initiate or cause self-sustained combustion without ignition from an external energy source.

Lower flammable limit (lower explosive limit) is the minimum concentration of vapor in air below which a flame is *not* propagated when an ignition source is present. Below this concentration, the mixture is too lean to burn.

Upper flammable limit (upper explosive limit) is the maximum concentration of vapor in air in which a flame can be propagated. Above this concentration, the mixture is too rich to burn.

Flammable range consists of all concentrations between the lower flammable limit and the upper flammable limit.

Specific gravity of a liquid is the ratio of its density to that of water under specified conditions. This term is important in that a material that does not mix with water will float if its specific gravity is less than 1 (one) and will sink and be covered with water if its specific gravity is greater than 1 (one).

Vapor density is expressed as the relative density of a vapor with respect to air at the same temperature. Thus, a vapor having a density less than 1 (one) will tend to rise, and a vapor with a density greater than 1 (one) will tend to sink.

Water solubility is sometimes important in determining whether water can be used effectively to flush away flammable liquids. Remember that a water solution of soluble solvents can give off sufficient vapors to burn. For example, a 5(five) percent solution of ethyl alcohol in water has a determinable flash point.

Classification of Flammable and Combustible Liquids

The following classification system for flammable and combustible liquids (from National Fire Prevention Association 321) is based on dividing liquids that will burn into three categories. In most areas the indoor temperature could reach 100° F at some time during the year. Therefore, all liquids with flash points below 100° F are called **Class I** liquids. In some areas the ambient temperature could exceed 100° F, or only a moderate degree of heating would be required to heat the liquid to its flash point. Based on this concept, an arbitrary division of 100° F to 140° F was established for liquids in this flash point range, to be known as **Class II** liquids. Liquids with flash points higher than 140° F requiring considerable heating from a source other than ambient temperatures, identified as **Class III** liquids.

Flammable Liquids

Flammable liquids have flash points below 100° F and vapor pressures not exceeding 40 psia at 100° F.

Class I liquids include those with flash points below 100° F and may be subdivided as follows:

Class IA includes those with flash points below 73° F and with boiling points below 100° F.

Class IB includes those with flash points below 73° F and with boiling points at

or above 100° F.
Class IC includes those flash points at or above 73° F and below 100° F.

Combustible Liquids

Liquids with flash points at or above 100° F are referred to as combustible liquids and may be subdivided as follows:
Class II liquids have flash points at or above 100° F and below 140° F.
Class IIIA liquids have flash points at or above 140° F and below 200° F.
Class IIIB liquids have flash points at or above 200° F.
Underwriters Laboratories Inc., Classification

Underwriters Laboratories Inc., has a classification system for grading the relative flammability hazards of various liquids, based on the following scale:

Ether class	100
Gasoline class	90 - 100
Alcohol (ethyl) class	60 - 70
Kerosene class*	30 - 40
Paraffin oil class	10 - 20

*A standard kerosene of 100° F closed cap flash point is rated 40

The flash point, although the commonly accepted and most important criterion of the relative hazard of flammable and combustible liquids, is by no means the only factor in evaluating the hazard. The ignition temperature, flammable range, rate of evaporation, reactivity when contaminated or exposed to heat, density, and rate of diffusion of the vapor are also important factors.

Source: *Clinical Laboratory Safety,* Susan L. Rose, U.S. Department of Energy, J. B. Lippincott Company, New York, 1985.

Toxic and Flammable Chemicals

Toxic To Skin	**Toxic Through Inhalation**	**Flammable or explosive**
Acetic acid	Acetone	Acetone
Acetone	Ammonia	Amyl alcohol
Acetyl chloride	Amyl alcohol	Benzene
Alkali, caustic	Aniline	Butyl acetate
Aniline	Benzene	Butyl alcohol
Bromine	Bromine	Carbon disulfide
Carbon Disulfide	Butyl acetate	Cellosolve
Chromic acid	Butyl alcohol	Cellosolve acetate
Chloroform	Carbon disulfide	Chloroform
Cresol	Carbon dioxide (dry ice)	Dichloroethylene
Ethylene oxide	Carbon tetrachloride	Ethyl acetate
Hydrochloric acid	Chlorine	Ethyl alcohol
Hydrofluoric acid	Chloroform	Ethyl chloride
Hydrogen peroxide (30%)	Cresol	Ethyl ether
Iodine	Dichlorethylene	Ethylene dichloride
Mercuric chloride	Ethyl chloride	Ethylene oxide
Nitrobenzene	Ethyl ether	Formic acid
Nitric acid	Ethylene dichloride	Hexane
Perchloric acid	Formaldehyde	Methyl alcohol
Phenol	Formic acid	Perchloric acid
Silver nitrate	Hydrochloric acid (fumes)	Toluene (toluol)
Sodium Hydroxide	Hydrogen sulfide	Trichlorethylene
Sodium hypochlorite (bleach)	Hydrofluoric acid	Xylene (xylol)
Sulfuric acid	Mercury	
Trichlorethylene	Methyl alcohol	
Tricresol	Methylene chloride	
Xylene (xylol)	Nitrobenzene	
	Nitric acid	
	Tetrachlorethylene	
	Toluene (toluol)	
	Xylene (xylol)	

APPENDIX D

Material Safety Data Sheet (Example)

Section 1. Material Identification

Material Name: METHYL ALCOHOL
Description: Industrial Solvent
Other Designations/Synonyms: Methanol, Wood alcohol, Wood naphtha, carbinol, CH_3OH, CAS #000 067 561
Manufacturer/Supplier: Available from many suppliers

Section II. Ingredients And Hazards

	%	HAZARD DATA
Methyl Alcohol	ca 100	8-hr TWA 200 ppm* (skin) or 260 mg/m^3
*Current OSHA Standard; ACGIH (1981) TLV adds (skin) notation. NIOSH has recommended a 10-hr TWA of 200 ppm with a ceiling of 800 ppm (15 minute sample)		Human Eye: 5 ppm Primary irritation dose Oral: LDLo 340 mg/kg Inhalation: TCLo 8600 mg/m^3 Toxic irritant effects (systemic)

Section III. Physical Data

Boiling point at 1 atm, deg C	64.5
Vapor density (Air = 1)	1.1
Vapor pressure @ 21.2°C, mm Hg	100
Water solubility	Total miscible
Viscosity @ 20°C, cps	0.59
Specific gravity (20°/4°C)	0.791
Melting point, deg C	-97.8
Volatiles, %	ca 100
Evaporation rate (n-BuAc=1)	4.6
Molecular weight	32.04

Appearance and Odor: A clear, colorless liquid with characteristic alcohol odor.

The odor recognition threshold (100% of test panel) is 53.3 ppm.

Section IV. Fire And Explosion Data

Flash Point and Method: 54°F (12°C) (closed cup)
Autoignition Temperature: 867°F (465°C)
Flammability Limits in Air: % by Volume: Lower = 6; Upper = 36.5

Extinguishing media: CO_2, dry chemical, alcohol foam, and water mist or fog. Methyl alcohol fires are Class IB fires, use a blanketing effect to smother fire.

It is a moderate explosion hazard and dangerous fire hazard when exposed to heat, sparks, or flames and can react vigorously with oxidizing agents.

Firefighters should use self-contained breathing apparatus with full facepiece operated in pressure-demand or other positive pressure mode. Wear full protective clothing.

Section V. Reactivity Data

Methyl alcohol is a flammable material, but it is stable under normal storage and use conditions. It does not undergo hazardous polymerization.

Avoid contact with strong oxidizing agents such as nitrates, perchlorates or sulfuric acid.

Oxidation products in air include oxides of carbon and nitrogen.

Section VI. Health Hazard Information

TLV 200 ppm (Skin) or 260 mg/m^3

Methanol is a poisonous, narcotic chemical that may exert its effects through inhalation, skin absorption or ingestion. Body elimination of methanol is slow, and the toxic effects can be compounded by repeated excessive exposures over several days. Toxic effects are exerted upon the CNS, especially the optic nerve. Ingestion can produce blindness. Symptoms of overexposure include dizziness, visual impairment, nausea, respiratory failure, muscular incoordination and narcosis. Prolonged or repeated skin contact will cause dermatitis, erythema, and scaling. Ingestion of 100-250 ml can be fatal.

FIRST AID:

Skin Contact: Remove contaminated clothing. Wash affected area with soap and water; apply lotions.

Eye Contact: Irrigate with running water for 15 minutes. Get medical help.

Inhalation: Remove victim to fresh air and prevent further exposure for 7 days. Obtain medical assistance if victim is not fully normal within 10 minutes.

Ingestion: Drink 3 glasses milk, water or 4% sodium bicarbonate Gastric lavage by medical personnel. Repeat $NaHCO_3$ treatment after lavage. (NIOSH recommends inducing vomiting if victim is conscious.)

Section VII. Spill, Leak, And Disposal Procedures

Notify safety personnel. Remove all sources of ignition; provide adequate ventilation. Absorb on vermiculite, paper or other absorbent. Burn in an approved incinerator or open pit away from buildings and people.

Spills in sensitive areas may be diluted and flushed to ground with a water spray. Do not flush to sewer.

Dispose of large quantities of waste via a licensed waste solvent disposal company, or reclaim via filtration and distillation procedures. It can be incinerated.

Follow Federal, state and local regulations.

Aquatic toxicity rating: TLm 96: over 1000 ppm.

Section VIII. Special Protection Information

Provide adequate ventilation to meet TLV requirements. Exhaust ventilation with 100 lfm minimum should be used where vapor exposure is likely. Engineering controls shall be sparkproof and explosion proof.

Use air-supplied or self-contained breathing apparatus when concentration is above TLV, but less than 2,000 ppm. A full facepiece is required above 10,000 ppm.

Prevent skin contact by wearing rubber gloves. Protective aprons, boots and face shields should be used where splashing may occur. Use safety glasses in other areas of use.

Eye wash stations and safety showers should be available in areas of use.

No smoking in areas of use.

Provide suitable training to those working with methanol. Monitor the workplace. Keep records.

Section IX. Special Precautions And Comments

Store in a well-ventilated, fire-proof area, away from sources of heat, open flame and ignition. Ground and electrically interconnect containers for transfer. Use sparkproof tools. Use with adequate ventilation. No smoking in areas of storage or use.

Avoid prolonged or repeated breathing of vapor or contact with skin. Avoid contact with eyes. This material is poisonous when introduced into the body metabolism. Do not ingest.

Provide pre-placement medical exams for industrially exposed workers, periodic medical surveillance, with emphasis on neurological and visual functions, liver and kidney systems.

DOT CLASSIFICATION: Flammable Liquid

LABEL: Flammable Liquid

DATA SOURCE(S) CODE: 2, 4-12, 16, 19, 20, 23-26, 31, 34, 37-39, 43, 47.

MEDICAL REVIEW: October 8, 1981

Judgements as to the suitability of information herein for purchaser's purposes are necessarily purchaser's responsibility. Therefore, although reasonable care has been taken in the preparation of such information, we extend no warranties, make no representations and assume no responsibility as to the accuracy or suitability of such information for application to purchaser's intended purposes or for consequences of its use.

APPENDIX E

Glossary

ABPA	Allergic Bronchopulmonary Aspergillosis. An allergy to Aspergillus.
ABSORPTION	The passage of a substance through some surface of the body into body fluids and tissues.
ACGIH	See American Conference of Governmental Industrial Hygienists.
ACID	A substance which dissolves in water and releases hydrogen ions (H+). An acid reacts with a metal to form a salt, neutralizes bases, and turns litmus paper red. Acids cause irritation, burns, or more serious damage to tissue depending on the strength of the acid. Acids are measured by pH of from 0 to 6.9. Most acids taste "sour".
ACS	See American Chemical Society.
ACTION LEVEL	The exposure level (concentration in air) at which OSHA regulations to protect employees take effect (29 CFR 1910.1001-1047); e.g., workplace air analysis, employee training, medical monitoring, and record keeping. Exposure at or above action level is termed occupational exposure. Exposure below this level can also be harmful. This level is *generally* half the TLV.

ACTIVE INGREDIENT	The ingredient of a product that actually does what the product is designed to do.
ACUTE EFFECT	An adverse effect, usually the result of a short term and high level exposure, with symptoms developing rapidly.
AEROSOL	A system of particles, solid or liquid, suspended in the air and dispersed as a gas, mist, smoke or fog.
AGENT	Any substance, force, radiation, organism, or influence affecting the body. The effects may be beneficial or harmful.
AIR PURIFYING RESPIRATOR	A device designed to protect the wearer from the inhalation of harmful atmospheres by removing the contaminants through a filtering media.
ALARA	Acronym for "as low as reasonably achievable."
ALLERGIC BRONCHOPULMONARY ASPERGILLOSIS	See ABPA
ALKALI	A strong base, especially the metallic hydroxides. Alkalies combine with acids to form salts; combine with fatty acids to form soap; neutralize acids; and turn litmus paper blue. Alkalies are measured by pH of from 7.1 to 14..
ALLERGIC REACTION	An abnormal physiological response to a chemical or physical stimulus by a sensitive person. The stimulus may be inhalants such as dusts, pollens, fungi, smoke, perfumes, odors of plastics; foods such as milk, chocolate, wheat; drugs such as aspirin, antibiotics, serums; infectius agents such as bacteria, viruses, fungi; contactants such as chemicals, animals, plants, metals; or physical agents such as heat, cold, light or pressure.

AMBIENT	Usual or surrounding conditions of temperatures, humidity, pressure, etc.
AMERICAN CHEMICAL SOCIETY	Professional society that establishes standards of purity for a number of reagents. Publishes *Chemical Abstracts* and other professional journals and magazines dealing with various areas of chemistry.
AMERICAN CONFERENCE OF GOVERNMENTAL INDUSTRIAL HYGIENISTS	An organization of professionals in governmental agencies or educational institutions engaged in occupational safety and health programs. ACGIH develops and publishes recommended occupational exposure limits for chemical substances and physical agents.
AMERICAN NATIONAL STANDARDS INSTITUTE	A privately funded organization that identifies industrial/public national consensus standards and coordinates their development. Many ANSI standards relate to safe design or performance of equipment and safe practices or procedures.
AMERICAN SOCIETY FOR TESTING AND MATERIALS	An organization that devises consensus standards for materials characterization and use.
ANESTHETIC EFFECT	The temporary loss of feeling caused by certain chemical agents which reduce the ability to feel pain or other sensations.
ANHYDRIDE	A compound derived from another compound (e.g. an acid) by removing the elements that compose water (hydrogen and oxygen).
ANHYDROUS	A term used to describe chemical compounds which do not contain water.
ANSI	See American National Standards Institute.
ANTIDOTE	A substance that neutralizes poisons or their effects.

APPEARANCE — A material's physical state (powder, gas or liquid), its color, and other visible attributes. There should not be a difference between a material's appearance and that listed on the MSDS.

AQUEOUS — Describes a water-based solution or suspension. Frequently describes a gaseous compound dissolved in water.

ASBESTOSIS — Lung disease resulting from the prolonged inhalation of airborne asbestos fibers.

ASPERGILLOSIS — Aspergillus infection in the tissues or on any mucous surface marked by inflammatory granular tumor or growth lesions. This condition may develop in the bronchi, lungs, aural (ear) canal, skin, or the mucous membranes of the eye,nose or urethra. It may extend through the various viscera (internal organs enclosed within a cavity, esp. the abdominal organs such as the heart, lungs and intestines) producing mycotic or fungus induced nodules in the lungs, liver, kidney, and other organs.

ASPERGILLUS — Group of molds that can pose pathogenic problems. *Aspergillus fumigatus* is found in soil and manure, and is the most common cause of aspergillosis in man. It has been found in the ear, nose and lungs.

ASPHYXIANT — A vapor or gas which can cause unconsciousness or death by suffocation (insufficient intake of oxygen). Many asphyxiants are harmful because they displace the available oxygen in the air (normally about 21%) to dangerous levels (18% or lower). Examples of these simple asphyxiants are carbon dioxide, nitrogen, hydrogen and helium. Chemical asphyxiants like carbon monoxide reduce the blood's ability to carry oxygen, or like cyanide interfere with the body's ability to use oxygen. Asphyxiation is one of the principal potential hazards of working in confined spaces.

ASPIRATION HAZARD	The danger of drawing material into the lungs, leading to an inflammatory response that can be fatal.
ASTHMA	A disease characterized by recurrent attacks of audible labored breathing, wheezing, and perhaps coughing caused by spasmodic contraction of the main airways in the lungs.
ASTM	See American Society for Testing and Materials.
ASYMPTOMATIC	Without symptoms.
ATM	See Atmosphere.
ATMOSPHERE	A unit of pressure equal to the average pressure the air exerts at sea level.
AUTOIGNITION TEMPERATURE	The approximate lowest temperature at which a flammable gas or vapor-air mixture will spontaneously ignite without spark or flame. Vapors and gases will spontaneously ignite at a lower temperature in oxygen than in air.
BACTERIAL TOXIN	Toxin (poison) produced by bacteria. Includes exotoxins, which diffuse from bacterial cells into surrounding medium and endotoxins, which are liberated only when the bacterial cell is destroyed.
BASE	Any substance that combines with hydrogen ions (H+). Strong bases feel slippery or slimy and are corrosive to human tissue. Also known as alkali. Bases are measured by pH of from 7.1 to 14.
BEI	See Biological exposure indexes.
BIODEGRADABLE	An organic material's capacity for decomposition as a result of attack by microorganisms. Sewage-treatment routines are based on this property. Biodegradable materials do not persist in nature but break down.

BIOLOGICAL EXPOSURE INDEXES	Biological Exposure Indexes. Numerical values based on procedures to determine the amount of a material the human body absorbs by measuring the material or its metabolic products in tissue, fluid,or exhaled air.
BIOLOGICAL MONITORING	Periodic examination of body substances, such as blood or urine, to determine the extent of hazardous material absorption or accumulation in the body.
BOILING POINT	The degree of heat required for a liquid to change into a vapor state at a given pressure; varies according to the chemicals present in different liquids.
BONDING	A safety practice where two objects (tanks, cylinders, etc.) are interconnected with clamps and wire. This equalizes the electrical potential between the objects and helps prevent static sparks that can ignite flammable materials.
BRONCHITIS	Inflammation of the mucous membranes of the bronchial tubes (breathing airways) of the lungs.
BUFFER	A substance, especially a salt of the blood, tending to preserve original hydrogen-ion concentration of its solution, upon adding an acid or base. A pH stabilizer.
°C	See Degrees Celsius (centigrade.)
CANCER, CARCINOMA	An abnormal multiplication of cells that tends to infiltrate other tissues and spread (metastasize). Each cancer is believed to originate from a single "transformed" cell that grows (splits) at a fast, abnormally regulated pace, no matter where it occurs in the body.
CARCINOGEN	A substance or agent that produces or increases the risk of developing cancer in humans or lower animals either from acute or chronic exposure.

CARTRIDGE	A small canister containing a filter solvent, or catalyst, or any combination of these elements, which removes specific contaminants from the air drawn through it.
CAS NUMBER	CAS Registration Number. An assigned number used to identify a chemical.
CATALYST	A substance that changes (slows, but usually speeds up) the rate of a chemical reaction without itself being permanently altered in the reaction.
CATARACT	Opacity in the lens of the eye that may obscure vision.
CAUSTIC	A substance, especially an alkali, that strongly irritates, corrodes or destroys living tissue.
CEILING LIMIT	The concentration of a hazardous material that should not be exceeded at any time (in terms of employee exposure.)
CELSIUS	See Degrees Celsius (Centigrade.)
CENTIGRADE	See Degrees Celsius (Centigrade.) Celsius is now this temperatures scale's preferred name.
CENTRAL NERVOUS SYSTEM	Brain and spinal cord, with their end organs that control voluntary and involuntary acts. A material's effect on the CNS may include headache, tremors, drowsiness, convulsions, hypnosis, anesthesia, nervousness, irritability, narcosis, dizziness, fatigue, memory loss, sleep disturbance, etc.
CFC	See Chlorofluorocarbon.
CFR	See Code of Federal Regulations.
CHELATING AGENT	A chemical compound capable of forming multiple chemical bonds to a metal ion. Used to treat metal poisoning and to avoid scale deposition from water.

CHEMICAL ASPHYXIANT:	A substance which prevents the body from receiving or using an adequate supply of oxygen.
CHEMICAL COMPOUND	A substance consisting of two or more chemical elements in definite proportions and in chemical combination and for which a chemical formula can be written. For example, water has two atoms of hydrogen and one of oxygen (H2O).
CHEMICAL FAMILY	A group of single elements or compounds of a common general type. For example, acetone and methyl ethyl ketone are of the ketone family.
CHEMICAL HYGIENE PLAN	A written program developed and implemented by the employer which sets forth standard operating procedures, equipment, engineering controls, personal protective equipment and specific work practices that are capable of protecting employees from hazardous chemicals used in that particular workplace. Established by 29 CFR 1910.1450.
CHEMICAL NAME	A chemical's scientific name. Complex chemicals may have more than one name, corresponding to different naming systems.
CHEMICAL REACTIVITY	A chemical's tendency to react with other materials. Undesirable and dangerous effects such as heat, explosions, or production of noxious substances can result.
CHEMI-LUMINESCENCE	Cold light or light produced as a result of a chemical reaction and without the production of heat.
CHLOROFLUORO-CARBON	Chemical associated with damage to the Earth's ozone layer.
CHP	See Chemical Hygiene Plan.
CHRONIC EFFECT	An adverse effect, usually the result of a long term and low-level exposure, with symptoms developing slowly.

CHRONIC EXPOSURE	Continuous or intermittent exposure over a long period of time, usually to relatively low material amounts or concentrations.
CNS	See Central nervous system.
CODE OF FEDERAL REGULATIONS	A collection of the regulations established by Congress, updated annually.
COMBUSTIBILITY	The capacity of a material to fuel a fire. The term is also used to classify certain liquids on the basis of their flash points. A chemical property defined by having a flash point greater than 100°F and below 200°F.
COMMON NAME	A designation for a material other than its chemical name, such as code name or code number or trade, brand, or generic name. For example, Arklone P-113 is a registered tradename for 1,1,2-Trichlorotrifluoroethane.
COMPRESSED GAS	Any material which is a gas at normal temperature and pressure and which is contained under pressure as a dissolved gas or liquefied by compression or refrigeration.
CONJUNCTIVA	The delicate mucous membrane that lines the eyelids and covers the eyeball.
CONJUNCTIVITIS	Inflammation of the conjunctiva.
CONTAMINANT	A harmful, irritating or nuisance material that is foreign to the natural atmosphere.
CONTAMINATION REDUCTION ZONE	Also known as the Warm Zone. Area at clandestine drug laboratories which provides a transition area between contaminated and clean zones. This is the area where decontamination stations are established and materials collected for removal by a licensed waste hauler.

CONTAMINATION ZONE	Also known as the Hot Zone or Exclusion Zone. Area at clandestine drug laboratories where contamination does or could occur. A boundary is established with barrier tape and entry and exit checkpoints created.
CONVULSION	Contortion of the body caused by violent, involuntary muscular contractions and relaxations.
CORNEA	Transparent membrane covering the front portion of the eyeball.
CORROSIVE	The capacity of a material to cause immediate and extensive damage to human tissue at the site of contact.
CUTANEOUS	Pertaining to the skin.
DEGREES CELSIUS (CENTIGRADE)	Metric temperature scale on which 0 = water's freezing point and 100 = its boiling point.
DEGREES FAHRENHEIT	Temperature scale on which 32 =water's freezing point and 212 its boiling point.
DENSITY	Ratio of weight (mass) to volume of a material, usually in grams per cubic centimeter or pounds per gallon.
DEPARTMENT OF TRANSPORTATION	Federal agency that regulates transportation of materials to protect the public as well as fire, law, and other emergency-response personnel. DOT classifications specify the use of appropriate warnings, such as "Flammable Liquid."
DERMAL	Pertaining to the skin.
DERMATITIS	Inflammation or irritation of the skin as evidenced by itching, redness and various skin lesions.

DOFF	To remove or take off, such as personal protective equipment.
DON	To put on, such as personal protective equipment.
DOT	See Department of Transportation.
DOT IDENT NUMBER	Four-digit number used to identify particular materials for regulation of their transportation.
DUST	Any minute fine, solid particle of earth or other matter with size varying from submicroscopic to visible.
ECZEMA	An acute or chronic inflammatory skin condition. May produce itching or burning sensation. Often includes scales, crusts, scabs or pustules which may be dry or with watery discharge. This word has become synonymous with dermatitis caused by a number of external and internal factors.
EDEMA:	A condition in which the body tissues contain an excessive amount of tissue fluid. Swelling.
ELECTROLYTE	A substance that, in solution, conducts an electric current and is decomposed by the passage of an electric current. Acids, bases and salts are common electrolytes. Electrolytes can be lost from the body through perspiration and can result in impairment of the central nervous system if not replaced.
EMBRYO	The young of any organism in an early stage of development. In humans, the pre-fetal product of conception up to the third month of pregnancy.
EMBRYOTOXIN	A material harmful to a developing embryo at a concentration that has no adverse effect on the pregnant female.
ENDOTHERMIC	A chemical reaction that absorbs heat.

ENDOTOXINS	Bacterial toxin (poison) confined within the body of a bacterium, freed only when the bacterium is broken down.
ENGINEERING CONTROLS	Engineering control systems reduce potential hazards by isolating the worker from the hazard or by removing the hazard from the work environment. Methods include substitution, ventilation, isolation, and enclosure. This is preferred over personal protective equipment.
ENVIRONMENTAL PROTECTION AGENCY	Federal agency responsible for environmental protection.
EPA	See Environmental Protection Agency.
EPIDEMIOLOGY	Science concerned with defining and explaining the interrelationships of factors that determine disease frequency and distribution in populations.
ERGONOMICS	Science concerned with how to fit a job to a human's anatomical, physiological, and psycho-logical characteristics in a way that will enhance efficiency and well-being.
ERYTHEMA	Reddening of the skin.
ETIOLOGY	All of the factors that contribute to the cause of a disease or an abnormal condition.
EVAPORATION	The rate at which a material vaporizes or evaporates from the liquid or solid state when compared to a known material's vaporization rate.
EXOTOXIN	A toxin (poison) produced by a microorganism and excreted into its surrounding medium.

EXPLOSIVE — A substance that causes a sudden, almost instantaneous release of pressure, gas and heat when subjected to sudden shock, pressure or high temperature.

EXPLOSIVE LIMIT — The range of concentrations (% by volume in air) of a flammable gas or vapor that can result in an explosion. Usually given as upper and lower explosive limits.

EXPOSURE — Any situation arising from a work operation where an employee may ingest, inhale, absorb through the skin or eyes, or otherwise come into contact with a hazardous substance.

EYE PROTECTION — Recommended personal protective equipment for protection of the eyes to be used when handling materials. These include safety glasses, chemical splash goggles and face shields.

EXOTHERMIC: — A chemical reaction that gives off heat.

°F — See Degrees Fahrenheit and Degrees Celsius.

FIRE DIAMOND — NFPA Hazard Rating. Per "NFPA 704" publication. Visual system that provides a general idea of the inherent hazards and their severity of materials relating to fire prevention, exposure and control.

FIRE POINT — The lowest temperature at which a liquid produces sufficient vapor to flash near its surface and continues to burn. Usually 10° to 30° higher than the flash point.

FLAMMABLE — Describes any solid, liquid, vapor, or gas that ignites easily and burns rapidly, perhaps violently.

FLAMMABLE LIMITS — Minimum and maximum concentrations of a flammable gas or vapor between which ignition can occur. Concentrations below the lower flammable limit (LFL) are too lean to burn, while concentrations above the upper flammable limit (UFL) are too rich. All concentrations in between are in the flammable range and require special precautions to avoid ignition or explosion.

FLASH POINT	Lowest temperature at which a flammable liquid gives off sufficient vapor to form an ignitable mixture with air near its surface or within a vessel. Combustion does not continue.
FOVEA	A depression or pit in the center of the macula of the eye; it is the area of clearest vision.
FUME	An airborne dispersion of minute solid particles arising from the heating of a solid. Heating is often accompanied by a chemical reaction where the particles react with oxygen to form an oxide.
GAS	A basic form of matter distinguished from the solid and liquid states. The molecules are free and move swiftly in all directions and take the shape of any containing vessel. It can be changed to its liquid or solid state only by increased pressure or decreased temperature.
GENERIC NAME	A common, possible chemical, name applied generally to a substance. For example, 1,1,2-Trichlorotrifluoroethane is the generic name, and "Freon" is a registered trademark name. A chemical name may be used as a generic name, but trade names are not generic names.
GENERATOR	Any person, company or organization that produces hazardous waste which is subject to regulation.
GROUNDING	A safety practice to conduct any electrical charge to the ground, preventing sparks that could ignite a flammable material. Also called "bonding".

HANTAVIRUS	Virus associated with the urine, saliva and feces of the deer mouse. Infection with the virus results in Hantavirus Pulmonary Syndrome (HPS) which can be fatal.
HAZARDOUS COMMUNICATION RULE	Requires chemical manufacturers and importers to assess the hazards associated with the materials in their workplace (29 CFR 1910.1200). MSDS's, labeling,and training are all required by this law.
HAZARDOUS SUBSTANCE	A substance or combination of substances which may cause injury or death because of its concentration, physical, chemical or infectious characteristics.
HEALTH SURVEILLANCE	The continuing medical evaluation of particular individuals for the purpose of identifying health problems which may relate to exposure to hazardous materials.
HEPA:	See High-efficiency particulate air filter.
HEPATITIS	Inflammation of the liver.
HERPES	An acute inflammation of the skin or mucous membranes.
HIGH-EFFICIENCY PARTICULATE AIR FILTER	Also called "absolute." Has a 99.97% removal efficiency for .03-micron particles.
HPS	Hantavirus Pulmonary Syndrome. See Hantavirus.
HYDROLYSIS	Decomposition of a chemical compound by reaction with water.
HYDROPHILIC	Describes materials which have an affinity for absorbing, tending to combine with, or capable of dissolving in water.

HYGROSCOPIC	Readily absorbing moisture, such as from the atmosphere.
IARC	See International Agency for Research on Cancer.
IDLH	See Immediately dangerous to life and health.
IGNITION TEMPERATURE:	The lowest temperature at which a combustible material ignites in air and continues to burn independently of the heat source.
IMMEDIATELY DANGEROUS TO LIFE AND HEALTH	The maximum concentration from which a person could escape within 30 minutes without irreversible health effects. Used to determine respirator selection.
IMPERVIOUS	Describes a material which is incapable of being penetrated by another substance.
INCOMPATIBLE	Describes materials that direct contact could cause to react dangerously and release energy.
INERT	Having little or no tendency or ability to react with other chemicals.
INERT INGREDIENTS	Any material other than the active ingredient in a product. These ingredients can be hazardous, e.g., the propellant gas in aerosol spray cans may be flammable.
INFLAMMABLE	See Flammable.
INFLAMMATION	Tissue reaction to injury, infection or irritation which results in localized heat, redness, swelling and pain.
INGESTION	Taking into the body through the mouth by swallowing.
INHALATION	Drawing in of breath, gas, vapor, fume, mist or dust into the lungs.

INHIBITOR	A material used to retard or halt an unwanted reaction.
INORGANIC MATERIALS	Compounds which are not animal or vegetable by nature and so do not contain carbon atoms. However, some simple carbon compounds such as carbonates, cyanides and carbon dioxide are considered inorganic.
INTERNATIONAL AGENCY FOR RESEARCH ON CANCER	One of three sources to which OSHA refers for data on carcenogenicity. Oversees the interpretation of results from cancer research.
IRRITANT	A substance that causes a local and reversible inflammatory reaction on living tissue by chemical action at the site of contact as a function of concentration or duration of exposure.
ISOMER	A compound having the same percentage composition and molecular weight as another compound but differing in chemical or physical properties.
KERATITIS	Inflammation of the cornea.
LABEL	Any written, printed, or graphic sign or symbol displayed on or affixed to containers of hazardous chemicals. Labels should identify the hazardous chemical, appropriate hazard warnings, and the name and address of the chemical manufacturer, importer, or other responsible party.
LABORATORY	29 CFR 1910.1450 defines as a facility where "laboratory use of hazardous chemicals" occurs, and/ or where relatively small quantities of hazardous chemicals are used on a non-production basis.

LABORATORY-TYPE HOOD	An enclosed laboratory cabinet with a moveable sash or fixed access port on the front connected to a ventilating system which may incorporate air scrubbing or filtering facilities. The hood draws in and then exhausts air from the laboratory to prevent or minimize the escape of air contaminants. Enables employee to work with materials in the hood using only his or her hands and arms.
LC50	See Lethal concentration 50.
LCLo	See Lethal concentration low.
LD50	See Lethal dose 50.
LDLo	See Lethal dose low.
LEL	See Lower explosive limit.
LENS (EYE)	A transparent biconvex body situated in between the front chamber (aqueous) and the rear chamber (vitreous) through which the light rays are further focused on the retina.
LESION	An abnormal change, injury, or damage to tissue or to an organ.
LETHAL CONCENTRATION 50	Median lethal concentration. The concentration of a material in air that on the basis of laboratory tests (respiratory route) is expected to kill 50% of a group of test animals when administered as a single exposure in a specific time period, usually 1 hour. LC50 is expressed as parts of material per million parts of air, by volume (ppm) for gases and vapors, as micrograms of material per liter of air (μg/l), or milligrams of material per cubic meter of air (mg/m^3) for dusts and mists, as well as for gases and vapors.

LETHAL CONCENTRATION LOW	The lowest concentration of a substance in air reported to have caused death in humans or animals. The reported concentrations may be entered for periods of exposure that are less that 24 hour (acute) or greater than 24 hour (subacute and chronic).
LETHAL DOSE 50	The single dose of a substance that causes the death of 50% of an animal population from exposure to the substance by any route other than inhalation. LD50 is usually expressed as milligrams or grams of material per kilogram of animal weight (mg/kg or g/kg). The animal species and means of administering the dose (oral, intraveneous, etc.) should also be stated.
LETHAL DOSE LOW	The lowest dose of a substance introduced by any route other than inhalation reported to have caused death in humans or animals.
LFL	Lower flammable limit, see Lower Explosive Limit.
LFM or lfm	Linear feet per minute.
LOWER EXPLOSIVE LIMIT (LEL)	Refers to the lowest concentration of gas or vapor (% by volume in air) that burns or explodes if an ignition source is present at ambient temperatures. Also called lower flammable limit.
LYME DISEASE	A recurrent inflammatory disorder accompanied by distinctive skin lesions, colored spots or skin area, polyarthritis and involvement of the heart and nervous system. Also known as Lyme Arthritis. Caused by a spirochete transmitted by small ticks.
LUPUS ERYTHEMATOSUS	A chronic disease of the skin characterized by remissions and exacerbations of a scaling, red rash.
MACULA (EYE)	An oval area in the center of the retina devoid of blood vessels; the area most responsible for color vision.

MALAISE — Discomfort, uneasiness, or indisposition, often indicative of infection.

MATERIAL SAFETY DATA SHEET — OSHA guidelines for descriptive data provided on a data sheet to serve as the basis for written hazard communication programs. Those who make, distribute, and use hazardous materials are responsible for effective communication.

MELTING POINT — The temperature above which a solid changes to a liquid.

MENINGES — The three membranes investing the spinal cord and brain.

MENINGITIS — An inflammation of the membranes of the spinal cord or brain caused by bacteria, viruses, or other organisms that reach the meninges from other foci in the body via blood or lymph, through trauma, or from adjacent bony structures (sinuses, mastoid cells).

MINE SAFETY AND HEALTH ADMINISTRATION — A federal agency within the US Dept. of Labor that devises and promotes mandatory safety and health rules for mines. This agency has tested and approved many of the respirators and respirator cartridges which are used in forensics.

MISCIBLE — Capable of being mixed. When two liquids or two gases are completely soluble in each other in all proportions. While gases mix with one another in all proportions, the miscibility of liquids depends on their chemical nature.

MIST — Suspended liquid droplets in the air generated by condensation from the gaseous to the liquid state or by mechanically breaking up a liquid by splashing or atomizing.

MIXTURE	A heterogeneous association of materials that cannot be represented by a chemial formula and that does not undergo chemical change because of interaction among the mixed materials. The constituent materials may or may not be uniformly dispersed and can usually be separated by mechanical means (as opposed to to a chemical reaction). Uniform liquid mixtures are called solutions.
MOLECULE	The smallest quantity into which a substance may be divided without loss of its characteristics. The chemical combination of two or more atoms that form a specific chemical compound.
MSDS	See Material safety data sheet.
MSHA	See Mine Safety and Health Administration.
MUCOUS MEMBRANE	The mucous-secreting membrane lining the hollow organs of the body, i.e. nose, mouth, stomach, intestine, bronchial tubes, and urinary tract.
MUTAGEN	Any agent that causes genetic mutations (permanent changes in chromosomes or the genetic code). Many medicines, chemicals, and physical agents such as ionizing radiations and ultraviolet light have this ability.
MYCOTOXINS	Substances, produced by mold growing in food or animal feed, that cause illness or death when ingested by man or animals.
NARCOSIS	A state of drowsiness or unconsciousness produced by a drug, organic chemical, heat, cold or electricity.
NATIONAL CANCER INSTITUTE	The part of the National Institutes of Health that studies cancer.

NATIONAL FIRE PROTECTION ASSOCIATION	An international organization to promote/improve fire protection and prevention and establish safeguards against loss of life and property by fire.
NATIONAL INSTITUTE OF OCCUPATIONAL SAFETY AND HEALTH	The agency of the Public Health Service that tests and certifies respiratory and air-sampling devices. It recommends exposure limits to OSHA for substances, investigates incidents, and researches occupational safety.
NATIONAL TOXICOLOGY PROGRAM	Federal activity overseen by the Department of Health and Human Services with resources from National Institutes of Health, the Food and Drug Administration, and the Center for Disease Control. Its goals are to develop tests useful for public health regulations of toxic chemicals, to develop toxicological profiles of materials, to foster testing of materials, and to communicate the results for use by others.
NAUSEA	An unpleasant sensation in the stomach which usually precedes vomiting.
NCI	See National Cancer Institute.
NEUTRALIZE	To render chemically harmless; to return the pH to the neutral level of 7 by adding acid (base) to a basic (acidic) compound.
NFPA	See National Fire Protection Association.
NIOSH	See National Institute of Occupational Safety and Health.
NONFLAMMABLE	Not combustible or easily set on fire. Does not burn, or burns very slowly.
NTP	See National toxicology program.

NUISANCE PARTICULATES	Dusts that do not produce significant organic disease or toxic effect from "reasonable" concentrations and exposures.
OCCUPATIONAL EXPOSURE	See Action Level.
OCCUPATIONAL SAFETY AND HEALTH ADMINISTRATION	Part of the US Department of Labor. The regulatory and enforcement agency for safety and health in most US industrial sectors.
ODOR THRESHOLD	The lowest concentration of a material's vapor (or a gas) in air that is detectable by odor.
ORGANIC MATERIALS	Compounds composed of carbon, hydrogen, and other elements with chain or ring structures. Almost all chemical constituents of living matter (plant and animal in nature) are of this type, but very many compounds of this type are manufactured and do not occur naturally.
OSHA	See Occupational Safety and Health Administration.
OSHA ACT	The Occupational Safety and Health Act of 1070. Effective April 28, 1971. Public Law 91-596. Found at 29 CFR 1910, 1915, 1918, 1926. OSHA jurisdiction. The regulatory vehicle to ensure the safety and health of workers in firms larger than 10 employees. Its goal is to set standards of safety that prevent injury and illness among the workers. Regulating employee exposure and informing employees of the dangers of materials are key factors. This act established the hazard communication rule (29 CFR 1910.1200).
OXIDATION	The process of a substance combining with oxygen or another oxidizer.

OXIDIZER	A substance that yields oxygen readily to stimulate the combustion (oxidization) of organic matter.
OXIDIZING AGENT	A chemical or substance that brings about an oxidation reaction. The agent may provide the oxygen to the substance being oxidized (in which case the agent has to be oxygen or contain oxygen) or receive electrons being transferred from the substance undergoing oxidation.
PAH	See Polycyclic aromatic hydrocarbons.
PARTICULATE	Small, separate pieces of an airborne material. Dusts, fumes, smokes, mists, and fogs are examples. Generally, anything airborne that is not a fiber.
PERMISSIBLE EXPOSURE LIMIT (PEL)	Established by OSHA. This measurement may be expressed as a time-weighted average (TWA) limit or as a ceiling exposure limit. A ceiling limit must never be exceeded instantaneously even if the TWA exposure limit is not violated. OSHA PELs have the force of law. Note that ACGIH TLVs and NIOSH RELs are recommended exposure limits that OSHA may or may not enact into law.
PERSONAL PROTECTIVE EQUIPMENT	Equipment or clothing used/worn to help insulate a worker from direct exposure to hazardous materials. Examples include laboratory coats, gloves, safety glasses, and respirators.
pH	Indicates how acidic or alkaline a solution or chemical is using a logarithmic scale of 1 to 14.
PHYSICAL HAZARD	A substance for which there is valid evidence that it is a combustible liquid, compressed gas, explosive, flammable, an organic peroxide, an oxidizer, pyrophoric, instable (reactive), or water reactive. In the general safety sense, a hazard of physical origin, such as a fall, a heat burn, etc., and not a chemical or infective disease hazard.

PHYSICAL STATE	The condition of a material: e.g., solid, liquid, or gas, at room temperature.
POISON	Any substance taken into the body by ingestion, inhalation, injection, or absorption that interferes with normal physiological functions. Virtually any substance can be poisonous if consumed in sufficient quantity; therefore, the term poison more often implies an excessive degree of dosage rather than a specific group of substances.
POISON IVY	A climbing vine, *Rhus Toxicodendron*, which on contact produces a severe form of dermatitis. *Rhus* species contain urushiol, an extremely irritating oily resin. Urushiol may also be a potent sensitizer since in many cases subsequent contacts produce increasingly severe reactions.
POISON OAK	A climbing vine, *Rhus radicans* or *R. diversiloba*, closely related to Poison Ivy and containing the same active principle. Symptoms and treatment are the same as for poison ivy dermatitis.
POISON SUMAC	A shrublike plant, *Toxicodendron vernix*, widely distributed in the U.S. Because it contains the same active principle as Poison Ivy, symptoms and treatment are the same as for poison ivy dermatitis.
POLYCYCLIC AROMATIC HYDROCARBONS	A family of chemical compounds containing only carbon and hydrogen, in which molecules consist of three or more carbon ring structures fused so that some carbon atoms are common to two or three rings. A large number of this chemical family's members are carcinogens, or are converted to carcinogens when metabolized by animals or humans. PAHs are formed during incomplete combustion of hydrocarbons. They are common in smoke, such as that of vehicle exhaust or tobacco, and are also important industrial contaminants in coal gas or coke manufacture and other processes involving heating of coal tar and pitch.

POLYMERIZATION — A chemical reaction in which one or more small molecules combine to form larger molecules. Hazardous polymerization takes place at a rate that releases large amounts of energy that can cause fires or exploxions or burst containers. Materials that can polymerize usually contain inhibitors that can delay reactions.

PPE — See Personal protective equipment.

REACTIVE MATERIAL — A chemical substance or mixture that vigorously polymerizes, decomposes, condenses, or becomes self-reactive due to shock, pressure, or temperature.

REAGENT — A substance used in analysis and synthesis of another substance because of the reaction it causes.

RECOMMENDED EXPOSURE LIMIT — The NIOSH recommended exposure limit is the highest allowable airborne concentration that is not expected to injure a worker. It may be expressed as a ceiling limit or as a time-weighted average (TWA), usually for 10-hour work shifts.

REDUCING AGENT — In a reduction reaction (which always occurs simultaneously with an oxidation reaction), the reducing agent is the chemical or substance that combines with oxygen or loses electrons to the reaction.

REGISTRY OF TOXIC EFFECTS OF CHEMICAL SUBSTANCES — Published by NIOSH. Presents basic toxicity data on thousands of materials. Its objective is to identify “all known toxic substances” and to reference the original studies.

REL — See Recommended exposure limit.

REPROCUCTIVE HEALTH HAZARD OR TOXIN — Any agent with a harmful effect on the adult male or female reproductive systems or on the developing fetus or child. Such hazards affect people in many ways, including loss of sexual drive, mental disorders, impotence, infertility, sterility, mutagenic effects on germ cells, teratogenic effects on the fetus, and transplacental carcinogenesis.

RESPIRATOR — A variety of devices that limit inhalation of toxic materials. They range from disposable dust masks to self-contained breathing apparatus (SCBA). All have specific uses and limitations. Their use is covered by 29 CFR 1910.134.

RETINA — The light-sensitive inner surface of the eye that receives and transmits the image formed by the lens.

ROUTES OF ENTRY — Methods of bodily contact. The routes of entry are absorption (eye or skin contact), ingestion, inhalation, and injection.

RTECS — See *Registry of Toxic Effects of Chemical Substances*.

SCBA — See Self-contained breathing apparatus.

SECONDARY CONTAINER — Any container which is used to contain and store any chemicals or prepared reagents. Not the original container in which the chemical was shipped and/or received.

SECONDARY LABEL — Any written, printed, or graphic sign or symbol displayed on or affixed to secondary containers of hazardous chemicals. A label should identify the hazardous material, appropriate hazard warnings, initials of the employee who mixed the chemcials, and the date the reagent was prepared.

SELF-CONTAINED BREATHING APPARATUS — A respirator which provides the user with a clean air source.

SEROCONVERSION — Development of evidence of antibody response to a disease or vaccine.

SOLUTION	A uniform liquid mixture comprised of two or more chemical components.
SOLVENT	A material that can dissolve other materials to form a solution. Water is the most common solvent. Many alcohols and ketones are also used for this purpose.
STABILITY	The ability of a material to remain unchanged. For MSDS purposes, a material is stable if it remains in the same form under expected and reasonable conditions of storage or use.
SUPPORT ZONE	Also known as the Cold Zone. Area at clandestine drug laboratory at the outermost part of the site. This is a non-contaminated or clean zone. Support equipment, vehicles, rest area and the command post are located in this zone.
TARGET ORGAN EFFECTS	Chemically caused effects from exposure to a material on specific listed organs and systems such as liver, kidneys, nervous system, lungs, skin, and eyes.
TCLo	See Toxic concentration low.
TDLo	See Toxic dose low.
TERATOGEN	An agent or material causing physical defects in a developing embryo.
THESHOLD LIMIT VALUE (TLV)	A term ACGIH uses to express the airborne concentration of a material to which *most* workers can be exposed during a normal daily and weekly work schedule without adverse effects.
TIME WEIGHTED AVERAGE (TWA)	The allowable concentration of airborne contaminants for a normal 8-hr workday or 40-hr week.

TITRE (TITER)	Standard of strength per volume of a volumetric test solution. Agglutination is the highest dilution of a serum that will cause clumping or agglutination of the bacteria being tested.
TOXIC	Describes a material's ability to injure biological tissue.
TOXIC CONCENTRATION LOW	The lowest concentration of a substance in air to which humans or animals have been exposed for any given period of time that has produced any toxic effect in humans or produced a tumorigenic or reproductive effects in animals or humans.
TOXIC DOSE LOW	Lowest dose of a substance introduced by any route other than inhalation over any given period of time and reported to produce any toxic effect in humans or to produce tumorigenic or reproductive effects in animals or humans.
TOXIN	A poisonous substance of animal or plant origin.
TRADE NAME	A name, usually not the chemical name, the manufacturer or supplier gives to a product and usually protected as a registered trade mark. The same or similar products can be marketed under different trade names by different companies.
TUBERCULOSIS	A contageous disease caused by infection with the bacterium *Mycobacterium tuberculosis*. It usually affects the lung, but bone, lymph glands, and other tissues may be affected.
TUMOR	A growth of tissue without physiological function. May be non-invasive or cancerous.
UEL	See Upper explosive limit.

UNSTABLE	Tending toward decomposition or other unwanted chemical change during normal handling or storage. An unstable chemical in its pure state, or as commonly produced or transported, polymerizes vigorously, decomposes, condenses, or becomes self-reactive under conditions of shock, pressure, or temperature.
UPPER EXPLOSIVE LIMIT	The highest concentration of a material in air that produces an explosion in fire or that ignites when it contacts an ignition source (high heat, electric arc, spark, or flame). A higher concentration of the material in a smaller percentage of concentration in air is too rich to be ignited.
VALLEY FEVER	A fungal infection caused by the inhalation of *Coccidioides immitis* transmitted in dust particles. The disease exists in two forms. The primary form is acute but self-limiting and involves only the lungs. The progressive form is chronic, may involve any part of the body and can be fatal. Also known as Coccidioidomycosis.
VAPOR	The gaseous state of a material normally encountered as liquid or solid.
VOLATILITY	Measure of a material's tendency to vaporize or evaporate at ambient routine conditions.
WATER REACTIVE	A material that reacts with water to release a flammable gas or to present a health hazard.
WAVELENGTH	The distance in the line of advance of a wave (of light) from any point to a like point on the next wave. It is usually measured in angstroms, microns, micrometers, or nanometers.

Sources of Information

Chemical Hygiene Plan, California Department of Justice, Office of the Attorney General, 1993.

Barbara A. Plog, Ed.
Fundamentals of Industrial Hygiene, 3rd Ed., National Safety Council: United States, 1988.

MSDS Pocket Dictionary, Genium Publishing Corporation: USA, 1993.

Thomas, Clayton L., Ed. Taber's Cyclopedic Medical Dictionary, 16th Edition. F.A. Davis Company: Philadelphia, 1989.

Webster's New World Dictionary of the American Language, 2nd Ed., World Publishing Company: New York, 1972.

APPENDIX F

Weights and Measures

Abbreviations/definitions:

atm	Atmosphere. A unit of pressure equal to the average pressure the air exerts at sea level.
Btu	British thermal unit. The quantity of heat required to raise the temperature of 1 lb of water from 63°F to 64°F.
cc, cm^3	Cubic centimeter, equals 1 milliliter.
Centimeter, cm	1/100 meter; approximately 0.4 inches.
cgs	Metric units of measure based upon centimeter, gram, and second.
cu ft, ft^3	Cubic foot. Usually expressed as cu ft.
cu m, m^3	Cubic meter. Usually expressed as m^3.
g	Gram. Metric unit of weight. One gram equals approximately 0.035 ounces.
kg	Kilogram. 1000 grams.
l	Liter. Basic metric unit of volume. One liter of water weighs 1 kg and is equal to 1.057 quarts.
m	Meter. Basic metric measure of length equal to 39.371 inches.
m^3, cu m	Cubic meter. Usually expressed as m^3.
mg	Milligram. Equals 1/1000 or 10^{-3} of a gram.

mg/kg	Milligram per kilogram. Dosage used in toxicology testing to indicate a dose administered per kg of body weight.
mg/m³	Milligram per cubic meter of air.
Microgram	One-millionth of a gram. Can be expressed as 10^{-6} of a gram. Is often expressed with the symbol "μ."
Micrometer	One-millionth of a meter. Can be expressed as 10^{-6} of a meter and is often referred to as a micron. Is expressed with the symbol "m."
Millimeter	Also seen as mm. Equals 1/1000 of a meter.
min	Minute
ml	Milliliter. Equals 1/1000 of a liter. A metric unit of capacity. For practical purposes is equal to 1 cubic centimeter. One cubic inch is about 16 ml. One ounce is equal to 30 milliliters.
mm Hg	A measure of pressure in millimeters of a mercury column above a reservoir, or difference of level in a U-tube.
mppcf	Millions of particles per cubic foot of air.
ng	Nanogram. One billionth, or 10^{-9}, of a gram.
nm	Nanometer. One billionth, or $10^{-9,}$ of a meter.
ppb	Parts per billion.
ppm	Parts per million.
ppt	Parts per trillion.
psia	Pounds per square inch absolute
psig	Pounds per square inch gauge (i.e., above atmospheric pressure).
torr	A unit of pressure, equal to 1 mm Hg.

Metric/U.S. Equivalents:

Length

Unit	Number of Meters		Approximate U. S. Equivalent
kilometer	1,000	0.621	mile
hectometer	100	109.361	yards
decameter	10	32.808	feet
meter	1	39.370	inches
decimeter	0.1	3.937	inches
centimeter	0.01	0.394	inch
millimeter	0.001	0.039	inch

Mass and Weight

Unit	Number of Grams		Approximate U. S. Equivalent
kilogram	1,000	2.205	pounds
hectogram	100	3.527	ounces
decagram	10	0.353	ounce
gram	1	0.035	ounce
decigram	0.1	1.543	grains
centigram	0.01	0.154	grain
milligram	0.001	0.015	grain

Temperature Conversions:

Familiarity with temperatures in degrees Celsius comes from experience using this system. People in countries which use the Celsius scale have as much difficulty and frustration in working with degrees Fahrenheit as Americans experience dealing with Celsius. To convert for the exact temperature from one scale to the other, use the following formula.

To find the Celsius temperature: ˚F - 32, x 5/9. Example: Start with 68˚F.
68 - 32 = 36 x 5 = 180 ÷ 9 = 20 ˚C.

To find the Fahrenheit temperature: ˚C x 9/5, + 32. Example: Start with 30˚C.
30 x 9 = 270 ÷ 5 = 54 + 32 = 86 ˚F.

Some of the following temperatures are frequently encountered and may offer a sense of familiarity with the more unfamiliar scale.

0˚ C ....Freezing point of water (32˚F)
10˚ C ....A warm winter day (50˚F)
20˚ C ....A mild spring day (68˚F)
30˚ C ....A hot summer day (86˚F)
37˚ C ....Normal body temperature (98.6˚F)
40˚ C ....Heat wave conditions (104˚F)
100˚ C ....Boiling point of water (212˚F)

Sources of Information

MSDS Pocket Dictionary, Genium Publishing Corporation: USA, 1993.

American Heritage Dictionary, 2nd College Ed., Houghton Mifflin Company: Boston, 1982: 778-79.

APPENDIX G

Laboratory Self-Inspection Checklist

EMPLOYER POSTING

__ Are emergency telephone numbers posted where they can be readily found in case of emergency?

__ Where employees may be exposed to any toxic substances or harmful physical agents, has appropriate information concerning employee access to medical and exposure records and Material Safety Data Sheets been posted or otherwise made readily available to affected employees?

__ Are signs concerning exiting from buildings, room capacities, floor loading, exposures to x-ray, microwave, or other harmful radiation or substances posted where appropriate?

__ Are other state or federal posters properly displayed, such as:

  __ Industrial Welfare Commission orders regulating wages, hours, and working conditions?

  __ Discrimination in employment prohibited by law?

  __ Notice to employees of unemployment and disability insurance?

  __ Payday notice?

  __ Notice of compensation carrier?

RECORD KEEPING

__ Are you recording all occupational injuries or illnesses, except minor injuries requiring only first aid, as required by law?

__ Are employees' medical records and records of employee exposure to hazardous substances or harmful physical agents current?

__ Have you made arrangements to maintain required records for the legal period of time for each specific type of record? (Some records must be maintained for at least 40 years.)

__ Are you filing carcinogen use reports as required by any regulating agencies?

__ Are you maintaining employee safety and health training records?

__ Are you maintaining records of safety inspections and corrections?

__ Are you maintaining the minutes of safety committee meeting?

INJURY AND ILLNESS PREVENTION PROGRAM

__ Do you have a written, effective injury and illness prevention program?

__ Do you have a person who is responsible and has authority for overall activities of the injury and illness prevention program?

__ Do you have a system for identifying and evaluating your workplace hazards?

__ Do you systematically correct these hazards in a timely manner?

__ Do you provide training in both general and specific safe work practices?

__ Do you encourage employee participation in health and safety matters?

__ Do you maintain an ongoing safety training program?

__ Do you have a system in place that ensures employees will be recognized for safe and healthful work practices?

__ Will you discipline employees for unsafe or unhealthy acts?

__ Is there a labor-management safety committee?

__ If there is no safety committee, do you have a system for communicating safety and health concerns to employees?

MEDICAL SERVICES AND FIRST AID

__ Do you require each employee to have a pre-employment physical examination?

__ Is there a hospital, clinic, or infirmary for medical care close to your workplace?

__ If medical and first aid facilities are not near your workplace, is at least one employee on each shift currently qualified to render first aid?

__ Are medical personnel readily available for advice and consultation on matters of employee health?

__ Are emergency phone numbers posted?

__ Do you keep first aid kits easily accessible to each work area, with necessary supplies available and periodically inspect and replenish them as needed?

__ Has a physician approved first aid kit supplies, indicating they are adequate for a particular area of operation?

__ Do you provide means for quick drenching or flushing of the eyes and body in areas where corrosive liquids or materials are handled?

FIRE PROTECTION

__ Do you have a fire prevention plan?

__ Does your plan describe the type of fire protection equipment and/or systems?

__ Have you established practices and procedures to control potential fire hazards and ignition sources?

__ Are employees aware of the fire hazards of the materials and processes to which they are exposed?

__ Is your local fire department well acquainted with your facilities, location and specific hazards?

__ If you have a fire alarm system, is it certified as required?

__ If you have a fire alarm system, do you test it at least annually?

__ If you have interior stand pipes and valves, do you inspect them regularly?

__ Are fire doors and shutters in good operating condition?

__ Are fire doors and shutters unobstructed and protected against obstructions, including their counterweights?

__ Do you check the automatic sprinkler system water control valves, air and water pressures weekly/periodically as required?

__ Do you assign maintenance of automatic sprinkler systems to responsible persons or to a sprinkler contractor?

__ Do metal guards protect sprinkler heads when they are exposed to physical damage?

__ Do you maintain proper clearance below sprinkler heads?

__ Do you provide portable fire extinguishers in adequate number and type?

__ Do you mount fire extinguishers in readily accessible locations?

__ Do you recharge fire extinguishers regularly and note it on the inspection log?

__ Do you periodically instruct employees in the use of extinguishers and fire portection procedures?

PERSONAL PROTECTIVE EQUIPMENT AND CLOTHING

__ Do you provide and make sure employees wear protective goggles or face shields where there is any danger of flying particles or corrosive materials?

__ Do you require employees to wear approved safety glasses at all times in areas where there is risk of eye injuries such as punctures, abrasion, contusions or burns?

__ Do you require employees who need corrective lenses (glasses, contact lenses) and work in environments with harmful exposures to wear only approved safety glasses, protective goggles or to use other medically approved precautionary prodcedures?

__ Do you provide protective gloves, aprons, shields, or other means against cuts, corrosive liquids and chemicals?

__ Do you provide approved respirators for regular or emergency use where needed?

__ Do you maintain all protective equipment in a sanitary condition and ready for use?

__ Do you have eye wash facilities and a quick drench shower within a work area where employees are exposed to injurious corrosive materials?

__ When lunches are eaten on the premises, do employees eat in areas where there is no exposure to toxic materials or other health hazards?

__ Do you provide protection against the effects of occupational noise exposure when sound levels exceed standards?

__ Do you provide adequate work procedures, protective clothing and equipment for employees to use when cleaning up spilled toxic or other hazardous materials or liquids?

GENERAL WORK ENVIRONMENT

__ Are all worksites clean and orderly?

__ Do you keep work surfaces dry or take appropriate means to ensure the surfaces are slip-resistant?

__ Do you clean up all spilled materials or liquids immediately?

__ Do you store combustible scrap, debris and waste safely and remove them promptly from the worksite?

__ Do you provide the minimum number of toilets and washing facilities?

__ Are all toilets and washing facilities clean and sanitary?

__ Do you light all work areas adequately?

WALKWAYS

__ Do you keep aisles and passageways clear?

__ Do you mark aisles and walkways as appropriate?

__ Do you cover wet surfaces with nonslip materials?

__ Do you clean up spilled materials immediately?

EXITS

__ Do you mark all exits with exit signs and light them by reliable light sources?

__ Do you mark the directions to exits, when not immediately apparent, with visible signs?

__ Do you mark doors, passageways or stairways that are neither exits nor access to exits and could be mistaken for exits appropriately, "NOT AN EXIT," "TO BASEMENT," "STOREROOM," and the like?

__ Do you provide exit signs with the word "EXIT" in lettering at least 5 inches high and the stroke of the lettering at least ½ inch wide?

__ Are exit doors side-hinged?

__ Do you keep all exits free of obstructions?

__ Do you provide at least two means of egress from elevated platforms, pits or rooms where the absence of a second exit would increase the risk of injury from hot, poisonous, corrosive, suffocating, flammable, or explosive substances?

__ Are there sufficient exits to permit prompt escape in case of emergency?

EXIT DOORS

__ Do you design and construct your exit doors so that the way of exit travel is obvious and direct?

__ Do you bar windows which could be mistaken for exit doors?

__ Can you open exit doors from the direction of exit travel without using a key or any special knowledge or effort when the building is occupied?

__ Do you prohibit a revolving, sliding or overhead door from serving as a required exit door?

__ Where panic hardware is installed on a required exit door, can you open it by applying a force of 15 pounds or fewer in the direction of the exit traffic?

__ Do you provide doors on cold storage rooms with an inside release mechanism which will release the latch and open the door even if it is padlocked or otherwise locked on the outside?

__ Do you provide doors with viewing panels when they swing in both directions and are located between rooms where there is frequent traffic?

PORTABLE LADDERS

__ Do you maintain all ladders in good condition, tighten joints between steps and side rails, attach securely all hardware and fittings, and keep moveable parts operating freely without binding or undue play?

__ Do you provide nonslip safety feet on each ladder?

__ Do you provide nonslip safety feet on each rung of metal ladder?

__ Are ladder rungs and steps free of grease and oil?

__ Do you forbid placing a ladder in front of doors opening toward the ladder, except when the door is blocked open, locked or guarded?

__ Do you forbid placing ladders on boxes, barrels, or other unstable bases to obtain additional height?

__ Do you instruct employees to face the ladder when ascending or descending?

__ Do you forbid employees to use ladders that are broken, missing steps, rungs, cleats, or have broken side rails or other faulty equipment?

__ Do you instruct employees not to stand on the top step of ordinary stepladders?

__ Do you mark portable metal ladders legibly with signs reading "CAUTION" "Do Not Use Around Electrical Equipment" or equivalent wording?

__ Do you inspect metal ladders for damage?

__ Are the rungs of ladders uniformly spaced at 12 inches, center to center?

FUEL GAS CYLINDERS

__ Do you keep cylinders, cylinder valves, couplings, regulators, hoses and apparatus free of oily or greasy substances?

__ Do you take care not to drop or strike cylinders?

__ Unless secured on special trucks, do you remove regulators and replace them with valve-protection caps before moving cylinders?

__ Do cylinders without fixed hand wheels have keys, handles, or nonadjustable wrenches on stem valves when in service?

__ Do you store and ship liquefied gases valve-end up with valve covers in place?

__ Do you instruct employees never to crack a fuel-gas cylinder valve near sources of ignition?

__ Before a regulator is removed, do you close the valve and release gas from the regulator?

__ Do you use pressure-reducing regulators only for the gas and pressures intended?

__ Is suitable fire extinguishing equipment available for immediate use?

COMPRESSORS AND COMPRESSED AIR

__ Do you equip compressors with pressure relief valves and pressure gauges?

__ Do you check safety devices on compressed air systems frequently?

__ Before any repair work is done on the pressure system of a compressor, is the pressure bled off and the system locked out?

__ Do you post signs to warn of the automatic starting feature of the compressors?

__ Is it strictly prohibited to direct compressed air towards a person?

__ Do you prohibit employees from using highly compressed air for cleaning purposes?

__ If compressed air is used for cleaning off clothing, is the pressure reduced to less than 10 psi?

__ When using compressed air for cleaning, do employees use personal protective equipment?

__ Do you check the safe working pressure of the container before compressed air is used to empty containers of liquid?

COMPRESSED GAS AND CYLINDERS

__ Do you equip cylinders with a water weight capacity over 30 pounds with means for connecting a valve protector device, or with a collar or recess to protect the valve?

__ Do you mark cylinders legibly to clearly identify the gas contained?

__ Do you store compressed gas cylinders in areas which are protected from external heat sources, such as flame impingement, intense radiant heat, electric arcs or high temperature lines?

__ Do you locate or store cylinders in areas where they will not be damaged by passing or falling objects, or subject to tampering by unauthorized persons?

__ Do you store or transport cylinders in a manner to prevent them tipping, falling or rolling?

__ Do you store or transport cylinders containing liquefied fuel gas in a position so that the safety relief device is always in direct contact with the vapor space in the cylinder?

__ Do you always place valve protectors on cylinders when the cylinders are not in use or connected for use?

__ Do you close all valves before moving a cylinder, after emptying a cylinder, and at the completion of each job?

__ Do you check low pressure fuel-gas cylinders periodically for corrosion, general distortion, cracks, or any other defect that might indicate a weakness or render them unfit for service?

__ Does the periodic check of low-pressure fuel-gas cylinders include a close inspection of the cylinder's bottom?

SPRAYING OPERATIONS

__ Do you ensure adequate ventilation before starting spray operations?

__ Do you provide mechanical ventilation when you spray in enclosed areas?

__ When providing mechanical ventilation during spraying operations, do you arrange not to circulate the contaminated air?

__ Is the spray area free of hot surfaces?

__ Is the spray area at least 20 feet from flames, sparks, operating electrical motors and other ignition sources?

__ Do you provide approved respiratory equipment to use when appropriate during spraying operations?

__ Do solvents used for cleaning have a flash point of 100°F or more?

__ Do you keep fire control sprinkler heads clean?

__ Do you post "NO SMOKING" signs in spray areas?

ENVIRONMENTAL CONTROLS

__ Do you light all work areas properly?

__ Do you instruct employees in proper first aid and other emergency procedures?

__ Do you identify hazardous substances which may cause harm by inhalation, ingestion, skin absorption or contact?

__ Do employees know of the hazards involved with the various chemicals to which they may be exposed in their work environment, such as ammonia, chlorine, epoxies, caustics?

__ Do you keep employee exposure to chemicals in the workplace within acceptable levels?

__ Can you use a less harmful method or product?

__ Is the work area's ventilation system appropriate for the work being performed?

__ Are noise levels in the facilities within acceptable levels?

__ Do you providem use and maintain personal protective equipment wherever required?

__ Are there written standard operating procedures for the selection and use of respirators?

__ Do you keep restrooms and washrooms clean and sanitary?

__ Do you instruct employees in the proper manner of lifting heavy objects?

__ Where heat is a problem, have you provided all fixed work areas with spot cooling or air conditioning?

__ Do you screen employees before assignemnt to areas of high heat to determine if their health might make them more susceptible?

__ Do you locate exhaust stacks and air intakes so that contaminated air will not be recirculated within a building or other enclosed area?

__ Do you sheild properly the equipment producing ultraviolet radiation?

FLAMMABLE AND COMBUSTIBLE MATERIALS

__ Do you practice proper storage to minimize risks of fire and spontaneous combustion?

__ Do you use approved containers for the storage and handling of flammable and combustible liquids?

__ Do you keep all flammable liquids in closed containers when not in use?

__ Do storage rooms for flammable and combustible liquids have explosion-proof lights?

__ Do storage rooms for flammable and combustible liquids have mechanical or gravity ventilation?

__ Do you keep all solvent wastes and flammable liquids in fire-resistant, covered containers until removed from the worksite?

__ Do you place fire separators between stacked containers of combustible or flammables to ensure support and stability?

__ Do you separate stored fuel gas cylinders and oxygen cylinders by distance, fire resistant barriers or other means?

__ Do you select and provide fire extinguishers for the types of materials, in areas where they are to be used?
Class A: Ordinary combustible material fires.
Class B: Flammable liquid, gas or grease fires.
Class C: Energized-electrical equipment fires.

__ If a Halon 1301 fire extinguisher is used, can employees evacuate within the specified time?

__ Do you mount appropriate fire extinguishers within 75 feet of outside areas containing flammable liquids and within 10 feet of any inside storage area for such materials?

__ Do trained personnel transfer/withdraw flammable or combustible liquids?

__ Do you mount fire extinguishers so that employees do not have to travel more than 75 feet for a class "A" fire or 50 feet for a class "B" fire?

__ Do you train employees in the use of fire extinguishers?

__ Are extinguishers free from obstructions or blockage?

__ Do you service, maintain and tag all extinguishers at intervals not to exceed one year?

__ Do you keep all extinguishers fully charged and in their designated places?

__ Do you maintain records of required monthly checks of extinguishers?

__ Where sprinkler systems are permanently installed, do you direct the nozzle heads so that water will not be sprayed into operating electrical switch boards and equipment?

__ Do you post "NO SMOKING" signs in areas where you use or store flammable or combustible materials?

__ Do you enforce "NO SMOKING" rules in areas involving storage and use of flammable materials?

__ Do you clean up all spills of flammable or combustible liquids promptly?

HAZARDOUS CHEMICAL EXPOSURES

__ Do you train employees in the safe handling practices of hazardous chemicals, such as acids, caustics, and the like?

__ Do employees know the potential hazards involving various chemicals stored or used in the workplace, such as acids, bases, caustics, epoxies, phenols?

__ Do you keep employee exposure to chemicals within acceptable levels?

__ Do you provide eye wash fountains and safety showers in areas where corrosive chemicals are handled?

__ Do you require all employees to use personal protective clothing and equipment when handling chemicals (e.g., gloves, eye protection, respirators)?

__ Do you keep flammable or toxic chemicals in closed containers when not in use?

__ Have you established standard operating procedures and are employees following them when cleaning up chemical spills?

__ Where needed for emergency use, do you store respirators in a convenient, clean and sanitary location?

__ Are respirators intended for emergency use adequate for the various uses for which they may be needed?

__ Do you prohibit employees from eating in areas where hazardous chemicals are present?

__ Do you provide, use and maintain personal protective equipment whenever necessary?

__ Do you have written standard operating procedures for the selection and use of respirators where needed?

__ If you have a respirator protection program, do you instruct your employees on the correct usage and limits of the respirators?

__ Are the respirators NIOSH approved for this particular application?

__ Do you regularly inspect, clean, sanitize and maintain respirators?

__ If hazardous substances are used in your processes, do you operate a medical or biological monitoring system?

__ Are you familiar with the threshold limit values or permissible exposure limits of airborne contaminants and physical agents used in your workplace?

__ Have you instituted control procedures for hazardous materials where appropriate such as respirators, ventilation systems, handling practices?

__ Whenever possible, do you handle hazardous substances properly in designated and exhausted booths or similar locations?

__ Do you use general dilution or local exhaust ventilation systems to control dusts, vapors, gases, fumes, smoke, solvents or mists which may be generated in your workplace?

__ Do employees complain about dizziness, headaches, nausea, irritation or other factors of discomfort when they use solvents or other chemicals?

__ Is there a dermatitis problem? Do employees complain about skin dryness, irritation, or sensitization?

__ Have you considered using an industrial hygienist or environmental health specialist to evaluate your operation?

__ Do you store materials which give off toxic asphyxiant, suffocating or anesthetic fumes in remote or isolated locations when not in use?

HAZARDOUS SUBSTANCES COMMUNICATION

__ Do you have a list of hazardous substances used in your workplace?

__ Have you written a hazard communication program dealing with Material Safety Data Sheets (MSDS), labeling and employee training?

__ Who is responsible for MSDS's, container labeling, employee training?

__ Do you label each container for a hazardous substance (bottles) with product identity and a hazard warning (communication of the specific health hazards and physical hazards)?

__ Do you have a Material Safety Data Sheet readily available for each hazardous substance used?

__ How will you inform other employers whose employees share the same work area?

__ Do you have an employee training program for hazardous substances?

__ Does this program include:

- __ An explanation of what an MSDS is and how to use and obtain one?
- __ MSDS contents for each hazardous substance or class of substances?
- __ Explanation of "Right to Know?"
- __ Place where employees can see the employer's written hazard communication program and where hazardous substances are present in their work area?
- __ Describe the physical and health hazards of substances in the work area, how to detect their presence, and specific protective measures to be used?
- __ Details of the hazard communication program, including how to use the labeling system and MSDS's?
- __ How employees will be informed of hazards of non-routine tasks?

ELECTRICAL

__ Do you specify compliance with all state safety mandates for all contract electrical work?

__ Do you require all employees to report as soon as practicable any obvious hazard to life or property observed in connection with electrical equipment or lines?

__ Are portable electrical tools and equipment grounded or of the doubly insulated type?

__ Are electrical appliances such as vacuum cleaners, polishers, and vending machines grounded?

__ Do extension cords have a grounding conductor?

__ Do you ban multiple plug adapters?

__ Do you promptly replace or repair exposed wiring and cords with frayed or deteriorated insulation?

__ Are flexible cords and cables free of splices or taps?

__ Are there clamps or other means of securing flexible cords and cables at plugs, receptacles, tools, equipment, and do they hold the cord jacket securely in place?

__ In wet or damp locations, are electrical tools and equipment appropriate for the use, or location, or otherwise protected?

__ Do you prohibit the use of metal ladders in areas where the ladder or the person using the ladder could come in contact with energized parts of equipment, fixtures or circuit conductors?

__ Do you label all disconnecting switches and circuit breakers to indicate their use or equipment served?

__ Do you always disconnect the circuit before replacing fuses?

__ Do all interior wiring systems include provisions for grounding metal parts or electrical raceways, equipment and enclosures?

__ Are all energized parts of electrical circuits and equipment guarded against accidental contact by approved cabinets or enclosures?

__ Do you close all unused openings (including conduit knockouts) in electrical enclosures and fittings with appropriate covers, plugs or plates?

__ Do you provide electrical enclosures such as switches, receptacles, and junction boxes with tight-fitting covers or plates?

__ Do you instruct employees who regularly work on or around energized electrical equipment or lines in cardiopulmonary resuscitation (CPR) methods?

NOISE

__ Are there areas in the workplace where continuous noise levels exceed 85 dBA?

__ Do you measure noise levels using a sound level meter or an octave band analyzer and keep records?

__ Have you tried isolating noisy machinery from the rest of your operation?

__ Have you used engineering controls to reduce excessive noise levels?

__ Where engineering controls are not feasible, are you using administrative controls (e.g., worker rotation) to minimize individual employee exposure to noise?

__ Do you have an ongoing preventative health program to educate employees in safe levels of noise and exposure, effects of noise on their health, and use of personal protection?

__ Do employees exposed to continuous noise above 85 dBA repeat training annually?

__ Do you provide approved hearing protective equipment (noise attenuating devices) to every employee working in areas where continuous noise levels exceed 85 dBA?

__ Do you fit employees properly with ear protectors and instruct them in their use and care?

__ Do you give employees exposed to continuous noise above 85 dBA periodic audiometric testing to ensure that you have an effective hearing protection system?

MATERIAL HANDLING

__ Does equipment have safe clearance through aisles and doorways?

__ Do you design, permanently mark, and keep aisles clear to allow unhindered passage?

TRANSPORTING EMPLOYEES AND MATERIALS

__ Do employees who operate vehicles on public thoroughfares have an operator's licenses?

__ Do you equip vehicles used to transport employees with lamps, brakes, horns, mirrors, windshields and turn signals in good repair?

__ Do you maintain a fully-charged fire extinguisher, in good condition, with at least 4 B:C rating in each employee transport vehicle?

__ Do you equip employee transport vehicles at all times with at least two reflective-type flares?

CONTROL OF HARMFUL SUBSTANCES BY VENTILATION

__ Is the volume and velocity of air in each exhaust system sufficient to gather the dusts, fumes, mists, vapors or gases to be controlled and to convey them to a suitable point of disposal?

__ Do you design, construct, and support exhaust inlets, ducts and plenums to prevent collapse or failure of any part of the system?

__ Do you provide clean-out ports or doors at intervals not to exceed 12 feet in all horizontal runs of exhaust ducts?

__ Where two or more different types of operations are being controlled through the same exhaust system, will the combination of substances being controlled constitute a fire, explosion or chemical reaction hazard in the duct?

__ Do you provide adequate makeup air to areas where exhaust systems are operating?

__ Do you locate the intake for makeup air so that only clean, fresh air will enter the work environment?

__ Can two or more ventilation systems serve a work area so that one will not hinder the functions of the other?

SANITIZING EQUIPMENT AND CLOTHING

__ Can employees easily clean or disinfect the required personal protective clothing or equipment?

__ Do you prohibit employees from interchanging personal protective clothing or equipment unless it has been properly cleaned?

__ Do you prohibit employees from smoking or eating in any area where contaminants are present?

__ When employees are required to change from street clothing into protective clothing, do you provide a clean change room with separate storage facility for street and protective clothing?

__ Do you require employees to shower and wash their hair as soon as possible after contacting a carcinogen?

__ Do you bring or remove equipment, materials or other items into or from a carcinogen-regulated area, in a manner that will not contaminate non-regulated areas or the external environment?

EMERGENCY ACTION PLAN

__ Are you required to have an emergency action plan?

__ Does the emergency action plan comply with requirements of state occupational health and safety mandates?

__ Have you developed and communicated emergency escape procedures and routes to all employees?

__ Does the employee alarm system provide a warning for emergency action that is recognizable and perceptible above ambient conditions?

__ Do you maintain and test alarm systems regularly?

__ Do you review and revise the emergency action plan periodically?

__ Do employees know their responsibilities:

  __ For reporting emergencies?

  __ During an emergency?

  __ For conducting rescue and medical duties?

INFECTION CONTROL

__ Are employees potentially exposed to infectious agents in body fluids?

__ Have you identified and documented occasions of potential occupational exposure?

__ Do you provide a training and information program for employees exposed to or potentially exposed to blood and/or body fluids?

__ Have you instituted infection control procedures such as ventilation, universal precautions, workplace practices, personal protective equipment?

__ Do employees know specific workplace practices to follow? (Hand washing, handling sharp instruments, handling of laundry, disposal of contaminated materials, reusable equipment.)

__ Do you provide personal protective equipment to employees in all appropriate locations?

__ Do you provide the necessary equipment (e.g., mouthpieces, resuscitation bags, other ventilation devices) for administering mouth-to-mouth resuscitation on potentially infected patients?

__ Do facilities/equipment comply with workplace practices, such as hand-washing sinks, biohazard tags and labels, needle containers, detergents/disinfectants to clean up spills?

__ Do you clean and disinfect all equipment and environmental and working surfaces after contact with blood or potentially infectious materials?

__ Do you place infectious waste in closable, leak-proof containers, bags or puncture-resistant holders with proper labels?

__ Have you made medical surveillance, including HBV evaluation, antibody testing and vaccination, available to potentially exposed employees?

__ How often is training done? Does it cover:

> __ Universal precautions?
>
> __ Personal protective equipment?
>
> __ Workplace practices, which should include blood drawing, room cleaning, laundry handling, cleanup of blood spills?
>
> __ Needlestick exposure/management?
>
> __ Hepatitis B vaccination?

ERGONOMICS

__ Can employees perform the work without eye strain or glare?

__ Does the task require employees to raise arms for a prolonged time?

__ Must employees stoop to view the task?

__ Do they feel pressure points on any parts of the body (wrists, forearms, back of thighs)?

__ Can they work using the larger muscles of the body?

__ Can they work without twisting or overly bending the lower back?

__ Do they have sufficient rest breaks, in addition to the regular rest breaks, to relieve stress from repetitive-motion tasks?

__ Do you shape, position and handle tools, instruments and machinery so that employees can work comfortably?

__ Do you adjust, position and arrange all pieces of furniture to minimize strain on all parts of the body?

Reprinted, in part, with permission of CAL/OSHA Consultation Service, State of California, Department of Industrial Relations, Division of Occupational Safety and Health, San Francisco, California.

Index

A

B

C

D

E

F

G

H

I

L

M

N

O

P

R

S

T

U

V

W

X

Z

NOTES